T0257804

Advanced Cancer Treatment

Advanced Cancer Treatment

Edited by **Karen Miles and Richard Gray**

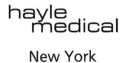

New York

Published by Hayle Medical,
30 West, 37th Street, Suite 612,
New York, NY 10018, USA
www.haylemedical.com

Advanced Cancer Treatment
Edited by Karen Miles and Richard Gray

International Standard Book Number: 978-1-63241-009-2 (Hardback)

Contents

Preface   VII

**Complementary / Alternative
Cancer Therapy Modalities**   1

Chapter 1   **Antioxidants in Cancer Treatment**   3
Júlio César Nepomuceno

Chapter 2   **Combination Chemotherapy in Cancer:
Principles, Evaluation and Drug Delivery Strategies**   31
Ana Catarina Pinto, João Nuno Moreira and Sérgio Simões

Chapter 3   **Cytotoxic Plants: Potential Uses
in Prevention and Treatment of Cancer**   53
Zahra Tayarani-Najaran and Seyed Ahmad Emami

Chapter 4   **Multimodal Therapies
for Upper Gastrointestinal Cancers
– Past, Now, and Future**   95
Shouji Shimoyama

Chapter 5   **Evidence-Based Usefulness of Physiotherapy
Techniques in Breast Cancer Patients**   131
Almir José Sarri and Sonia Marta Moriguchi

Chapter 6   **The Evolving Role of Tissue
Biospecimens in the Treatment of Cancer**   147
Wilfrido D. Mojica

Chapter 7   **Negative Impact of Paclitaxel Crystallization
on Hydrogels and Novel Approaches
for Anticancer Drug Delivery Systems**   175
Javier S. Castro, Lillian V.Tapia, Rocio A. Silveyra,
Carlos A. Martinez and Pierre A. Deymier

Permissions

List of Contributors

Preface

This book has been a concerted effort by a group of academicians, researchers and scientists, who have contributed their research works for the realization of the book. This book has materialized in the wake of emerging advancements and innovations in this field. Therefore, the need of the hour was to compile all the required researches and disseminate the knowledge to a broad spectrum of people comprising of students, researchers and specialists of the field.

There are many modern techniques and mechanisms available for use in cancer treatment today. This reflects that an ultimate treatment has not yet been found, and it needs more time and research to develop more effective methods for cancer treatment. This book will serve not just physicians but also patients with an overview on new research and developments in this area. This book is a comprehensive and valuable account discussing various therapeutic methods in cancer treatment comprising of some rare classic treatment approaches like treatment of metastatic liver disease of colorectal origin, breast and ovarian cancer treatment, radiation treatment of skull and spine chordoma, changing the face of adjuvant therapy for early breast cancer and laser photo chemotherapy as an alternative treatment.

At the end of the preface, I would like to thank the authors for their brilliant chapters and the publisher for guiding us all-through the making of the book till its final stage. Also, I would like to thank my family for providing the support and encouragement throughout my academic career and research projects.

Editor

Complementary / Alternative Cancer Therapy Modalities

Antioxidants in Cancer Treatment

Júlio César Nepomuceno

Universidade Federal de Uberlândia/Instituto de Genética e Bioquímica
Brazil

1. Introduction

There are many different chemotherapeutic agents used in cancer treatment. Most of the chemotherapeutic drugs can be divided into alkylating agents, antimetabolites, anthracyclines, plant alkaloids, topoisomerase inhibitors, and other antitumour agents. All of these drugs affect cell division or DNA synthesis and function in some way. Several classes of chemotherapy work by producing a reactive oxygen compound or free radical.

Alkylating agents work to add alkyl groups to negatively-charged groups. They are known to stop tumor growth through cross-linking guanine nucleobases in strands of DNA, which directly damages the DNA by making it unable to uncoil and separate. The cell, when attacked in this way, is unable to replicate. While it may not die, it also cannot grow. Cyclophosphamide, a cytotoxic alkylating agent, is extensively used as an antineoplastic agent for the treatment of haematological malignancies and a variety of solid tumours, including leukaemia, ovarian cancer and small-cell lung cancer. Cyclophosphamide is bioactivated by hepatic cytochrome P450 enzymes resulting in the formation of phosphoramide mustard and acrolein. The therapeutic effect of cyclophosphamide is attributed to phosphoramide mustard, while the other metabolite, acrolein is associated with toxic side effects. The cellular mechanism of cyclophosphamide toxicity is due to the production of highly reactive oxygen free radicals by these metabolites. It is obvious that high levels of ROS within the body could culminate in oxidative stress.

Anthracyclines (or anthracycline antibiotics) are a class of drugs used in cancer chemotherapy derived from Streptomyces bacteria. Anthracycline has three mechanisms of action: inhibits DNA and RNA synthesis by intercalating between base pairs of the DNA/RNA strand, thus preventing the replication of rapidly-growing cancer cells: inhibits topoisomerase II enzyme, preventing the relaxing of supercoiled DNA and thus blocking DNA transcription and replication: creates iron-mediated free oxygen radicals that damage the DNA and cell membranes.

Radiation therapy is another type of cancer treatment that uses ionizing radiation to produce cell death through free radical formation. The cell death occurs by damaging the DNA of cancerous cells. This DNA damage is caused by one of two types of energy: photon or charged particle, directly or indirectly ionizing the atoms which make up the DNA chain. Indirect ionization happens as a result of the ionization of water, forming free radicals, notably hydroxyl radicals, which then damage the DNA.

The oxidative stress produced during cancer treatment induces a range of side effects such as hair loss, nausea or vomiting and cardiotoxicity. Several authors believe that the use of antioxidants during cancer treatment can reduce these side effects. However, there is a concern that antioxidants might reduce oxidizing free radicals created by radiotherapy and some forms of chemotherapy, and thereby decrease the effectiveness of the therapy. The authors that support the idea that administration of oral antioxidants is contraindicated during cancer therapeutics, suggest that a drug's ability to destroy micrometastases may be impaired by the addition of antioxidants and, this may result in an improved short-term tolerance to treatment followed by an increased long-term chance for recurrence. On the other hand, there are several articles showing no evidence of significant decreases in the efficacy of chemotherapy with antioxidant supplementation and that supplementation of antioxidant vitamins during cancer treatment is effective, increasing quality and life expectancy.

Considering that the use of antioxidants during treatment is a very contentious issue, the purpose of this chapter is to review studies in humans to evaluate the use of these antioxidants as a therapeutic intervention in cancer patients, and their interactions with radiation therapy and chemotherapy.

2. Classes of agents used in cancer treatment that produce a reactive oxygen compound or free radical

The ultimate clinical effectiveness of any anti-cancer drug requires that it kill malignant tumor cells *in vivo* at doses that allow enough cells in the patient's critical tissues (e.g., bone marrow, gastrointestinal tract) to survive so that recovery can occur. This is difficult to accomplish because, in general, anticancer drugs are most useful against malignant tumor with a high proportion of dividing cells, and some normal tissues such as the bone marrow and GI tract also have a high cell-proliferation rate. Anticancer drugs used by themselves are primarily effective against high-growth-fraction tumors such as the leukemias and lymphomas. The most common malignant tumors, however, are "solid" tumors, including those of the colon, rectum, lung and breast. These tumors usually have a low proportion of dividing cells and therefore are less susceptible to treatment by drugs alone (Pratt, 1994).

There are some standard methods of cancer treaments: surgery, chemotherapy, radiation therapy, immunotherapy and biologic therapy. Undoubtedly, chemotherapy and radiotherapy are the treatments to fight cancer with more side effects.

Chemotherapy agents can be divided into several categories: alkylating agents (e.g., cyclophosphamide, ifosfamide), antibiotics which affect nucleic acids (e.g., doxorubicin, bleomycin), platinum compounds (e.g., cisplatin), mitotic inhibitors (e.g., vincristine), antimetabolites (e.g., 5-fluorouracil), camptothecin derivatives (e.g., topotecan), biological response modifiers (e.g., interferon), and hormone therapies (e.g., tamoxifen). The agents most noted for creating cellular damage by initiating free radical oxidants are the alkylating agents, the tumor antibiotics, and the platinum compounds (Lamson & Brignall, 1999).

2.1 Alkylating agents

Inhibiting DNA replication, therefore, affords a logical approach for retarding tumour growth. For this reason, DNA has become a critical target in cancer chemotherapy. Indeed, many of the antitumour agents currently in the cancer armamentarium are DNA-interactive. Among them, the DNA alkylators or cross-linkers, which include the platinum-based drugs, are the most active available for effective cancer management. By virtue of their high chemical reactivity, either intrinsic or acquired in a biological environment, all alkylating agents form covalent linkages with macromolecules having nucleophilic centres. They have no specificity, but the chance reaction with DNA forms the basis for the antitumour effects. Bifunctional alkylating agents form covalent bonds at two nucleophilic sites on different DNA bases to induce interstrand (between two opposite strands) and/or intrastrand (on same strand) cross-links (Fig. 1). Monofunctional agents have only one alkylating group and, therefore, cannot form crosslinks (Siddik, 2002).

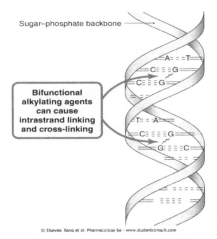

Fig. 1. The effects of bifunctional alkylating agents on DNA. Note the cross-linking of two guanines (www.studentconsult.com).

According to Siddik (2002), the end effect of these DNA-interactive agents is to inhibit DNA replication, which in turn may affect the production of RNA and protein. Such changes in the superhelical structure are then processed as distinct signals that determine whether a cell lives or dies.

The cyclophosphamide (CP) is a nitrogenous mustard pertaining to this group of substances named alkylating agents, which are effective against slow-growing tumors that damage cells at any phase of cellular growth. Cyclophosphamide is inactive per se and requires microsomal mixed function oxidase-mediated metabolism to activated metabolites capable of binding covalently to nucleic acids and proteins. The commonly accepted scheme of cyclophosphamide metabolism involves intermediate formation of 4-hydroxy-CP which undergoes ring-opening to form aldophosphamide, an isomer of 4-hydroxy-CP (Gurtoo et al., 1985). Aldophosphamide is metabolized to phosphoramide mustard and acrolein (Murgo & Weinberger, 1993).

Phosphoramide mustard forms DNA crosslinks between (interstrand crosslinkages) and within (intrastrand crosslinkages) DNA strands at guanine N-7 positions. This is irreversible and leads to cell death (Dong et al., 1995). According to Shanmugarajan et al. (2008), the therapeutic effect of cyclophosphamide is attributed to phosphoramide mustard and acrolein is associated with toxic side effects.

Adams and Klaidman (1993) showed that acrolein and its glutathione adduct, glutathionylpropionaldehyde, induce oxygen radical formation. Acrolein was oxidized by xanthine oxidase to produce acroleinyl radical and $O_2(\cdot-)$. Aldehyde dehydrogenase metabolized acrolein to form $O_2\cdot-$ but not acroleinyl radical. The fact that glutathionylpropionaldehyde is a more potent stimulator of oxygen radical formation than acrolein indicates that glutathionylpropionaldehyde is a toxic metabolite of acrolein and may be responsible for some of the *in vivo* toxicity of acrolein (Adams & Klaidman, 1993). In this regard, evidences reveal that oxidative stress plays a key role in the pathogenesis of cyclophosphamide induced cardiotoxicity (Shanmugarajan et al., 2008).

2.2 Anthracyclines (antibiotics)

Anthracyclines attack cancer cells by multiple mechanisms, inhibiting replication and cells damaging in ways that promote cell death. They work primarily by DNA intercalation. In order for a cell to divide, the DNA in the cell's nucleus must be unravelled and then duplicated (a process known as transcription). Anthracyclines bind to portions of the unwound strand of nuclear DNA, halting the transcription process, which in turn prevents cell replication. Among other details, scientists have found that anthracyclines inhibit the action of topoisomerase II ("Topo II"), an enzyme that unzips the DNA molecule for replication. It is anthracycline's interference with topoisomerase II that is credited with both its cardiotoxicity and mutagenic effects, since its Topo II inhibition leaves DNA breaks at even low concentrations, resulting in an accumulation of DNA damage following prolonged, repeated, or higher exposures (Pratt, 1999).

The biological activity of several well-known and widely used anthracycline antibiotics such as daunomycin and doxorubicin is thought to be associated to the hydroxyquinone structure (Young et al., 1981). Quinones are classified by the aromatic moieties present in their structure and naphthoquinone constitutes the naphtalenic ring (Silva et al., 2003).

The naphthoquinones are a class of compounds having cytotoxic properties that can be advantageous in treating cancer. Two essential mechanisms are linked to the effects of naphthoquinone, oxidative stress and nucleophilic alkylation (Bolton et al., 2000). These substances are able to accept electrons and generate reactive oxygen species (O_2-., HO., H_2O_2), whose oxidative effects could explain the cytotoxicity produced by these compounds (Boveris et al., 1978; Silva et al., 2003; Witte et al., 2004).

Bolton et al. (2000) suggested that quinones are highly reactive molecules and can reduce the redox cycle using semi-quinine radicals, generating reactive oxygen species (ROS) that include superoxide radicals, peroxide radicals, hydrogen peroxide and hydroxyl radicals. ROS production can cause severe oxidative cell stress, forming oxidative macromolecule cells, affecting lipids, proteins and DNA.

Rajagopalan et al. (1988) demonstrated that Adriamycin, an anthracycline drug with a wide spectrum of clinical antineoplastic activity, stimulates the formation of OH in the isolated rat heart and suggests that this mechanism may be significant in Adriamycin-induced cardiotoxicity.

According to Minotti, Cairo and Monti (1999) the cardiotoxicity of anthracyclines is mediated by mechanisms that are distinct from those underlying the antitumor effects of these drugs. For these authors a major role in the development of cardiotoxicity has been assigned to iron, presumably because this metal can catalyze free radical reactions that overrule the antioxidant defenses of cardiomyocytes. For them some investigators have proposed mechanisms of cardiotoxicity that are independent altogether of both iron and free radicals. In an attempt to bridge the two extremes of this field, other studies have maintained a role for iron but not for free radicals, suggesting that anthracycline cardiotoxicity reflects disturbances in iron homeostasis within cardiomyocytes rather than the outcome of iron-catalyzed free radical injury.

2.3 Platinum compounds

The application of inorganic chemistry to medicine is a rapidly developing field, and novel therapeutic and diagnostic metal complexes are now having an impact on medical practice. Cisplatin, as one of the leading metal-based drugs, is widely used in the treatment of cancer. Significant side effects and drug resistance, however, have limited its clinical applications. Biological carriers conjugated to cisplatin analogs have improved specificity for tumor tissue, thereby reducing side effects and drug resistance (Kostova, 2006).

The history of platinum in cancer treatment began 150 years ago with the first synthesis of cisplatin, but it was not used in the clinic before 30 years ago. Then 3000 derivatives were synthesised and tested, with poor successes: three other derivatives only are available today. Clearly they are not more active, but they are less toxic than cisplatin, although two, carboplatin and nedaplatin, yield a cross-resistance, while one, oxaliplatin, does not. Their mechanisms of action are similar: these four pro-drugs form adducts with DNA, impairing DNA synthesis and repair then (Fig. 2). Their pharmacokinetics are complicated since we always measure two overlapping pharmacokinetics: those of the parent compound and of the bound platinum. Cisplatin is now recommended for few cancers, it is replaced by less-toxic carboplatin, and therefore more easily used in combination. Oxaliplatin give interesting results in a number of cancers (Desoize & Madoulet, 2002).

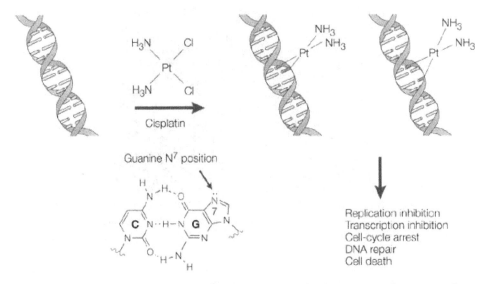

Fig. 2. The platinum atom of cisplatin binds covalently to the N7 position of purines to form 1,2- or 1,3-intrastrand crosslinks, and interstrand crosslinks. Cisplatin–DNA adducts cause various cellular responses, such as replication arrest, transcription inhibition, cell-cycle arrest, DNA repair and apoptosis (Wang & Lippard, 2005).

According to Boulikas and Vougiouka (2003) Cisplatin, carboplatin, oxaliplatin and most other platinum compounds induce damage to tumors via induction of apoptosis. Apoptosis is responsible for the characteristic nephrotoxicity, ototoxicity and most other toxicities of the drugs. The severity of cisplatin nephrotoxicity is related to platinum concentration in the kidneys. There is a growing amount of evidence that cisplatin-induced nephrotoxicity is ascribed to oxidative damage resulting from free radical generation (Antunes & Bianchi, 2004). Reactive oxygen metabolites (superoxide, hydrogen peroxide, hydroxyl radical, and hypochlorous acid) are important mediators of renal damage in acute renal failure and glomerular and tubulointerstitial diseases (Klahr, 1997).

2.4 Radiation therapy

Radiation therapy has been used in cancer treatment for many decades. The primary focus in radiotherapy is to increase DNA damage in tumor cells, as double strand breaks are important in cell death. Another course of action is to alter cellular homeostasis, modifying signal transduction pathways, redox state, and disposition to apoptosis. The cellular changes ideally would enhance the killing of tumor cells while reducing the probability of normal cell death. Radiation damages cells by direct ionization of DNA and other cellular targets and by indirect effect through ROS. Indirect ionization happens as a result of the ionization of water, forming free radicals, notably hydroxyl radicals, which then damage the DNA (Fig. 3). Therefore, exposure to ionizing radiation produces oxygen-derived free radicals in the tissue environment; these include hydroxyl radicals (the most damaging), superoxide anion radicals and other oxidants such as hydrogen peroxide. Additional destructive radicals are formed through various chemical interactions (Borek, 2004a).

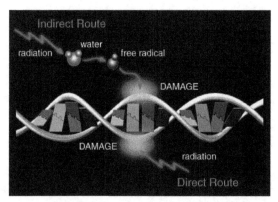

Fig. 3. There are two main ways radiation can damage DNA inside living cells. Radiation can strike the DNA molecule directly, ionizing and damaging it. Alternately, radiation can ionize water molecules, producing free radicals that react with and damage DNA molecules. Source unknown.

3. Antioxidants nutrients in cancer treatment

Cancer survivors receive a wide range of advice from many sources about foods they should eat, foods they should avoid, how they should exercise, and what types of supplements or herbal remedies they should take. Unfortunately, this advice is often conflicting (Doyle et al., 2006). Antioxidants vitamins show promise in cancer therapy by their palliative action, reducing painful side effects associated with treatment.

Examples of dietary antioxidants are vitamins A, C and E, selenium and flavonoids such as quercetin and genistein. In several *in vitro* and animal studies the hypothesis has been tested that antioxidants benefit patients receiving chemotherapy. In principle two opposing mechanistic arguments could be advanced supporting or refuting this notion. On the one hand, antioxidants might protect cancer cells against the oxidative damage induced by chemotherapy, which would mitigate against their use. On the other hand they may enhance drug-induced cytotoxicity by blocking reactive oxidant species. (D'Incalci et al., 2007).

Antioxidants nutrients such as vitamin E, vitamin C, vitamin A, and Beta-carotene are involved in detoxification of the Reactive oxygen species (ROS). Vitamin E, A, and Beta-carotene are lipophilic antioxidants whereas vitamin C is hydrophilic antioxidant. Vitamin E function as a free radical chain breaker particularly it interferes with the propagation step of lipid peroxidation. The vitamin A and Beta-carotene have actions by quenching both singlet oxygen and other free radicals generated by photochemical reactions (Peerapatdit et al., 2006).

Simone II et al. (2007) wrote a review which showed that since the 1970s, 280 peer-reviewed *in vitro* and *in vivo* studies, including 50 human studies involving 8,521 patients, 5,081 of whom were given nutrients, have consistently shown that those non-prescription antioxidants and other nutrients do not interfere in therapeutic modalities of cancer. Furthermore, they enhance the killing of therapeutic modalities of cancer, decrease their side effects, and protect normal tissue. For them in 15 human studies, 3,738 patients who took non-prescription antioxidants and other nutrients actually had increased survival.

3.1 Vitamin A and carotenoids

Some studies show that vitamin A supplementation, during cancer treatment, shows no benefit in terms of survival (Meyskens et al., 1994; Culine et al. 1999; van Zandwijk et al., 2000). However, the term "vitamin A" commonly refers to either of two very different families of substances: retinol, or preformed vitamin A, and its synthetic analogues (retinoic acid and the carotenoids). It is important to understand that retinoids and carotenoids behave very differently in the body, each may act via a different mechanism even if they both have an anticancer effect (Hennekens et al., 1986).

A study involving a total of 18,314 smokers, former smokers, and workers exposed to asbestos evaluated the effects of a combination of 30 mg of beta carotene per day and 25,000 IU of retinol (vitamin A) in the form of retinyl palmitate per day on the primary end point, the incidence of lung cancer. After an average of four years of supplementation, the combination of beta carotene and vitamin A had no benefit and may have had an adverse effect on the incidence of lung cancer and on the risk of death from lung cancer, cardiovascular disease, and any cause in smokers and workers exposed to asbestos (Omenn et al., 1996). Other findings confirm of a lack of any benefit from administration of large doses of synthetic β-carotene in cancer prevention (Klerk et al., 1998). On the other hand the adjuvant effect of high-dose vitamin A was tested on 307 patients with stage I non-small-cell lung cancer. After curative surgery, patients were randomly assigned to either a group prescribed retinol palmitate administration (orally 300,000 IU daily for 12 months). The authors concluded that daily oral administration of high-dose vitamin A is effective in reducing the number of new primary tumors related to tobacco consumption and may improve the disease-free interval in patients curatively resected for stage I lung cancer (Pastorino et al., 1993). Antioxidants, when added adjunctively, to first-line chemotherapy, may improve the efficacy of chemotherapy and may prove to be safe (Drisko et al., 2003).

136 patients with advanced non-small cell lung cancer were randomized to receive chemotherapy (paclitaxel and carboplatin) alone or chemotherapy in combination with

ascorbic acid 6100 mg/day, dl-alpha-tocopherol (vitamin E) 1050 mg/day and beta-carotene 60 mg/day. The results do not support the concern that antioxidants might protect cancer cells from the free radical damage induced by chemotherapy (Pathak et al., 2005). The authors suggest that high-dose multiple antioxidants in conjunction with chemotherapy increase the response rates and/or survival time in advanced lung cancer.

A phase III randomized study, comparing treatment with fluorouracil, epidoxorubicin and methotrexate (FEMTX) with the best supportive care, was conducted in patients with unresectable or metastatic gastric cancer. During treatment, these patients received tablets containing vitamins A and E. This study concluded that treatment with fluorouracil, epidoxorubicin and methotrexate combined with vitamin A and E is a fairly well-tolerated treatment, giving a response rate of 29% in patients with advanced gastric cancer, and also prolonging patients' survival (Pyrhönen et al., 1995).

Alpha- and beta-carotene have been examined for *in vitro* tumor inhibitory activity against human neuroblastoma cell lines, and alpha-carotene was found to have 10 times the anti-tumor activity of beta-carotene (Murakoshi et al., 1989).

Twenty patients with advanced squamous cell carcinoma of the mouth, who received 60 Gy telecobalt therapy given in 30 daily fractions with synchronous chemotherapy comprising vincristine, methotrexate and bleomycin, were randomized to receive standard diet with supplemental beta carotene. The results reported suggest that a protective action of beta-carotene is exerted on the mucosal membrane within the radiation fields used (Mills, 1988).

Kucuk et al. (2002) conducted a clinical trial to investigate the biological and clinical effects of lycopene supplementation in patients with localized prostate cancer. Twenty-six men with newly diagnosed prostate cancer were randomly assigned to receive a tomato oleoresin extract containing 30 mg of lycopene or no supplementation for 3 weeks before radical prostatectomy. This study suggested that lycopene may have beneficial effects in prostate cancer. The authors state that preparation that was used in this study was a mixture of tomato carotenoids and other tomato phytochemicals. Although lycopene was the predominant carotenoid in the capsules, there were significant amounts of phytoene and phytofluene and other bioactive compounds. It is possible that the combination of the phytochemicals present in the tomato extract was responsible for the observed clinical effects rather than lycopene alone.

Because of the poor response of pancreatic cancer to conventional therapy Recchia et al. (1998) performed a phase II pilot study to evaluate whether beta-interferon and retinoids, added to active chemotherapeutic agents, could increase response rate and survival in a group of patients who had metastatic disease. Twenty-three chemotherapy-naive patients were treated with epirubicin, mitomycin C, and 5-fluorouracil. Beta-Interferon, 1 x 10(6) IU/m2, subcutaneously three times a week, and retinol palmitate, 50,000 IU orally twice a day, were given between chemotherapy cycles. Eight patients responded (35%) and 8 (35%) had stable disease.

Prasad et al. (1999) has reviewed several studies showing the use of vitamin A and its analogs and its importance in cancer treatment. In this review the authors present a table (Table 1) on these studies. For them vitamins A derivatives at high doses, variable extents of tumor size reduction have been reported. Retinoids have been shown to have very little or no effect on several human tumors which included melanoma, non-small cell lung carcinoma, prostate cancer, breast cancer and neuroblastoma.

Tumor type	Design	Agents	Patient no.	Response
Actinic keratoses	Phase III (randomized)	Etretinate	54	84%
Advanced squamous cell carcinoma		13 cRA	4	50%
	Phase II	13 cRA	28	80%
Mycosis fungoides	No record	13 cRA	123	60%
Laryngeal papillomatosis	Phase II	13 cRA	6	60%
Oral leukoplakia	Phase II	b-carotene (synthetic)	24	71%
	Phase III randomized	13 cRA (high dose)	44	Marked regression
Cervical cancer (CIN II or III)	Phase II	tRA (topical)	20	50%
Cervical cancer (CIN II or III)	Phase III randomized	tRA (topical)	301	Increased regression of CIN II but not CIN III
Cervical cancer (CIN II or III)	Phase II	13 cRA + INFa	23	53%
Advanced cervical cancer	Phase II	13 cRA + INFa	26	50%
Advanced cervical cancer	Phase II	13 cRA + INFa	24	30%

Data from Prasad et al. (1999).
13 cRA513-cis Retinoic acid.
INFa5Interferon a.

Table 1. Efficacy of Retinoids in the Treatment of Human Tumors

13-cis-retinoic acid, even in short-term use, appears to be an effective treatment for oral leukoplakia and has an acceptable level of toxicity. 44 patients with this disease to receive 13-cis-retinoic acid (24 patients) or placebo (20), 1 to 2 mg per kilogram of body weight per day for three months, and followed them for six months. There were major decreases in the size of the lesions in 67 percent of those given the drug and in 10 percent of those given placebo. Dysplasia was reversed in 54 percent of the drug group (Hong et al., 1986).
Some of the analogs of retinoids produce extreme toxicity. The use of single antioxidant vitamins which require very high doses for its effectiveness has no significant value in the

treatment of cancer, even though such doses may cause tumor regression of variable degrees (Prasad et al, 1999). The antitumor activity demonstrated for retinoids (especially retinoic acid) alone and in combination with other agents supports the need for targeted phase II trials to define the spectrum of responsive tumors and for laboratory studies to further delineate the biologic mechanisms associated with therapeutic responses. High priority should then be given to phase III trials to delineate optimal strategies for improving outcome by combining retinoid-based treatments with conventional chemotherapy and radiotherapy regimens (Smith et al., 1992).

Addition of nutrition supplements such as lycopene may have potential therapeutic benefit in the adjuvant management of high-grade gliomas. The results verified in fifty patients with high-grade gliomas were treated with surgery followed by adjuvant radiotherapy and concomitant paclitaxel. Patients were randomized to receive either oral lycopene 8 mg daily with radiotherapy (Puri et al., 2010).

Docetaxel is currently the most effective drug for the treatment of castration-resistant prostate cancer (CRPC), but it only extends life by an average of 2 months. Tang et al. (2011) proposed a study of the interaction between docetaxel and lycopene in CRPC models. Lycopene, an antioxidant phytochemical, has antitumor activity against prostate cancer in several models and is generally safe. In this study, the authors demonstrated that lycopene enhances the effect of docetaxel on the growth of CRPC cell lines both *in vitro* and *in vivo*. These data provide a rationale for the clinical investigation of the efficacy and safety profile of lycopene in combination with docetaxel in CRPC patients. In particular, combining lycopene with docetaxel may provide clinical benefit for men with metastatic CRPC, for whom morbidity and mortality remain high despite wide use of docetaxel chemotherapy.

3.2 Vitamin C

It has been claimed that high-dose vitamin C is beneficial in the treatment of patients with advanced cancer, especially patients who have had no prior chemotherapy. The possibility that this compound may be useful in the treatment of cancer was first raised by Cameron and Pauling (1976) that published research suggesting a survival benefit from vitamin C in cancer treatment. The results of this clinical trial were made in 100 terminal cancer patients that were given supplemental ascorbate, by intravenous infusion for 10 days and orally thereafter, as part of their routine management. This study was compared with 1000 similar patients treated identically, but who received no supplemental ascorbate. The mean survival time was more than 4.2 times as great for the ascorbate subjects (more than 210 days) as for the controls (50 days). In the same journal Cameron and Pauling (1978) published, 2 years later, additional cases, and in this paper the authors confirm the idea that patients who had ascorbate treatment benefited with enhanced quality and prolongation of life. However, in a double-blind study 100 patients with advanced colorectal cancer were randomly assigned to treatment with either high-dose vitamin C (10 g daily) (the same dose that Pauling and Cameron recommended), using oral doses only, or placebo. None had received any previous treatment with cytotoxic drugs. Vitamin C therapy showed no advantage over placebo therapy with regard to either the interval between the beginning of treatment and disease progression or patient survival (Moertel et al., 1985). Saul (2010) and González et al. (2010) contest the work of Moertel et al. (1985). For Saul (2010) it is important to note that the negative results in Moertel studies were not true replications of Cameron and Pauling's work, as A) they used oral doses only, and B) vitamin C was discontinued at the first sign of disease progression.

D'Andrea (2005) believes that the antioxidant perhaps most widely used for treating cancer is vitamin C. For the author neither study was able to show any objective improvement in disease progression or survival over placebo. However, Maciocia (2010) contest D'Andrea's conclusions. Maciocia (2010) reported that there is no evidence of significant decreases in efficacy from antioxidant supplementation during chemotherapy. For him many of the studies indicated that antioxidant supplementation resulted in either increased survival times, increased tumor responses, or both, as well as fewer toxicities than controls. He concluded that trials that assessed chemotherapy toxicities, including diarrhea, weight loss, nerve damage and low blood counts, showed that the antioxidant group suffered similar or lower rates of these side effects than the control group.

Cabanillas (2010) after trials which have included at least 1,609 patients over 33 years concluded that we still do not know whether Vitamin C has any clinically significant antitumor activity. Nor does he know which histological types of cancers, if any, are susceptible to this agent. He doesn't know with certainty which is the required plasma ascorbic acid level that will result in antitumor effects. Assuming that this level is 10 mM/L then the recommended dose of Vitamin C appears to be in the range of 1.5 g/kg three times weekly. According to Ohno et al. (2009) the administration of more than 10 g of ascorbate is proposed to achieve plasma concentrations of 1 to 5 mM. At this time, vitamin C at high plasma concentration may function as a pro-oxidant. This occurs in the presence of free transition metals, such as copper and iron, which are reduced by ascorbate and, in turn, react with hydrogen peroxide (H_2O_2), leading to the formation of highly reactive and damaging hydroxyl radicals. As normal tissue receives adequate blood flow and is rich in antioxidant enzymes (e.g. catalase, glutathione peroxidase) in the blood, any H_2O_2 formed will be immediately destroyed. Meanwhile, tumor tissue is often associated with reduced blood flow and antioxidant enzymes, and consequently formed H_2O_2 remains active leading to cell damage and death. González et al. (2010) says that doses of 50-100 g given intravenously may result in plasma concentrations of about 14,000 micromol/L. At concentrations above 1000 micromol/L, vitamin C is toxic to cancer cells but not to normal cells *in vitro*. However, it is important that when referring to the plasma concentrations necessary to achieve antineoplastic activity there are other numerous factors involved that will affect the specific response. Some of these include sensitivity of tumor, hypoxia inducible factor, intracellular Redox signal transduction and gene expression, apoptosis, autoschizis, effect of collagen on tumor encapsulation and others.

Simone II et al. (2007) affirms that antioxidants and other nutrients do not interfere with cancer therapeutic modalities, enhance their killing capabilities, decrease their side effects, or protect normal tissues, and in 15 human studies, 3,738 patients actually had prolonged survival. Antioxidant and other nutrient food supplements are safe and can help to enhance cancer patient care.

Adriamycin (ADR) is effective against a wide range of human neoplasms. However, its clinical use is compromised by serious cardiac toxicity, possibly through induction of peroxidation in cardiac lipids. Ascorbic acid, a potent antioxidant, was examined for effect in reducing ADR toxicity in mice and guinea pigs. Ascorbic acid had no effect on the antitumor activity of ADR in mice inoculated with leukemia L1210 or Ehrlich ascites carcinoma, but it significantly prolonged the life of animals treated with ADR. The significant prevention of ADR-induced cardiomyopathy in guinea pigs by ascorbic acid was proved by electron microscopy. Ascorbic acid and the derivatives may delay general toxicity of ADR and also prevent the cardiac toxicity (Shimpo et al., 1991).

Borek (2004a) says in his studies that the antioxidants do protect against radiation-induced oncogenic transformation in experimental systems. However, she does not have comparable human studies that show the same association. Antioxidants do reduce the painful side effects of radiation therapy, thus supporting the beneficial effects of antioxidants in protecting normal cells in radiation therapy and in being used in conjunction with treatment for certain cancers. When considering antioxidant supplementation during treatment, it is doubtful whether high doses of radiation given in certain treatments would be rendered less effective if patients took a daily supplement of antioxidants.

Twenty consecutive symptomatic outpatients with endoscopically documented radiation proctitis seen in a single gastroenterology clinic were given a combination of vitamin E (400 IU tid) and vitamin C (500 mg tid). These patients presented with one or more of the following symptoms: rectal bleeding, rectal pain, diarrhea, or fecal urgency. There was a significant ($p < 0.05$; Wilcoxon rank) improvement in the symptom index (before treatment vs after treatment with vitamins E and C) for bleeding, diarrhea, and urgency. Patients with rectal pain did not improve significantly. Bleeding resolved in four of 11 patients, diarrhea resolved in eight of 16 patients, fecal urgency resolved in three of 16 patients, and rectal pain resolved in two of six patients. Lifestyle improved in 13 patients, including seven patients who reported a return to normal (Kennedy et al., 2001).

Cancer treatment by radiation and anticancer drugs reduces inherent antioxidants and induces oxidative stress, which increases with disease progression. Vitamins E and C have been shown to ameliorate adverse side effects associated with free radical damage to normal cells in cancer therapy, such as mucositis and fibrosis, and to reduce the recurrence of breast cancer. While clinical studies on the effect of anti-oxidants in modulating cancer treatment are limited in number and size, experimental studies show that antioxidant vitamins and some phytochemicals selectively induce apoptosis in cancer cells but not in normal cells and prevent angiogenesis and metastatic spread, suggesting a potential role for antioxidants as adjuvants in cancer therapy (Borek, 2004b).

3.3 Vitamin E

Vitamin E comprises a group of compounds possessing vitamin E activity. alpha-Tocopherol is the compound demonstrating the highest vitamin E activity, which is available both in its natural form as RRR-alpha-tocopherol isolated from plant sources, but more common as synthetically manufactured all-rac-alpha-tocopherol. Synthetic all-rac-alpha-tocopherol consists of a racemic mixture of all eight possible stereoisomers (Jensen & Lauridsen, 2007).

The ability of the vitamin E (RRR-α-tocopherol) derivatives α-tocopheryl succinate (α-TOS) and α-tocopheryloxyacetic acid (α-TEA) to suppress tumor growth in preclinical animal models has recently led to increased interest in their potential use for treating human cancer (Hahn et al., 2006).

With aim to evaluate the neuroprotective effect of antioxidant supplementation with vitamin E in patients treated with cisplatin chemotherapy Pace et al. (2003) evaluated, between April 1999 and October 2000, forty-seven patients assigned to either group one, which received vitamin E supplementation during cisplatin chemotherapy, or to group two, which received cisplatin chemotherapy alone. Alpha-tocopherol (vitamin E; 300 mg/d) was administered orally before cisplatin chemotherapy and continued for 3 months after the treatment suspension. The severity of neurotoxicity, measured with a comprehensive neurotoxicity score based on clinical and neurophysiological parameters, was significantly lower in patients who were supplemented with vitamin E than in patients who were not supplemented with vitamin E. Thirty-one patients with cancer treated with six courses of cumulative cisplatin, paclitaxel, or their combination regimens were randomly assigned in two groups and followed by neurologic examination and electrophysiologic study. Patients assigned in Group I (n = 16) received oral vitamin E at a daily dose of 600 mg/day during chemotherapy and 3 months after its cessation were compared to patients of Group II (n = 15), who received no supplementation and served as controls. This study showed significantly that the vitamin E supplementation in cancer patients may have an important neuroprotective effect (Argyriou et al., 2005). Contradicting the idea of these authors, Kottschade et al. (2010) published new data where two-hundred seven patients were enrolled between December 1, 2006 and December 14, 2007, producing 189 evaluable cases for analysis. A phase III, randomized, double-blind, placebo-controlled study was conducted in patients undergoing therapy with neurotoxic chemotherapy (cytotoxic agents included: taxanes, cisplatin, carboplatin, oxaliplatin, or combination), utilizing twice daily dosing of vitamin E (400 mg)/placebo. The authors concluded that Vitamin E did not appear to reduce the incidence of sensory neuropathy in the studied group of patients receiving neurotoxic chemotherapy.

Prasad et al. (2003) showed in their review article that alpha-Tocopheryl Succinate is the most Effective Form of Vitamin E for Adjuvant Cancer Treatment. For them alpha-Tocopheryl Succinate inhibits the proliferation of rodent and human cancer cells without affecting the proliferation of most normal cells. In addition, they also show that alpha-Tocopheryl Succinate when used in combination with some standard and experimental cancer therapeutic agents may enhance their growth-inhibitory effect on cancer cells, while protecting normal cells against some of their toxicities.

Chemotherapy- and radiotherapy-induced oral mucositis represents a therapeutic challenge frequently encountered in cancer patients. This side effect causes significant morbidity and may delay the treatment plan, as well as increase therapeutic expenses (Köstler et al., 2001). A randomized, double-blind, placebo-controlled study was performed to evaluate the efficacy of topical vitamin E in the treatment of oral mucositis in patients receiving chemotherapy for various types of malignancy. A total of 18 patients, 17 of whom had solid tumors and one with acute leukemia, were included in this study. Lesions were observed daily prior to and 5 days after topical application of either vitamin E or placebo oil. Six of nine patients receiving vitamin E had complete resolution of their oral lesions. In eight of nine patients who received placebo, complete resolution of their oral lesions was not observed. This difference is statistically significant (p = 0.025 by Fisher's exact test). No toxicity was observed in this study. These results suggest that vitamin E may be an effective therapy in patients with chemotherapy-induced mucositis (Wadleigh et al., 1992).

Women with breast carcinoma were asked to complete a questionnaire that recorded their use of dietary supplements. Blood samples were obtained for the assessment of serum vitamin B12 and folate levels before and after the first cycle of chemotherapy and for weekly complete blood counts. Toxicity was evaluated by measuring absolute neutrophil counts and the frequency and severity of oral mucositis. Of the 49 women who submitted questionnaires, 35 (71%) took a combined total of 165 supplements. The decrease in neutrophil count caused by chemotherapy was ameliorated by dietary supplementation with a multivitamin or vitamin E. However, neither multivitamin use nor vitamin E use appeared to be associated with the severity of mucositis. (Branda et al., 2004).

Conditioning therapy preceding bone marrow transplantation usually consists of high-dose chemotherapy and total body irradiation. It has acute and delayed toxic effects on several tissues, possibly related to peroxidation processes and exhaustion of antioxidants (Clemens et al., 1997). Blood from 19 patients was examined for the essential antioxidants alpha-tocopherol and beta-carotene before, during, and after bone marrow transplantation (BMT). Marrow ablation and immunosuppression for BMT conditioning was achieved by treatment with high-dose chemotherapy, mostly combined with total body irradiation. All patients required total parenteral nutrition beginning 1 wk before BMT. After conditioning therapy the concentration of absolute and lipid- standardized alpha-tocopherol and beta-carotene in plasma decreased significantly, presumably as a result of an enhanced breakdown of these antioxidants. The loss of these lipid-soluble antioxidants has to be considered as a possible cause for early posttransplant organ toxicity (Clemens et al., 1990). Therefore, the antioxidant supplementation prior to conditioning therapy reduces peroxidation processes induced by conditioning therapy in bone marrow recipients.

In the Women's Health Study conducted between 1992 and 2004, 39 876 apparently healthy US women aged at least 45 years were randomly assigned to receive vitamin E or placebo and aspirin or placebo, using a 2 × 2 factorial design, and were followed up for an average of 10.1 years (Lee et al., 2005). The data from this large trial indicated that 600 IU of natural-source vitamin E taken every other day provided no overall benefit for major cardiovascular events or cancer, did not affect total mortality, and decreased cardiovascular mortality in healthy women. Therefore, these data do not support recommending vitamin E supplementation for cardiovascular disease or cancer prevention among healthy women.

On the other hand, Nechuta et al. (2011) conducted a population-based prospective cohort study of 4,877 women aged 20 to 75 years diagnosed with invasive breast cancer in Shanghai, China, between March 2002 and April 2006. Women were interviewed approximately 6 months after diagnosis and followed up by in-person interviews and record linkage with the vital statistics registry. Women who used antioxidants (vitamin E, vitamin C, multivitamins) had 18% reduced mortality risk and 22% reduced recurrence risk. Therefore, Vitamin supplement use in the first 6 months after breast cancer diagnosis may be associated with reduced risk of mortality and recurrence.

Bladder cancer is one of the most aggressive epithelial tumors characterized by a high rate of early systemic dissemination. Patients with metastatic bladder cancer are routinely treated with systemic chemotherapy such as methotrexate, vinblastine, doxorubicin, and cisplatin regimen, particularly in the setting of unresectable, diffusely metastatic, measurable disease. In a study was investigated the cytotoxic effect of vitamin E succinate (α-TOS) and the enhancement of chemosensitivity to paclitaxel by α-TOS in bladder cancer. KU-19-19 and 5637 bladder cancer cell lines were cultured in α-TOS and/or paclitaxel *in vitro*. For *in vivo* therapeutic experiments, pre-established KU-19-19 tumors were treated with α-TOS and/or paclitaxel. The results demonstrated the efficacy and therapeutic potential of α-TOS and its enhancement of chemosensitivity to paclitaxel in bladder cancer cells. α-TOS inhibits NF-κB activity resulting in the promotion of apoptotic mechanisms in bladder cancer cell lines and also reduces activated NF-κB induced by paclitaxel resulting in enhanced apoptosis *in vitro*.α-TOS displayed an antitumor effect and α-TOS in combination with paclitaxel demonstrated dramatic tumor inhibition in an *in vivo* s.c. KU-19-19 tumor model (Kanai et al., 2010). For these authors additional studies are needed to confirm its safety for use in clinical trials, the cytotoxic effect of α-TOS and its enhancement of paclitaxel treatment might provide a novel strategy for advanced or metastatic bladder cancer patients.

3.4 Selenium

Selenium was recognized as a nutritional essential only in the late 1950s. That it might also be anticarcinogenic was first suggested a decade later based on ecological relationships of cancer mortality rates and forage crop selenium contents in the United States. Since that time, a substantial body of scientific evidence indicated that selenium can, indeed, play a role in cancer prevention. This is supported by a remarkably consistent body of findings from studies with animal tumor and cell culture models, and by some, but not all epidemiologic observations (Combs Jr., 2005). Selenium is an essential element that is specifically incorporated as selenocystein into selenoproteins. It is a potent modulator of eukaryotic cell growth with strictly concentration-dependant effects. Lower concentrations are necessary for cell survival and growth, whereas higher concentrations inhibit growth and induce cell death (Selenius et al., 2010). The protective effect of this mineral is especially associated with its presence in glutathione peroxidase and thioredoxin reductase, enzymes that protect the DNA and other cellular components against oxidative damage caused by ROS. Several studies have demonstrated reduced expression of these enzymes in various types of cancer, especially when associated with a low intake of selenium, which may exacerbate the damage (Almondes et al., 2010).

A total of 1312 patients (mean age, 63 years; range, 18-80 years) with a history of basal cell or squamous cell carcinomas of the skin were randomized from 1983 through 1991. Patients were treated for a mean (SD) of 4.5 (2.8) years and had a total follow-up of 6.4 (2.0) years. The patients were treated with oral administration of 200 µg of selenium per day or placebo. After a total follow-up of 8271 person-years, selenium treatment did not significantly affect the incidence of basal cell or squamous cell skin cancer. Therefore, Selenium treatment did not protect against development of basal or squamous cell carcinomas of the skin. However, results from secondary end-point analyses support the hypothesis that supplemental selenium may reduce the incidence of, and mortality from, carcinomas of several sites (Clark et al., 1996). Selenium treatment was associated with a significant (63%) reduction in the secondary endpoint of prostate cancer incidence during 1983-93 (Clark et al., 1998). A total of 974 men with a history of either a basal cell or squamous cell carcinoma were randomized to either a daily supplement of 200 microg of selenium or a placebo. Supplementation with a nutritional dose of the essential trace element selenium significantly reduced the incidence of prostate cancer in a population of patients with non-melanoma skin cancer. For the authors this was the first completed double-blind randomized controlled trial to specifically test if a dietary supplement can prevent prostate cancer. These results require confirmation in independent trials, but suggest that selenium supplementation may be important for both the primary and secondary prevention of prostate cancer.

A prospective study included 209 breast cancer patients treated by external beam radiotherapy from December 2007 until August 2008. Plasma selenium concentrations were determined before and at the end of the radiotherapeutic treatment. Sixty patients (28.7%) were in clinical stage I, 141 (67.5%) in clinical stage II and 8 (3.8%) in clinical stage III. At the beginning of radiotherapy, the mean selenium value for all patients was 86.4 µg/l and after radiation this value dropped to 47.8 µg/l. Multivariate analysis showed statistically significant difference in the plasma selenium concentration before and after radiotherapy. Therefore, significant reduction in plasma levels of selenium is recorded in patients undergoing radiotherapy, suggesting attention to the nutritional status of this micronutrient and other antioxidant agents (Franca et al., 2010).

However, a phase 2 randomized, double-blind, placebo-controlled clinical trial was conducted in men with localized nonmetastatic prostate cancer who had elected to forgo active treatment and be followed by active surveillance. A total of 140 men were randomized to placebo (n = 46), 200 µg/d (n = 47), or 800 µg/d (n = 47) selenium p.o. (as selenized yeast) and followed every 3 months for up to 5 years. Prostate-specific antigen (PSA) velocity was used as a marker of prostate cancer progression and was estimated using mixed-effects regression. Selenium supplementation did not show a protective effect on PSA velocity in subjects with localized prostate cancer. On the contrary, supplementation with high-dose selenium was observed to be a risk factor for increased PSA velocity in men with high baseline plasma selenium concentrations (Stratton et al., 2010).

3.5 Flavonoids

Flavonoids and their polymers constitute a large class of food constituents, synthesized by plants, many of which alter metabolic processes and have a positive impact on health. Flavonoids are a subclass of polyphenols (Beecher, 2003). Polyphenols are abundant micronutrients in our diet, and evidence for their role in the prevention of degenerative diseases such as cancer and cardiovascular diseases is emerging. The health effects of polyphenols depend on the amount consumed and on their bioavailability (Manach et al., 2004). The capacity of flavonoids to act as antioxidants *in vitro* has been the subject of several studies in the past years, and important structure–activity relationships of the antioxidant activity have been established. The antioxidant efficacy of flavonoids *in vivo* is less documented, presumably because of the limited knowledge on their uptake in humans (Pietta, 2000).

Sadzuka et al. (1998) investigated the effects of green tea and tea components on the antitumor activity of doxorubicin. We carried out the combined treatment of doxorubicin and green tea on Ehrlich ascites carcinoma tumor-bearing mice. The oral administration of green tea enhanced 2.5-fold the inhibitory effects of doxorubicin on tumor growth. The doxorubicin concentration in the tumor was increased by the combination of green tea with doxorubicin. In contrast, the increase in doxorubicin concentration was not observed in normal tissues after green tea combination. Furthermore, the enhancement of antitumor activity of doxorubicin induced by green tea was observed in M5076 ovarian sarcoma, which has low sensitivity to doxorubicin. These results suggest that drinking green tea can encourage cancer chemotherapy and may improve the quality of life of clinical patients.

A study demonstrates, for the first time, that cancer preventive effects of epigallocatechin gallate (EGCG) and quercetin can inhibit the self-renewal capacity of prostate cancer stem cells. In this study Tang et al. (2010) present data indicating that human prostate cancer cell lines contain a small population of CD44+CD133+ cancer stem cells and their self-renewal capacity is inhibited by EGCG. Furthermore, EGCG inhibits the self-renewal capacity of CD44+a2b1+CD133+ CSCs isolated from human primary prostate tumors, as measured by spheroid formation in suspension. EGCG induces apoptosis by activating capase-3/7 and inhibiting the expression of Bcl-2, survivin and XIAP in CSCs. Furthermore, EGCG inhibits epithelial-mesenchymal transition by inhibiting the expression of vimentin, slug, snail and nuclear b-catenin, and the activity of LEF-1/TCF responsive reporter, and also retards CSC's migration and invasion, suggesting the blockade of signaling involved in early metastasis. Interestingly, quercetin synergizes with EGCG in inhibiting the self-renewal properties of prostate CSCs, inducing apoptosis, and blocking CSC's migration and invasion. These data suggest that EGCG either alone or in combination with quercetin can eliminate cancer stem cell-characteristics.

Resistance of cancer cells to multiple chemotherapeutic drugs (a mechanism termed MDR) is a major obstacle to the success of cancer chemotherapy and has been closely associated with treatment failure. One of the most studied mechanisms of drug resistance is characterized by a decrease in drug accumulation resulting from over-expression of the 170 kDa plasma membrane, P-glycoprotein (Pgp). P-glycoprotein (Pgp), causes the efflux of chemotherapeutic drugs from cells and is believed to be an important mechanism in multidrug resistance (MDR) in human cancer (Khantamat et al., 2004). Khantamat et al. (2004) demonstrated that the flavonoid, i.e. kaempferol, could reverse the vinblastine resistant phenotype by inhibiting Pgp activity in KB-V1 cells, and the ability to affect the Pgp activity could be of relevance to the chemosensitization of this flavonoid towards anticancer drugs.

3.6 Melatonin

Melatonin, a derivative of an essential amino acid, tryptophan, was first identified in bovine pineal tissue and subsequently it has been portrayed exclusively as a hormone. Recently accumulated evidence has challenged this concept. Melatonin is present in the earliest life forms and is found in all organisms including bacteria, algae, fungi, plants, insects, and vertebrates including humans. Several characteristics of melatonin distinguish it from a classic hormone such as its direct, non-receptor-mediated free radical scavenging activity. As melatonin is also ingested in foodstuffs such as vegetables, fruits, rice, wheat and herbal medicines, from the nutritional point of view, melatonin can also be classified as a vitamin. It seems likely that melatonin initially evolved as an antioxidant, becoming a vitamin in the food chain, and in multicellular organisms (Tan et al., 2003).

Melatonin was found to be a potent free radical scavenger in 1993, since then over 800 publications have directly or indirectly confirmed this observation. Melatonin scavenges a variety of reactive oxygen and nitrogen species including hydroxyl radical, hydrogen peroxide, singlet oxygen, nitric oxide and peroxynitrite anion. The mechanisms of melatonin's interaction with reactive species probably involves donation of an electron to form the melatoninyl cation radical or through an radical addition at the site C3. Other possibilities include hydrogen donation from the nitrogen atom or substitution at position C2, C4 and C7 and nitrosation. Melatonin also has the ability to repair damaged biomolecules as shown by the fact that it converts the guanosine radical to guanosine by electron transfer. Unlike the classical antioxidants, melatonin is devoid of prooxidative activity and all known intermediates generated by the interaction of melatonin with reactive species are also free radical scavengers. This phenomenon is defined as the free radical scavenging cascade reaction of the melatonin family. Due to this cascade, one melatonin molecule has the potential to scavenge up to 4 or more reactive species. This makes melatonin very effective as an antioxidant. Under in vivo conditions, melatonin is often several times more potent than vitamin C and E in protecting tissues from oxidative injury when compared at an equivalent dosage (mmol / kg) (Tan et al., 2002).

Physiologic and pharmacologic concentrations of the pineal hormone melatonin have shown chemopreventive, oncostatic, and tumor inhibitory effects in a variety of in vitro and in vivo experimental models of neoplasia. Multiple mechanisms have been suggested for the biological effects of melatonin. Not only does melatonin seem to control development alone but also has the potential to increase the efficacy and decrease the side effects of chemotherapy when used in adjuvant settings (Jung & Ahmad, 2006).

Melatonin has a variety of functions in human physiology and is involved in a number of pathological events including neoplastic processes. The tissue protective actions of melatonin are attributed to its antioxidant activity though, under certain conditions, melatonin might also exert oxidant effects, particularly in cancer cells. Büyükavcı et al. (2006) verified that these pro-oxidant actions of melatonin may assist in limiting leukemic cell growth. A similar study (Bejarano et al., 2011) evaluated the pro-oxidant effects of melatonin in tumour cell lines of human haematopoietic origin. Melatonin treatment was able to stimulate production of intracellular reactive oxygen species (ROS), as revealed by the increase in rhodamine-123 fluorescence, which was associated with significant cytotoxicity and activation of caspase activities. According to authors, this pro-oxidant action of melatonin may assist in limiting tumour cell growth. An increase in the activation of caspase-3, -8, -9 was also observed when melatonin was combined with vincristine in Ewing sarcoma cell line (Casado-Zapico et al., 2010).

A study was done with 14 women with metastatic breast cancer who did not respond to tamoxifen (TMX) therapy or progressed after initial disease stabilization. The study evaluated the biological and clinical effects of a concomitant melatonin therapy in women with metastatic breast cancer who had progressed in response to TMX alone. Melatonin was given orally at 20 mg day in the evening, every day starting 7 days before TMX, which was given orally at 20 mg day at noon. The authors concluded that this preliminary phase II study would suggest that the pineal hormone melatonin may amplify the therapeutic efficacy of TMX in women with metastatic breast cancer and induce objective tumour regressions in patients who have not responded to previous therapy with TMX alone (Lissoni et al., 1995).

A study included 70 consecutive advanced non-small cell lung cancer patients (NSCLC), with poor clinical status, were randomized to receive chemotherapy alone with cisplatin (20 mg/m2/day i.v. for 3 days) and etoposide (100 mg/m2/day i.v. for 3 days) or chemotherapy plus melatonin (20 mg/day orally in the evening). Cycles were repeated at 21-day intervals. Clinical response and toxicity were evaluated according to World Health Organization criteria. The percent of 1-year survival was significantly higher in patients treated with melatonin plus chemotherapy than in those who received chemotherapy alone. Finally, chemotherapy was well tolerated in patients receiving melatonin, and in particular the frequency of myelosuppression, neuropathy, and cachexia was significantly lower in the melatonin group. This study shows that the concomitant administration of melatonin may improve the efficacy of chemotherapy, mainly in terms of survival time, and reduce chemotherapeutic toxicity in advanced NSCLC, at least in patients in poor clinical condition (Lissoni et al., 1997).

Lissoni et al. (1999) evaluated effects of concomitant melatonin administration on toxicity and efficacy of several chemotherapeutic combinations in advanced cancer patients with poor clinical status. The study included 250 metastatic solid tumour patients (lung cancer, 104; breast cancer, 77; gastrointestinal tract neoplasms, 42; head and neck cancers, 27), who were randomized to receive melatonin (20mg/day orally every day) plus chemotherapy, or chemotherapy alone. Chemotherapy consisted of cisplatin (CDDP) plus etoposide or gemcitabine alone for lung cancer, doxorubicin alone, mitoxantrone alone or paclitaxel alone for breast cancer, 5-FU plus folinic acid for gastro-intestinal tumours and 5-FU plus CDDP for head and neck cancers. The 1-year survival rate and the objective tumour regression rate were significantly higher in patients concomitantly treated with melatonin than in those who received chemotherapy alone. The concomitant administration of melatonin significantly reduced the frequency of thrombocytopenia, neurotoxicity, cardiotoxicity, stomatitis and asthenia. This study indicates that the pineal hormone melatonin may enhance the efficacy of chemotherapy and reduce its toxicity, at least in advanced cancer patients of poor clinical status.

A clinical trial was performed in locally advanced or metastatic patients with solid tumours other than renal cell cancer and melanoma. The study included 80 consecutive patients, who were randomized to be treated with interleukin 2 (IL-2) alone subcutaneously (3 million IU day-1 at 8.00 p.m. 6 days a week for 4 weeks) or IL-2 plus melatonin (40 mg day-1 orally at 8.00 p.m. every day starting 7 days before IL-2). Tumour objective regression rate was significantly higher in patients treated with IL-2 and melatonin than in those receiving IL-2 alone. The mean increase in lymphocyte and eosinophil number was significantly higher in the IL-2 plus melatonin group than in patients treated with IL-2 alone; on the contrary, the mean increase in the specific marker of macrophage activation neopterin was significantly higher in patients treated with IL-2 alone. The treatment was well tolerated in both groups of patients. This study shows that the concomitant administration of the pineal hormone melatonin may increase the efficacy of low-dose IL-2 subcutaneous therapy (Lissoni et al., 1994).

3.7 Dexrazoxane

Dexrazoxane received FDA approval in 1995 for reducing the incidence and severity of cardiomyopathy associated with doxorubicin administration in women with metastatic breast cancer who have received a cumulative doxorubicin dose of 300 mg/m2 and who continue to receive doxorubicin therapy. For this use, dexrazoxane is given immediately before doxorubicin i.v. in a ratio (in milligrams) of 10:1 dexrazoxane: doxorubicin. In Europe, a 20:1 ratio is used. Thus, in Europe, a typical schedule for cardioprotection in a patient receiving 50 mg/m2 of doxorubicin includes a single dose of 1,000 mg/m2 of dexrazoxane given immediately prior to doxorubicin. From this experience, the sponsor selected the 3-day schedule used in the clinical studies. Renal excretion of dexrazoxane is substantial; based on a model of systemic exposure, the dose should be reduced by 50% in patients with creatinine clearance values <40 ml/minute. The possible benefit of alternative dose schedules has not been examined. The sponsor is conducting a population pharmacokinetic analysis to compare population parameter estimates and interindividual variability with literature values for dexrazoxane. There are no known drug interactions (Kane et al., 2008).

It has been proposed that dexrazoxane may act through its rings-opened hydrolysis product ADR-925, which can either remove iron from the iron-doxorubicin complex or bind to free iron, thus preventing iron-based oxygen radical formation. However, it is not known whether the antioxidant actions of dexrazoxane are totally dependent on its metabolization to its rings-opened hydrolysis product and whether dexrazoxane has any effect on the iron-independent oxygen free radical production. However, Junjing et al. (2010) demonstrated that dexrazoxane was an antioxidant that could effectively scavenge these free radicals and the scavenging effects of dexrazoxane did not require the enzymatic hydrolysis. In addition, dexrazoxane was capable to inhibit the generation superoxide and hydroxyl radicals in iron free reaction system, indicating that the antioxidant properties of dexrazoxane were not solely dependent on iron chelation. Thus the application of dexrazoxane should not be limited to doxorubicin-induced cardiotoxicity. Instead, as an effective antioxidant that has been clinically proven safe, dexrazoxane may be used in a broader spectrum of diseases that are known to be benefited by antioxidant treatments.

Between January, 1996, and September, 2000, children with high-risk acute lymphoblastic leukaemia (ALL) were enrolled from nine centres in the USA, Canada, and Puerto Rico. Patients were assigned by block randomisation to receive ten doses of 30 mg/m2 doxorubicin alone or the same dose of doxorubicin preceded by 300 mg/m2 dexrazoxane. In this study was established the long-term effect of dexrazoxane on the subclinical state of cardiac health in survivors of childhood high-risk ALL 5 years after completion of doxorubicin treatment. 100 children were assigned to doxorubicin (66 analysed) and 105 to doxorubicin plus dexrazoxane (68 analysed). 5 years after the completion of doxorubicin chemotherapy, mean left ventricular fractional shortening and end-systolic dimension Z scores were significantly worse than normal for children who received doxorubicin alone but not for those who also received dexrazoxane. The protective effect of dexrazoxane, relative to doxorubicin alone, on left ventricular wall thickness and thickness-to-dimension ratio were the only statistically significant characteristics at 5 years. Subgroup analysis showed dexrazoxane protection for left ventricular fractional shortening at 5 years in girls, but not in boys. Similarly, subgroup analysis showed dexrazoxane protection for the left ventricular thickness-to-dimension ratio at 5 years in girls, but not in boys. With a median follow-up for recurrence and death of 8·7 years, event-free survival was 77% for children in the doxorubicin-alone group, and 76% for children in the doxorubicin plus dexrazoxane group (Lipshultz et al., 2010). The authors concluded that dexrazoxane provides long-term cardioprotection without compromising oncological efficacy in doxorubicin-treated children with high-risk ALL. Dexrazoxane exerts greater long-term cardioprotective effects in girls than in boys.

Lopez et al. (1998) conducted a randomized trial to evaluate primarily the cardioprotective effect of dexrazoxane in patients with advanced breast cancer and soft tissue sarcomas treated with high-dose epirubicin. Patients with breast cancer (n = 95) or STS (n = 34) received epirubicin 160 mg/m2 by intravenous (I.V.) bolus every 3 weeks with or without dexrazoxane 1,000 mg/m2 I.V. In either disease, antitumor response rates, time to progression, and survival did not significantly differ between the two arms. There was little difference in noncardiac toxicity for the two treatment groups. All methods of cardiac evaluation clearly documented the cardioprotective effect of dexrazoxane. Dexrazoxane significantly protects against the development of cardiotoxicity when high single doses of epirubicin are used. Apparently, there was no evidence of an adverse impact of dexrazoxane on antitumor activity.

Choi et al. (2010) enrolled patients who were diagnosed as having solid tumors and treated them with the same chemotherapeutic regimen. Doxorubicin was administered at a dose of 30 mg/m2 in combination with cisplatin 60 mg/m2, cyclophosphamide 60 mg/kg, and etoposide 200 mg/m2 at intervals of 4 weeks with or without chest radiation therapy. Doxorubicin was administered intravenously as a bolus infusion. Dexrazoxane was administered intravenously 30 min prior to each dose of doxorubicin in the 10:1 ratio dexrazoxane: doxorubicin. There was no clinically significant side effect associated with dexrazoxane administration. The authors concluded that dexrazoxane reduces the incidence and severity of early and late cardiotoxicity in children with solid tumors receiving doxorubicin chemotherapy. Administration of dexrazoxane was well tolerated and no second malignant neoplasm was observed during the follow-up period, which might be contributed by the limited follow-up period. For them, this study supports the benefit of dexrazoxane as a cardioprotective agent in children who are vulnerable to cardiac damage by anthracycline.

4. Conclusion

Until the present moment studies have shown that the association of antioxidant vitamins for the treatment of cancer is still a controversial issue. However, with few exceptions, we can say that most studies have reported positive findings from the interaction of antioxidants during cancer treatment. The majority of conventional chemotherapeutic agents cause cell death by directly inhibiting the synthesis of DNA or interfering with its function. Adverse effects such as cardiotoxicity of many drugs in cancer treatment are mediated by mechanisms that are distinct from those underlying the antitumor effects of these drugs. Most agents do not really depend that much on free radical damaging mechanisms of action. Thus, free radical generation would arise with an adverse effect and not as a primary mechanism of action. Although further studies are needed, the predominance of evidence supports a provisional conclusion that dietary antioxidants do not conflict with the use of chemotherapy in the treatment of a wide variety of cancers and may significantly mitigate the adverse effects of that treatment.

5. References

Adams, J.D. Jr. & Klaidman, L.K. (1993). Acrolein-induced oxygen radical formation, *Free Radic Biol Med* 15(2): 187-93.

Almondes, K.G.S., Leal, G.V.S., Cozzolino, S.M.F.; Philippi, S.T. & Carvalho, P.H.R. (2010). O papel das selenoproteínas no câncer, *Rev Assoc Med Bras* 56(4): 484-488.

Antunes, L.M.G. & Bianchi, M.L.P. (2004). Dietary antioxidants as inhibitors of cisplatin-induced nephrotoxicity, *Rev Nutr* 17(1): 89-96.

Argyriou, A.A., Chroni, E., Koutra, A., Ellul, J., Papapetropoulos, S., Katsoulas, G., Iconomou, G., & Kalofonos, H.P. (2005). Vitamin E for prophylaxis against chemotherapy-induced neuropathy - A randomized controlled trial, *Neurology* 64(1) 26-31.

Beecher, G.R. (2003). Overview of dietary flavonoids: nomenclature, occurrence and intake, *J Nutr* 133(10):3248S-3254S.

Bejarano, I., Espino, J., Barriga, C., Reiter, R.J., Pariente, J.A. & Rodríguez, A.B. (2011) Pro-oxidant effect of melatonin in tumour leucocytes: relation with its cytotoxic and pro-apoptotic effects, *Basic Clin Pharmacol Toxicol* 108(1): 14-20.

Bolton, J.L., Trush, M.A., Penning, T.M., Dryhurst, G, & Monks, T.J. (2000). Role of quinones in toxicology, *Chem Res Toxicol* 13: 135-160.

Borek, C. (2004a). Antioxidants and Radiation Therapy, *J Nutr* 134(11): 3207S-3209S.

Borek, C. (2004b). Dietary Antioxidants and Human Cancer, *Integr Cancer Ther* 3 (4): 333-341.

Boulikas, T. & Vougiouka, M. (2003). Cisplatin and platinum drugs at the molecular level, *Oncology reports* 10(6): 1663-1682.

Boveris, A., Docampo. R., Turrens. J.F. & Stoppani, A.O. (1978). Effect of B-Lapachone on Superoxide Anion and Hydrogen Peroxide Production in Trypanosoma cruzi, *Biochem J* 175: 431-439.

Branda, R.F., Naud, S.J., Brooks, E.M., Chen, Z. & Muss, H. (2004) Effect of vitamin B12, folate, and dietary supplements on breast carcinoma chemotherapy–induced mucositis and neutropenia, *Cancer* 101(5): 1058–1064.

Büyükavci, M., Ozdemir, O., Buck, S., Stout, M., Ravindranath, Y., Savaşan, S. (2006) Melatonin cytotoxicity in human leukemia cells: relation with its pro-oxidant effect, *Fundam Clin Pharmacol* 20(1): 73-79.

Cabanillas, F. (2010). Vitamin c and cancer: what can we conclude - 1,609 Patients and 33 Years later? *PRHSJ* 29(3): 215-217.

Cameron, E. & Pauling, L. (1976). Supplemental ascorbate in the supportive treatment of cancer: Prolongation of survival times in terminal human cancer, *Proc Natl Acad Sci U S A* 73(10): 3685-3689.

Cameron, E. & Pauling, L. (1978). Suplementar ascorbato no tratamento do câncer de apoio: reavaliação de prolongamento dos tempos de sobrevida no câncer humano terminal, *Proc Natl Acad Sci U S A* 75(9): 4538-4542.

Casado-Zapico S., Rodriguez-Blanco, J., García-Santos, G., Martín, V., Sánchez-Sánchez, A.M., Antolín, I. & Rodriguez, C. (2010). Synergistic antitumor effect of melatonin with several chemotherapeutic drugs on human Ewing sarcoma cancer cells: potentiation of the extrinsic apoptotic pathway, *J Pineal Res* 48(1): 72-80.

Choi, H. S., Park, E.S., Kang, H.J., Shin, H.Y., Noh, C., Yun, Y.S., Ahn, H.S. & Choi, J.Y. (2010). Dexrazoxane for Preventing Anthracycline Cardiotoxicity in Children with Solid Tumors, *J Korean Med Sci* 25(9): 1336–1342.

Clark, L.C., Combs Jr, G.F., Turnbull, B.W., Slate, E.H., Chalker, D.K., Chow, J., Davis, L.S., Glover, R.A., Graham, G.F., Gross, E.G., Krongrad, A., Lesher Jr, J.L., Park, H.K., Sanders Jr, B.B., Smith, C.L. & Taylor, J. R. (1996). Effects of Selenium Supplementation for Cancer Prevention in Patients With Carcinoma of the SkinA Randomized Controlled Trial, *JAMA* 276(24): 1957-1963.

Clark, L.C, Dalkin, B., Krongrad, A., Combs, G.F. Jr, Turnbull, B.W., Slate, E.H., Witherington, R., Herlong, J.H., Janosko, E., Carpenter, D., Borosso, C., Falk, S. & Rounder, J. (1998). Decreased incidence of prostate cancer with selenium supplementation: results of a double-blind cancer prevention trial, *Br J Urol* 81(5): 730-734.

Clemens, M.R., Ladner, C., Ehninger, G., Einsele, H., Renn, W., Buhler, E., Waller, H.D. & Gey, K.F. (1990). Plasma vitamin E and beta-carotene concentrations during radiochemotherapy preceding bone marrow transplantation, *Am J Clin Nutr* 51(2): 216-219.

Clemens, M.R., Waladkhani, A.R., Bublitz, K., Ehninger, G. & Gey, K.F. (1997). Supplementation with antioxidants prior to bone marrow transplantation, *Wien Klin Wochenschr* 109(19): 771-776.

Combs, G.F. Jr. (2005). Current Evidence and Research Needs to Support a Health Claim for Selenium and Cancer Prevention, *J Nutr* 135(2): 343-347.

Culine, S., Kramar, A., Droz, J.P. & Theodore, C. (1999). Phase II study of all-trans retinoic acid administered intermittently for hormone refractory prostate cancer, *J Urol* 161: 173-175.

D'Andrea, G.M. (2005) Use of Antioxidants During Chemotherapy and Radiotherapy Should Be Avoided, *CA Cancer J Clin* 55: 319-321.

Desoize, B. & Madoulet, C. (2002). Particular aspects of platinum compounds used at present in cancer treatment, *Oncology Hematology* 42(3): 317-325.

Dong, Q., Barsky, D., Colvin, M.E., Melius, C.F., Ludeman, S.M., Moravek, J.F. Colvin, O.M., Bigner, D.D., Modrich, P. & Friedman, H.S. (1995). A Structural Basis for a

Phosphoramide Mustard-Induced DNA Interstrand Cross-Link at 5'-d(GAC), *Proc Natl Acad Sci USA* 92: 12170-12174.

Doyle, C., Kushi, L.H., Byers, T., Courneya, K. S., Demark-Wahnefried, W., Grant, B., McTiernan, A., Rock, C.L., Thompson, C., Gansler, T. & Andrews, K.S. (2006). Nutrition and Physical Activity During and After Cancer Treatment: An American Cancer Society Guide for Informed Choices, *CA Cancer J Clin* 56: 323-353.

Drisko, J.A., Chapman, J. & Hunter, V.J. (2003). The Use of Antioxidants with First-Line Chemotherapy in Two Cases of Ovarian Cancer, *Journal of the American College of Nutrition* 22(2): 118-123.

Franca C. A. S., Nogueira C. R., Ramalho A., Carvalho A. C. P., Vieira S. L. & Penna A. B. R. C. Serum levels of selenium in patients with breast cancer before and after treatment of external beam radiotherapy. Doi: 10.1093/annonc/mdq547.

González, M.J., Miranda-Massari, J.R. & Duconge J. (2010). Vitamin C and Cancer: What can we Conclude - 1,609 Patients and 33 Years Later: comment on the article by Cabanillas, *PRHSJ* 29(4): 410-411.

Gurtoo, H.L., Bansal, S.K., Pavelic Z. & Struck, R.F. (1985). Effects of the induction of hepatic microsomal metabolism on the toxicity of cyclophosphamide, *Br J Cancer* 51: 67-75.

Hahn, T., Szabo, L., Gold, M., Ramanathapuram, L., Hurley, L.H. & Akporiaye, E.T. (2006). Dietary Administration of the Proapoptotic Vitamin E Analogue α-Tocopheryloxyacetic Acid Inhibits Metastatic Murine Breast Cancer, *Cancer Res* 66: 9374-9378.

Hennekens, C.H., Mayrent, S.L. & Willet, W. (1986). Vitamin A, Carotenoids, and Retinoids, *Cancer* 58: 1837-1841.

Hong, W.K., Endicott, J., Itri, L.M., Doos, W., Batsakis, J.G., Bell, R., Fofonoff, S., Byers, R., Atkinson, N., Vaughan, C., Toth, B.B., Kramer, A., Dimery, I.W., Skipper, P. & Strong, S. (1986). 13-Cis-Retinoic Acid in the Treatment of Oral Leukoplakia, *N Engl J Med* 315: 1501-1505.

D'Incalci, M., Steward, W.P., & Gescher, A.J. (2007). Modulation of response to cancer chemotherapeutic agents by diet constituents-: Is the available evidence sufficiently robust for rational advice for patients? *Cancer treatment reviews* 33(3): 223-229.

Jensen, S.K. & Lauridsen, C. (2007). Alpha-tocopherol stereoisomers, *Vitam Horm* 76: 281-308.

Jung, B. & Ahmad, N. (2006). Melatonin in Cancer Management: Progress and Promise, *Cancer Res* 66(20): 9789-9793.

Junjing, Z., Yan, Z., Baolu, Z. (2010). Scavenging effects of dexrazoxane on free radicals, *J Clin Biochem Nutr* 47(3): 238-245.

Kanai, K., Kikuchi, E., Mikami, S., Suzuki, E., Uchida, Y., Kodaira, K., Miyajima, A., Ohigashi, T., Nakashima, J. & Oya, M. (2010). Vitamin E succinate induced apoptosis and enhanced chemosensitivity to paclitaxel in human bladder cancer cells *in vitro* and *in vivo*, *Cancer Science* 101(1): 216–223.

Kane R.C., McGuinn, W.D.Jr., Dagher, R., Justice, R. & Pazdur, R. (2008) Dexrazoxane (Totect™): FDA Review and Approval for the Treatment of Accidental Extravasation Following Intravenous Anthracycline Chemotherapy, *The Oncologist*, 13(4): 445-450.

Kennedy, M., Bruninga, K., Mutlu, E.A., Losurdo, J., Choudhary, S. & Keshavarzian, A. (2001). Successful and sustained treatment of chronic radiation proctitis with antioxidant vitamins E and C, *Am J Gastroenterol* 96(4): 1080-1084.

Khantamat, O., Chaiwangyen, W. & Limtrakul, P. (2004). Screening of flavonoids for their potential inhibitory effect on P-glycopotrein activity in human cervical carcinoma KB cells, *Chiang Mai Med Bull* 43(2): 45-56.

Klahr, S. (1997). Oxygen radicals and renal diseases, *Miner Electrolyte Metab* 23(3-6): 140-143.

Klerk, N.H., Musk, A.W., Ambrosini, G.L., Eccles, J.L., Hansen, J., Olsen, N., Watts, V.L., Lund, H.G., Pang, S.C., Beilby, J. & Hobbs, M.S.T. (1998). Vitamin A and cancer prevention II: Comparison of the effects of retinol and β-carotene, *International Journal of Cancer* 75(3): 362-367.

Köstler, W.J., Hejna, M., Wenzel, C. & Zielinski, C.C. (2001). Oral Mucositis Complicating Chemotherapy and/or Radiotherapy: Options for Prevention and Treatment, *CA: A Cancer Journal for Clinicians* 51(5): 290–315.

Kostova, I. (2006). Platinum Complexes as Anticancer Agents, *Recent Patents on Anti-Cancer Drug Discovery* 1: 1-22.

Kucuk, O., Sarkar, F.H., Djuric, Z., Sakr, W., Pollak, M.N., Khachik F., Banerjee, M., Bertram, J. S. & Wood, D.P. Jr. (2002). Effects of Lycopene Supplementation in Patients with Localized Prostate Cancer, *Exp Biol Med* 227:881–885.

Lamson, D.W. & Brignall, M.S. (1999). Antioxidants in cancer therapy; their actions and interactions with oncologic therapies, *Altern Med Rev* 4(5): 304-29.

Lee, I-Min, Cook, N.R., Gaziano, M., Gordon, D., Ridker, P.M., Manson, J.E., Hennekens, C.H. & Buring, J.E. (2005). Vitamin E in the Primary Prevention of Cardiovascular Disease and Cancer The Women's Health Study: A Randomized Controlled Trial, *JAMA* 294(1): 56-65.

Lipshultz, S.E., Scully, R.E., Lipsitz, S.R., Sallan, S.E., Silverman, L.B., Miller, T.L., Barry, E.V. Asselin, B.L., Athale, U., Clavell, L.A., Larsen, E., Moghrabi, A., Samson, Y., Michon, B., Schorin, M.A., Cohen, H.J., Neuberg, D.S., Orav, E.J. & Colan, S.D. (2010). Assessment of dexrazoxane as a cardioprotectant in doxorubicin-treated children with high-risk acute lymphoblastic leukaemia: long-term follow-up of a prospective, randomized, multicentre trial, *The Lancet Oncology* 11(10): 950 – 961.

Lissoni, P., Barni, S., Mandalà, M., Ardizzoia, A., Paolorossi, F., Vaghi, M., Longarini, R., Malugani, F. & Tancini, G. Decreased toxicity and increased efficacy of cancer chemotherapy using the pineal hormone melatonin in metastatic solid tumour patients with poor clinical status, *European Journal of Cancer* 35(12): 1688-1692.

Lissoni, P., Barni, S., Meregalli, S., Fossati, V., Cazzaniga, M., Esposti, D. & Tancini, G. (1995). Modulation of cancer endocrine therapy by melatonin: a phase II study of tamoxifen plus melatonin in metastatic breast cancer patients progressing under tamoxifen alone, *British Journal of Cancer* 71: 854-856.

Lissoni, P., Barni, S., Tancini, G., Ardizzoia, A., Ricci, G., Aldeghi, R., Brivio, F., Tisi, E., Rovelli, F. & Rescaldani, R. (1994). A randomized study with subcutaneous low-dose interleukin 2 alone vs interleukin 2 plus the pineal neurohormone melatonin in advanced solid neoplasms other than renal cancer and melanoma, *Br J Cancer* 69(1): 196–199.

Lissoni, P., Paolorossi, F., Ardizzoia, A., Barni, S., Chilelli, M., Mancuso, M., Tancini, G., Conti, A. & Maestroni, G.J.M. (1997). A randomized study of chemotherapy with cisplatin plus etoposide versus chemoendocrine therapy with cisplatin, etoposide and the pineal hormone melatonin as a first-line treatment of advanced non-small cell lung cancer patients in a poor clinical state, *Journal of Pineal Research* 23(1): 15–19.

Lopez, M., Vici, P., Di Lauro, K., Conti, F., Paoletti, G., Ferraironi, A., Sciuto, R., Giannarelli, D. & Maini, C.L. (1998). Randomized prospective clinical trial of high-dose epirubicin and dexrazoxane in patients with advanced breast cancer and soft tissue sarcomas, *Journal of Clinical Oncolog* 16: 86-92.

Kottschade, L.A., Sloan, J.A., Mazurczak, M.A., Johnson, D.B., Murphy, B.P., Rowland K.M., Smith, D.A., Berg, Alan R., Stella, P.J. & Loprinzi, C.L. (2010). The use of vitamin E for the prevention of chemotherapy-induced peripheral neuropathy: results of a randomized phase III clinical trial, *Support Care Cancer* DOI: 10.1007/s00520-010-1018-3.

Maciocia, G. (2010). *The three treasures news. Chemotherapy and antioxidants*, Available from http://www.biospharm.de/fileadmin/bios/img/Three_Treasure_News_Spring_2 010.pdf.

Manach, C., Scalbert, A., Morand, C., Rémésy, C. & Jiménez, L. (2004). Polyphenols: food sources and bioavailability, *Am J Clin Nutr* 79(5): 727-47.

Meyskens, F.L., Jr., Liu, P.Y., Tuthill, R.J., Sondak, V.K., Fletcher, W.S., Jewell, W.R., Samlowski, W., Balcerzak, S.P., Rector, D.J. & Noyes, R.D. (1994). Randomized trial of vitamin A versus observation as adjuvant therapy in high-risk primary malignant melanoma: a Southwest Oncology Group study, *J Clin Oncol* 12: 2060-2065.

Mills, E.E.D. (1988). The modifying effect of beta-carotene on radiation and chemotherapy induced oral mucositis, *Br J Cancer* 57: 416-417.

Minotti, G., Cairo, G. & Monti, E. (1999). Role of iron in anthracycline cardiotoxicity: new tunes for an old song?, *The FASEB Journal* 13(2): 199-212.

Moertel, C.G., Fleming, T.R., Creagan, E.T., Rubin, J. & O'Connell, M.J. (1985). High-Dose Vitamin C versus Placebo in the Treatment of Patients with Advanced Cancer Who Have Had No Prior Chemotherapy — A Randomized Double-Blind Comparison. *N Engl J Med* 312: 137-141.

Murakoshi, M., Takayasu, J., Kimura, O., Kohmura, E., Nishino, H., Iwashima, A., Okuzumi, J., Sakai, T., Sugimoto, T. & Imanishi, J. (1989). Inhibitory effects of alpha-carotene on proliferation of the human neuroblastoma cell line GOTO, *J Natl Cancer Inst* 81: 1649-1652.

Murgo, A.J. & Weinberger, B.B. (1993). Pharmacological bone marrow purging in autologous transplantation: Focus on the cyclophosphamide derivatives, *Crit Rev Oncol Hematol* 14(1): 41-60.

Nechuta, S., Lu, W., Chen, Z., Zheng, Y., Gu, K., Cai, H., Zheng, W. & Shu, X. (2011). Vitamin Supplement Use During Breast Cancer Treatment and Survival: A Prospective Cohort Study, *Cancer Epidemiol Biomarkers Prev* 20(2): 262-271.

Ohno, S., Ohno, Y., Suzuki, N., Soma, G. & Inoue, M. (2009). High-dose Vitamin C (Ascorbic Acid) Therapy in the Treatment of Patients with Advanced Cancer, *Anticancer Research* 29(3) 809-815.

Omenn, G.S., Goodman, G.E., Thornquist, M.D., Balmes, J., Cullen, M.R., Glass, A., Keogh, J.P., Meyskens, Jr F.L., Valanis, B., Williams, Jr J.H., Barnhart, S., & Hammar, S.

(1996). Effects of a Combination of Beta Carotene and Vitamin A on Lung Cancer and Cardiovascular Disease, *N Engl J Med* 334: 1150-1155.

Pace, A., Savarese, A., Picardo, M., Maresca, V., Pacetti, U., Del Monte, G., Biroccio, A., Leonetti, C., Jandolo, B., Cognetti, F. & Bove, L. (2003). Neuroprotective Effect of Vitamin E Supplementation in Patients Treated With Cisplatin Chemotherapy, *Journal of Clinical Oncology* 21(5): 927-931.

Pastorino, U., Infante, M., Maioli, M., Chiesa, G., Buyse, M., Firket, P., Rosmentz, N., Clerici, M., Soresi, E. & Valente, M. (1993). Adjuvant treatment of stage I lung cancer with high-dose vitamin A, *J Clin Oncol* 11(7): 1204-1207.

Pathak, A.K., Bhutani, M., Guleria, R., Bal, S., Mohan, A., Mohanti, B.K., Sharma, A., Pathak, R., Bhardwaj, N.K., Prasad, K. & Kochupillai, V. (2005). Chemotherapy Alone vs. Chemotherapy Plus High Dose Multiple Antioxidants in Patients with Advanced Non Small Cell Lung Cancer, *Journal of the American College of Nutrition*, 24(1): 16-21.

Peerapatdit, T., Patchanans, N., Likidlilid, A., Poldee, S. & Sriratanasathavorn, C. (2006). Plasma lipid peroxidation and antioxidiant nutrients in Type 2 Diabetic patients, *J Med Assoc Thai* 89(5): S147-155.

Pietta, Pier-Giorgio (2000). Flavonoids as Antioxidants, *J Nat Prod* 63(7): 1035-1042.

Prasad, K.N., Kumar, A., Kochupillai, V., & Cole, W.C. (1999). High Doses of Multiple Antioxidant Vitamins: Essential Ingredients in Improving the Efficacy of Standard Cancer Therapy, *Journal of the American College of Nutrition* 18(1): 13-25.

Prasad, K.N., Kumar, B., Yan, X., Hanson, A.J. & Cole, W.C. (2003). α-Tocopheryl Succinate, the Most Effective Form of Vitamin E for Adjuvant Cancer Treatment: A Review, *Journal of the American College of Nutrition* 22(2): 108-117.

Pratt, W. B. *The Anticancer Drugs*, 2ed. New York: Oxford Univ. Press USA, 1994.

Puri, T., Goyal. S., Julka, P.K., Nair, O., Sharma, D.N. & Rath, G.K. (2010). Lycopene in treatment of high-grade gliomas: A pilot study, *Neurol India* 58: 20-23.

Pyrhönen, S., Kuitunen, T., Nyandoto, P., Kouri, M. (1995). Randomized comparison of fluorouracil, epidoxorubicin and methotrexate (FEMTX) plus supportive care with supportive care alone in patients with non-resectable gastric cancer, *Br J Cancer* 71(3): 587-91.

Rajagopalan, S., Politi, P.M., Sinha, B.K. & Myers, C.E. (1988). Adriamycin-induced Free Radical Formation in the Perfused Rat Heart: Implications for Cardiotoxicity, *Cancer Res* 48(17): 4766-4769.

Recchia, F., Sica, G., Casucci, D., Rea, S., Gulino, A., Frati, L. (1998). Advanced carcinoma of the pancreas: phase II study of combined chemotherapy, beta-interferon, and retinoids, *Am J Clin Oncol* 21(3): 275-278.

Sadzuka, Y., Sugiyama, T. & Hirota, S. (1998). Modulation of cancer chemotherapy by green tea, *Clin Cancer Res* 4: 153-156.

Saul, A.W. (2010). Vitamin C and Cancer: What can we Conclude - 1,609 Patients and 33 Years Later: comment on the article by Cabanillas (Letters), *PRHSJ* 29(4): 409.

Selenius, M., Rundlöf, A., Olm, E., Fernandes, A.P. & Björnstedt, M. (2010). Selenium and the Selenoprotein Thioredoxin Reductase in the Prevention, Treatment and Diagnostics of Cancer, *Antioxidants & Redox Signaling* 12(7): 867-880.

Shanmugarajan, T.S., Arunsundar, M., Somasundaram, I., Krishnakumar, E., Sivaraman, D. & Ravichandiran, V. (2008). Cardioprotective effect of Ficus hispida Linn. on cyclophosphamide provoked oxidative myocardial injury in a rat model, *Int J Pharmacol* 4: 78-87.

Shimpo, K., Nagatsu, T., Yamada, K., Sato, T., Niimi, H., Shamoto, M., Takeuchi, T., Umezawa, H. & Fujita, K. (1991). Ascorbic acid and adriamycin toxicity, *Am J Clin Nutr* 54(6): 1298S-1301S.

Siddik, Z.H. (2002). Mechanisms of Action of Cancer Chemotherapeutic Agents: DNA-Interactive Alkylating Agents and Antitumour Platinum-Based Drugs. *The Cancer Handbook* 1st Edition. Edited by Malcolm R. Alison.

Silva, M.N., Ferreira, V.F. & Souza, M.C.B.V. (2003). An overview of the chemistry and pharmacology of naphthoquinone with emphasis on β-lapachone and derivatives. *Quim Nova* 26: 407-416.

Simone II, C.B. Simone, N.L. Simone, V. & Simone, C.B. (2007). Antioxidants and other nutrients do not interfere with chemotherapy or radioation therapy and can increase kill and increase survival. Part 1, *Alternative Therapies in Health and Medicine* 13: 22-28.

Smith, M.A., Parkinson, D.R., Cheson, B.D. & Friedman, M.A. (1992). Retinoids in cancer therapy, *Journal of Clinical Oncology* 10(5): 839-864.

Stratton, M.S., Algotar, A.M., Ranger-Moore, J, Stratton, S.P., Slate, E.H., Hsu, C.H., Thompson, P.A., Clark, L.C. & Ahmann, F.R. (2010). Oral Selenium Supplementation Has No Effect on Prostate-Specific Antigen Velocity in Men Undergoing Active Surveillance for Localized Prostate Cancer, *Cancer Prev Res* 3(8): 1035-1043.

Tan, D-x., Manchester, L.C., Hardeland, R., Lopez-Burillo, S., Mayo, J.C., Sainz, R.M. & Reiter, R.J. (2003). Melatonin: a hormone, a tissue factor, an autocoid, a paracoid, and an antioxidant vitamin, *Journal of Pineal Research* 34(1): 75–78.

Tan, D-x., Reiter, R.J., Manchester, L.C., Yan, M-t., El-Sawi, M., Sainz, R.M., Mayo, J.C., Kohen, R., Allegra, M.C. & Hardelan, R. (2002). Chemical and Physical Properties and Potential Mechanisms: Melatonin as a Broad Spectrum Antioxidant and Free Radical Scavenger, *Current Topics in Medicinal Chemistry* 2(2): 181-197.

Tang, Su-Ni, Singh, C., Nall, D., Meeker, D., Shankar, S. & Srivastava, R.K. (2010). The dietary bioflavonoid quercetin synergizes with epigallocathechin gallate (EGCG) to inhibit prostate cancer stem cell characteristics, invasion, migration and epithelial-mesenchymal transition, *Journal of Molecular Signaling* 5(14): 1-15.

Tang, Y., Parmakhtiar, B., Simoneau, A.R., Xie, J., Fruehauf, J., Lilly, M. & Zi, X. (2011) Lycopene Enhances Docetaxel's Effect in Castration-Resistant Prostate Cancer Associated with Insulin-like Growth Factor I Receptor Levels, *Neoplasia* 13(2): 108–119.

van Zandwijk, N., Dalesio, O., Pastorino, U., de Vries, N. & van Tinteren, H. (2000). EUROSCAN, a Randomized Trial of Vitamin A and N-Acetylcysteine in Patients With Head and Neck Cancer or Lung Cancer For the European Organization for Research and Treatment of Cancer Head and Neck and Lung Cancer Cooperative Groups, *J Natl Cancer Inst* 92(12): 977-986.

Wadleigh, R.G., Redman, R.S., Graham, M.L., Krasnow, S.H., Anderson, A. & Cohen, M.H. (1992) Vitamin E in the treatment of chemotherapy-induced mucositis, *The American Journal of Medicine* 92(5): 481-484.

Wang, D. & Lippard, S.J. (2005). Cellular processing of platinum anticancer drugs, *Nature Reviews Drug Discovery* 4: 307-320.

Witte, N.V., Stoppani, A.O. & Dubin, M. (2004). 2-Phenyl-betalapachone can affect mitochondrial function by redox cycling mediated oxidation, *Arch Biochem Biophys* 432: 129-135.

Young, R.C., Ozols, R.F. & Myers, C.E. (1981). The anthracycline antineoplasic drugs. *New Engl J Med* 305: 139-153.

Combination Chemotherapy in Cancer: Principles, Evaluation and Drug Delivery Strategies

Ana Catarina Pinto[1], João Nuno Moreira[2,3] and Sérgio Simões[1,2,3]
[1]Bluepharma, Indústria Farmacêutica S.A., S. Martinho do Bispo, Coimbra
[2]Laboratory of Pharmaceutical Technology, Faculty of Pharmacy,
University of Coimbra, Coimbra
[3]Center for Neurosciences and Cell Biology, University of Coimbra, Coimbra
Portugal

1. Introduction

Cancer is a major public health problem since it is the second leading cause of illness-related death, only exceeded by heart disease (American Cancer Society [ACS], (2010)). Cancer results from structural and quantitative alterations in molecules that control different aspects of cell behavior. Genetic alterations probably represent the most common mechanisms for molecular changes that cause the development and progression of cancer (Dong, 2006). Great efforts have been made to identify common genetic modifications and the underlying target genes. Genetic alterations can be inherited, as in hereditary cancers, or induced by endogenous and exogenous carcinogenic factors as in most sporadic cancers (Dong, 2006). The six essential changes in cell physiology suggested to collectively dictate malignant growth are self-sufficiency in growth signals, insensitivity to anti-growth signals, tissue invasion and metastasis, limitless replicative potential, sustained angiogenesis and evading apoptosis (Hanahan & Weinberg, 2000).

Chemotherapeutic agents used in current clinical practice have played a significant role in reducing mortality/morbidity and in increasing patient's quality of life (Suggit & Bibby, 2005). Despite the recent advances in early diagnosis and in clinical protocols for cancer treatment, the development of antineoplastic agents that combine efficacy, safety and convenience for the patient remains a great challenge (Ismael et al., 2008).

Most anticancer drugs have narrow therapeutic index, develop multidrug resistance (MDR) and present unspecific biodistribution upon intravenous administration leading to unacceptable side effects to healthy tissues, mainly bone marrow and gastrointestinal tract. These limitations of conventional chemotherapeutic strategies frequently result in suboptimal dosing, treatment delay or discontinuance and reduced patient compliance to therapy (Ismael et al., 2008).

2. Combination chemotherapy

2.1 Principles and advantages

Combination therapy has been the standard of care, especially in cancer treatment, since it is a rationale strategy to increase response and tolerability and to decrease resistance.

Currently, there is a growing interest in combining anticancer drugs aiming at maximizing efficacy while minimizing systemic toxicity through the delivery of lower drug doses (Mayer & Janoff, 2007; Ramsey et al., 2005; Zoli et al., 2001).

The fundamentals of combination chemotherapy development have remained largely unchanged over the last decades. The general principles have been to: i) use drugs with non-overlapping toxicities so that each drug can be administered at near-maximal dose; ii) combine agents with different mechanisms of action and minimal cross-resistance in order to inhibit the emergence of broad spectrum drug resistance; iii) preferentially use drugs with proven activity as single drugs and iv) administer the combination at early stage disease and at a schedule with a minimal treatment-free period between cycles but still allowing the recovery of sensitive target tissues (Mayer & Janoff, 2007; Harasym et al, 2007; Ramsey et al., 2005; Zoli et al., 2001). The advantages attributed to combination chemotherapy include improved patient compliance due to the reduced number of administrations, emergence of additive or synergistic interaction effects, ability to overcome or delay MDR and reduction of drug dose with consequent diminishing of toxicity to healthy tissues (Chou, 2010, 2006; Ramsey et al., 2005).

As an example, multimodal combination treatments for hormone refractory prostate cancer (HRPC) have gained support in the clinical setting over the last decade (De la Taille et al., 2001). Given the complexity, heterogeneity, resistance and recurrence features of prostate cancer, rationally-designed drug combinations are necessary to achieve significant therapeutic progress (Armstrong & Carducci, 2006).

2.2 Preclinical vs. clinical drug combination studies

The majority of clinical protocols for cancer combination therapies are mainly obtained empirically, in the absence of supporting experimental data, or based on results derived from retrospective analysis of clinical trials (Zoli et al, 2001; Goldie, 2001). These studies investigate the sequencing and scheduling of drugs rather than determining the optimal drug interactions. Information obtained from clinical protocols is valuable, but is time-consuming, expensive and does not provide data on the biochemical and molecular mechanisms of drug interaction at cellular level resulted from combined treatments (Zoli et al., 2001). It is very difficult to determine whether drug combinations are acting in a synergistic, additive or antagonistic fashion in cancer patients. Ultimately, one can only determine whether a new combination provides a statistically significant increase in a specific end point such as response rate, time to progression or survival (Mayer, 2007).

Preclinical drug interaction studies allow a more rational design of clinical combination chemotherapy protocols, which are generally based on the empiric assumption that maximal efficacy will be achieved by co-administering each drug at their maximum tolerated doses (MTDs) (Mayer & Janoff, 2007; Harasym et al., 2007; Mayer et al., 2006). This "more-is-better" philosophy applied to anticancer combinations may result in higher toxicity with minimal therapeutic benefit due to concentration-dependent drug interactions (Mayer et al, 2006; Ramsey et al., 2005). Undoubtedly, there are several molecular and pharmacological factors that determine the effectiveness of drug combinations. A rationally-designed fixed drug combination is required since certain drug ratios can be synergistic, while others are additive or even antagonistic (Mayer & Janoff, 2007; Mayer et al., 2006).

The design of preclinical drug combination studies on established cell lines, primary cell cultures or animal models has to take into account several factors such as drug concentration, exposure time, drug administration schedule and analytic method for evaluating the drug interaction (Zoli et al., 2001).

2.3 In vitro vs. in vivo drug combination studies

Evaluation of drug ratio-dependent effects in combination chemotherapy is frequently conducted in cell culture systems. During the course of the experiment, concentration and duration of administered drug(s) can be tightly controlled and the inhibition of tumor cell growth can be easily measured (Mayer & Janoff, 2007; Harasym et al., 2007; Chou et al., 2006). For the last two decades, in vitro experimentation with tumor-derived cell lines has been the most important resource for investigating molecular mechanisms of cancer pathogenesis (Mitchell et al., 2000). There are a number of advantages associated with the use of cell culture systems, e.g. availability of a wide range of human tumor cell lines, flexibility of culture conditions and easiness of protein/nucleic acid quantification (Harasym et al., 2007). Additionally, in vitro tests not only evaluate antiproliferative effects of tested drugs but also assess interference on cell cycle, induction of apoptosis and existence of molecular or biochemical interactions (Zoli et al., 2001).

Unfortunately, cell culture studies are of limited usefulness because the conditions are artificial, do not reflect the heterogeneity of clinical malignant disease and, hence, are unable to evaluate the therapeutic index (Budman et al., 2002). Unlike in vitro studies where drug concentration is relatively constant, in vivo models represents a dynamic system, where drug molecules undergo absorption, distribution, metabolism and elimination, thus leading to plasma drug concentration changes over time (Merlin, 1994). Nevertheless, when compared to in vitro studies, the determination of synergism or antagonism in vivo using animal models is more time consuming, more expensive and greater variability in measurements occurs. Therefore, in vivo drug combination studies are usually carried out, only for selected drugs, after in vitro evaluation and before clinical trials (Chou, 2010, 2006).

3. Drug interaction effects in combination chemotherapy

3.1 Definition and in vitro quantitative evaluation

A drug combination can result in synergistic, antagonistic or additive interaction effects at different concentration ratios. Synergy, additivity and antagonism are defined as the interaction between two or more components such that the combined effect is superior, equal or inferior, respectively, to the expected sum of individual effects. Additivity means that each constituent contributes to the effect in accordance with its own potency (Chou, 2006; Merlin, 1994).

Systematic screening analysis of drug combinations can identify additive or synergistic relationships previously unrecognized (Mayer & Janoff, 2007). In vitro synergistic activity is strongly dependent on drug:drug ratio and that dependence has profound implications on clinical application, since in vivo activity relies on the maintenance of those therapeutic ratios at the disease site (Mayer & Janoff, 2007; Harasym et al., 2007; Mayer et al., 2006). Therefore, in order to achieve maximal therapeutic efficacy in vivo, dosing schedule is essential to allow exposure of tumor cells to defined drug concentrations (Zhao et al., 2008).

Several methods for the quantitative evaluation of drug-combined interaction effects have been used and were comparatively reviewed elsewhere (Zoli et al., 2001; Merlin, 1994). A brief description of the principles and limitations of the different methods is compiled in Table 1. However, in the present book chapter only the median effect analysis is extensively reviewed in the next section.

Method	Author	Principle	Limitations
Fractional product	Webb (1963)	Summation of the effects of two inhibitors is expressed by the product of the fractional activities	Method does not take into account the possible sigmoidicity of the dose response curves (m > 1 or m < 1) and is not applicable in the case of two mutually exclusive drugs or second-order mutually non-exclusive drugs
Classical isobologram	Loewe (1957)	Lines join doses or dose-combinations exerting the same effect (iso-effect)	Method requires a large number of data points, has poor computer software, the statistical approach is incomplete and only two-drug combinations can be evaluated. Method is not applicable in the case of two mutually non-exclusive drugs
Isobologram modified	Stell and Peckham (1979)	Envelope of additivity: a region delimited by confidence limits in which the cytotoxic agents are not significantly interacting	
Median effect analysis	Chou and Talalay (1984)	Enzyme kinetic system: mass action law, Michaelis–Menten and Hill equations	Method should not be applied when the dose–response curves are not sigmoidal because of the difficulty of applying linear regression analysis
Three-dimensional	Fraser (1972) Carter and Wampler (1986) Kanzawa (1997)	Michaelis–Menten equations Median effect principle	Model requires several mathematical functions and software for each different type of response surface. The complex execution prevents it from being widely used in preclinical studies

Table 1. Methods for the quantitative evaluation of drug combination effects. Data was adapted and compiled from several literature references (Chou, 2006, 1994; Chou & Talalay, 1984; Zoli et al., 2001; Merlin, 1994).

3.2 The median effect analysis

By far the most prevalent method used for quantitative evaluation of drug combinations is the median effect analysis proposed by Chou and Talalay (Chou, 2010, 2006, 1994; Chou & Talalay, 1984). The fundamental equations of this method were derived from mass action enzyme kinetic models, previously established for enzyme-substrate interactions and then extended to multiple drug combinations (Chou, 1976). The equations underlying the median effect principle can be considered as a generalized form including the concepts of fractional product and isobologram analysis (Table 1) (Merlin, 1994; Chou & Talalay, 1984).

Regardless of the shape of the dose-effect curve or the drug mechanism of action, the median effect equation correlates drug dose and corresponding effect (cell growth inhibition) and is given by:

$$f_a / f_u = (D/D_m)^m \tag{1}$$

Where f_a and f_u are the fractions of cells affected and unaffected, respectively, by a dose (D); D_m is the dose causing the median effect and m the coefficient traducing the shape of the dose effect curve (m = 1, >1 and < 1, indicate hyperbolic, sigmoidal and negative sigmoidal, respectively). The m and D_m parameters are easily determined from the median effect plot since they correspond to the slope and to the antilog of the x-intercept, respectively (Chou 2006, 1994; Chou et al. 1994). When m and D_m are determined, the entire dose-effect relationship is described since for a given dose (D) it is possible to calculate the effect (f_a) and vice-versa (Chou, 2010, 1994). Application of equation 1 allows the linearization of hyperbolic (m = 1) as well as sigmoidal curves (m ≠ 1) which are often encountered in chemotherapy treatment data (Merlin, 1994; Chou & Talalay, 1984). Plotting x = log(D) vs. y = $\log(f_a/f_u)$ based on the logarithm form of equation 1 is called the median effect plot (Chou, 2010, 2006) (Fig. 1).

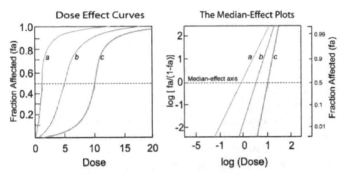

Fig. 1. Graphical representations executed in the median effect analysis method. Three sigmoidal dose-effect curves (a, b, c) (left graph) and respective transformation into the corresponding linear forms by the median effect plot (right graph), where y = log(fa/fu) vs. x = log(D). Adapted from reference (Chou, 2006).

The conformity of the data to the median effect principle can be readily manifested by the linear correlation coefficient (r) of the plot, in which r = 1 indicates perfect conformity (Chou, 2010, 2006, 1994). The fractional effect associated with a range of concentrations is determined for each individual drug and for their combination. The median effect plot gives parallel lines if the drugs have the same or similar modes of action and the effects are then considered mutually exclusive; if the plots for single drugs are parallel but the mixture plot is concave upward with the tendency to intersect the plot of the more potent drug, the drugs act independently and their effects are considered mutually non-exclusive (Chou & Talalay, 1984).

The combination index (CI) quantitatively evaluates the nature of drug interaction and is defined by the following equation:

$$CI = \frac{(D)_1}{(D_x)_1} + \frac{(D)_2}{(D_x)_2} + \alpha \frac{(D)_1(D)_2}{(D_x)_1(D_x)_2} \qquad (2)$$

Where α = 0 and α = 1, for drugs with mutually exclusive or non-exclusive mechanisms of action, respectively (Chou, 2010, 2006, 1994; Chou & Talalay, 1984). Denominators $(D_x)_1$ and $(D_x)_2$ are drug doses required to achieve a given effect level (f_a). Numerators $(D)_1$ and $(D)_2$ are doses of each drug in a given mixture which originates the same f_a. For three-drug combinations, a third term $(D)_3/(D_x)_3$ is added to equation 2. A plot of CI as a function of effect level (f_a) is represented in Fig. 2. CI values reflect synergism, additivity or antagonism when inferior, equal or superior to 1, respectively.

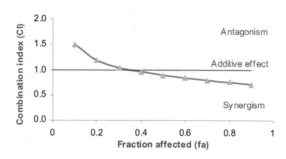

Fig. 2. Graphical representation of an exemplificative CI - fa plot. Combination index (CI) < 1, = 1, > 1 indicate synergism, additivity and antagonism, respectively.

If the nature of drug mechanisms is not clear, the authors of the method suggest that CI value must be determined by both mutually exclusive ($\alpha = 0$) and mutually non-exclusive ($\alpha = 1$) assumptions. The later approach is more conservative as the addition of a third term in equation 2 results in higher CI values than the former one (Chou, 2006, 1994, Chou & Talalay, 1984). Even though the CI value can be expressed for any effect level, the most accurate determination is for $f_a = 0.5$ since the median effect plot may be unreliable at the extremes as it represents a linear approximation of a non-linear function (Kreis et al., 2001).

The median effect analysis is a simple quantitative method that takes into account not only the potency (D_m) of each drug and of their combination but also the shape (hyperbolic or sigmoidal) of their dose-effect curves (Chou, 1994; Chou et al., 1994). Furthermore, this method evaluates interaction effects at different drug ratios, at different effect levels and up to three agents can be evaluated simultaneously (Chou et al., 1994; Chou & Talalay, 1984). It is recommended that an experiment should be carried out using a constant equipotency ratio (e.g. $(IC_{50})_1 / (IC_{50})_2$) so that the effect contribution of each drug to the combination can be roughly equal (Chou, 2010, 2006; Chou & Talalay, 1984). When evaluating anticancer drug combinations, the dose range administered must be wide enough to allow extrapolation of the results up to high levels of activity, i.e. $f_a \geq 0.5$, owing to the fact that tumor growth inhibition below that level is not clinically meaningful (Chou, 2010; Harasym et al., 2007; Merlin, 1994).

Dose reduction index (DRI) is a measure of how many folds the dose of a combined drug may be reduced at a given effect level as compared to the dose of the drug alone (Chou, 2006; Mayer et al., 2006). DRI is an important parameter in clinical practice because a favorable value (> 1) may lead to reduced systemic toxicity toward healthy tissues while maintaining therapeutic efficacy (Chou, 2010, 2006, 1998, 1994; Chou & Talalay, 1984).

4. Nanoparticles as drug delivery systems

In face of the difficulties and high costs inherent to the development of new therapeutic molecules, the strategy of most pharmaceutical companies seems to rely on the optimization of the existing drugs, namely those characterized by a low therapeutic index. In particular, the application of nanotechnology-based drug delivery systems, such as liposomes, to cancer chemotherapy has been an exciting and promising area of research and constitutes an important ongoing effort to improve specificity and efficacy of anticancer drugs.

4.1 Different types of nanoparticles

Several drugs have physical and biological properties which hinder their clinical applicability, namely poor water solubility, rapid metabolism, instability under physiological conditions, unfavorable pharmacokinetics and unspecific biodistribution to healthy tissues (Allen, 1998). Particularly, in the case of anticancer drugs, such features ultimately lead to inadequate delivery of effective therapeutic drug concentrations to tumor tissue and/or unacceptable toxic effects (Andresen et al., 2005; Cattel et al., 2003). Therefore, it is crucial to develop nanotechnology-based platforms (lipid or polymer-based nanocarriers such as liposomes, micelles, polymeric nanoparticles or dendrimers) to promote and control delivery of some anticancer drugs to tumors (Devalapally et al., 2007; Peer et al., 2007; Dutta, 2007) (Fig. 3).

Nanoparticles with medical applications differ in terms of structure, size and composition, thus resulting in different characteristics, namely drug loading capacity, physical stability and targeted delivery ability (Haley & Frenkel, 2008). It is beyond the scope of this chapter to review the current drug delivery nanocarriers since they have been widely reviewed in recent publications (Devalapally et al., 2007; Peer et al., 2007; Dutta, 2007; Haley & Frenkel, 2008; Lammers et al., 2008; Cho et al., 2008; Alexis et al., 2008). Therefore, in this chapter an overview will be restricted to liposomes, since these are probably the most used drug delivery system for small drug molecules.

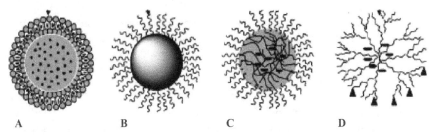

A   B   C   D

Fig. 3. Schematic representation of exemplificative nanocarriers for drug delivery. A Liposome; B Polymeric nanoparticle; C Micelle; D Dendrimer. Adapted from reference (Devalapally et al., 2007).

4.2 Liposomes
4.2.1 General definition and main features

Liposomes were firstly described by Bangham *et al.* (Bangham et al., 1965) and were originally called phospholipid spherules. Liposomes are self-assembling closed colloidal lipid vesicles (Fig. 4) with considerable potential for delivery of therapeutic agents due to several features: biodegradability, biocompatibility, simplicity, scaled-up production, low inherent toxicity, weak immunogenicity, versatility in structure and in physicochemical properties (lipid composition, size and surface charge) and ability to undergo surface engineering towards conjugation of polymers and targeting ligands (Immordino et al., 2006; Hofheinz et al., 2005; Cattel et al., 2003). Due to those specific attributes, liposomes have the ability to modulate in vivo behavior (pharmacokinetics and biodistribution profile) and/or solubility properties of drugs and to protect them from premature degradation or inactivation after intravenous administration (Fenske et al., 2008; Immordino et al., 2006; Drummond et al., 1999; Allen, 1998). In general, when a drug is encapsulated within a carrier, such as liposome (Fig. 4) the plasma clearance and volume of distribution decrease while the plasma circulation half-life ($t_{1/2}$) and area under the plasma concentration *vs.* time curve (AUC) increase (Gabizon et al., 2003).

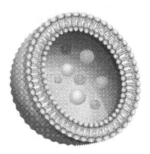

Fig. 4. Schematic representation of a liposome vehicle with drug molecules encapsulated in the aqueous internal compartment.

The pharmacokinetics, biodistribution and biological activity of a liposomal drug formulation are influenced by size, surface charge, lipid and drug doses, lipid composition, steric stabilization and route of administration (Charrois & Allen, 2004, 2003; Nagayasu et al., 1999; Mayer et al., 1989).

The development of a successful therapeutic liposomal drug formulation must comply with three fundamental requisites: i) clear knowledge of the biology and physiology of the disease to be treated; ii) good understanding of the physicochemical properties of both the carrier and the drug and iii) determination of the pharmacokinetic and biodistribution changes induced in the drug by the liposomal vehicle (Allen, 1998).

Liposome structural types, physicochemical composition and preparation methods will not be overviewed in the present chapter since they have been thoroughly reviewed over the last two decades, in particular by Dr. Allen (Allen, 1998, 1997, 1994) and Dr. Lasic (Lasic et al., 1999) research groups.

4.2.2 Medical applications

In the past decades there have been major advances in the development of liposomal drug formulations suitable for several medical applications. In addition to their feature as drug delivery systems in the treatment of cancer, bacterial infections or ophthalmic disorders, current clinical applications of liposomes also include gene delivery, diagnostic imaging, vaccine adjuvant, photodynamic therapy, dermatology, hemoglobin or chelating agent transporter and enzyme replacement therapy (Fenske et al., 2008; Torchillin, 2007; Immordino et al., 2006; Torchillin, 2005; Gregoriadis & Florence, 1993). The ultimate goal of an anticancer liposomal formulation is to improve overall therapeutic index of encapsulated drugs by increasing the antitumor activity and/or by reducing the toxicity profile, due to preferential delivery and accumulation at tumor tissue as compared to free drugs (Drummond et al., 1999; Gabizon, 1992).

4.2.3 In vivo behavior: From conventional to sterically stabilized liposomes

Ideally, liposomal drug formulations should have a mean diameter centered on 100 nm, a high drug-to-lipid ratio, an excellent retention of encapsulated drug(s) (while circulating in the blood) and a long circulation lifetime (from hours to days) (Fenske & Cullis, 2005). In general, the short blood residence time and in vivo drug leakage profile of conventional liposomes hinder their clinical applicability. Liposomes are recognized and bounded by serum proteins (opsonins) (Fig. 4) and by complement system after which they are cleared from systemic circulation by reticulo-endothelial system (RES) cells of the liver, spleen and bone marrow (Immordino et al., 2006; Chonn et al., 1992; Papadjopolous et al., 1991). The physicochemical properties of liposomes, such as net surface charge, hydrophobicity, size, fluidity and packing of the lipid bilayer, influence their stability and the type of proteins that bind to them (Chonn et al., 1992). Moreover, lipid exchange with plasma lipoproteins can destabilize liposomes and lead to their rupture with release of entrapped content (Immordino et al., 2006). The use of saturated phospholipids with high phase transition temperature associated with cholesterol, but mostly surface coating with a synthetic hydrophilic polymer such as poly(ethylene glycol) – PEG (Fig. 4) or with ganglioside G_{M1}, significantly extend bloodstream circulation time to several days and reduces RES clearance (Immordino et al., 2006; Gabizon et al., 2003; Allen, 1994, Papahadjopoulos et al., 1991; Gabizon & Papahadjopoulos, 1988). Nevertheless, there are some disadvantages associated with PEG coating. There is some evidence that pegylated liposomes are not completely inert and can still induce activation of complement system (Immordino et al., 2006). Furthermore, the presence of PEG may hinder drug release to the target cell population (Harrington et al., 2002). Attempts have been made to solve these limitations by generating liposomes that are reversibly pegylated as described in detail elsewhere (Immordino et al., 2006; Harrington et al., 2002).

Pegylated liposomes are named sterically stabilized liposomes (SSL) or Stealth® due to a highly hydrated surface, constituted by the hydrophilic PEG and water molecules, that acts as a steric barrier and prevents protein adsorption and opsonization (Fig. 5) (Immordino et al., 2006; Andresen et al., 2005; Gabizon et al., 2003).

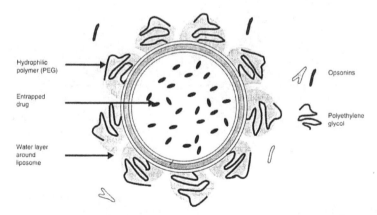

Fig. 5. Graphical representation of PEG-coated liposome (Stealth®). Extent of opsonization of pegylated liposomes is significantly diminished due to their highly hydrated surface. Adapted from reference (Allen, 1997).

4.2.4 The enhanced permeability and retention effect in tumor tissues

Most solid tumors possess unique pathophysiological characteristics that are absent in normal tissues, such as extensive and unregulated angiogenesis, defective vascular architecture, enhanced vascular permeability, dysfunctional lymphatic drainage and increased production of a number of permeability mediators (Gabizon et al., 2006; Maeda et al., 2000). This enhanced permeability and retention effect (EPR) inherent to solid tumors (Fig. 6) (Maeda et al., 2000; Drummond et al., 1999) has been described in several experimental tumors and depends mainly on tumor volume, vascularization and leakage from blood vessels (Gabizon et al., 2006; Yuan et al., 1995). Long-circulating liposomal drug formulations with size diameter within the range of 100-150 nm demonstrate preferential extravasation through leaky tumor vasculature and passively accumulate in the interstitial space due to the EPR effect. The release of drug molecules from liposomes into the tumor interstitium provides locally drug delivery at therapeutic dose levels (Abraham et al., 2005; Drummond et al., 1999; Gabizon & Papahadjopoulos, 1988). Interestingly, a particular study on tumor xenograft animal models reported that liposomes up to 400 nm can extravasate across tumor vessels and penetrate into tumor interstitium, suggesting that the threshold vesicle size of the pores is generally between 400 and 600 nm in diameter (Yuan et al., 1995). Nevertheless it is important to emphasize that the cut-off range mostly depends on tumor type. The extent of accumulation within the tumor is largely determined by the circulation lifetime of the liposomes (Song et al., 2006). Moreover, the impaired lymphatic drainage in the tumor interstitium favors the retention of liposomal formulations at the extravasation site, accentuating the passive targeting to solid tumors (Fig. 5) (Gabizon et al., 2006; Maeda et al., 2000; Drummond et al., 1999).

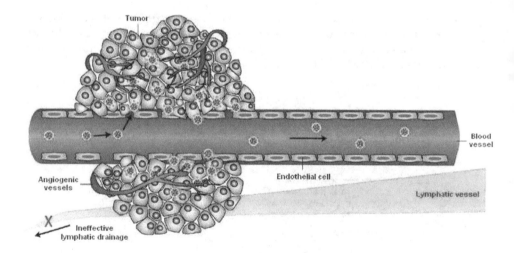

Fig. 6. Enhanced permeability and retention effect (EPR). Liposomes are shown as representative nanoparticles. Tumor targeting is achieved by passive extravasation of liposomes, from blood to tumor interstitium through highly permeable vasculature, and by accumulation in interstitial space due to non-functional lymphatic system in solid tumors. Adapted from reference (Peer et al., 2007).

4.2.5 Liposomal single drug formulations approved for clinical use or under clinical evaluation

The success of liposomes as drug delivery systems has been reflected by the significant number of formulations which are FDA or EMA-approved for clinical use (Table 2) or undergoing clinical evaluation (Table 3).

Representative examples of liposomal single drug formulations that have gained regulatory approval for clinical use are Doxil® and Myocet®. These LUV formulations encapsulating doxorubicin are being marketed for the treatment of several cancers, either as an individual formulation or in combination treatments (Table 2). Liposomal anthracyclines, namely doxorubicin, have raised significant interest due to their ability to decrease drug-related toxicity (cardiomyopathy, which can lead to congestive heart failure and death, bone marrow suppression, alopecia or nausea) with no associated loss of therapeutic activity (Abraham et al., 2005; Gabizon et al., 2003, 1998).

Formulation brand name	Drug name	Dosage form / route	Therapeutic indication	Date	Company name
Abelcet®		Lipid complex /injection	Systemic fungal infection	1995	Enzon
AmBisome®	Amphotericin B	Liposomal/ injection	Systemic fungal infection	1997	Astellas Pharma
Amphotec®		Lipid complex /injection	Systemic fungal infection	1996	Three Rivers Pharms
DaunoXome®	Daunorubicin citrate	Liposomal/ injection	AIDS-related Kaposi's sarcoma Breast cancer and other solid tumors	1996	Diatos S.A.
DepoCyt®	Cytarabine	Liposomal/ injection	Lymphomatous meningitis (intrathecal application)	1999	Pacira Pharmaceuticals Inc.
DepoDur®	Morphine sulfate	Liposomal/ epidural	Post-surgical pain reliever	2004	Pacira Pharmaceuticals Inc.
Doxil®(USA)			AIDS-related Kaposi's sarcoma	1995	Centocor Ortho Biotech Inc.
Caelyx® (Europe)	Doxorubicin.HCl	Liposomal/ injection	Advanced ovarian cancer Metastatic breast cancer Multiple myeloma (combination with bortezomib)	1996	Schering Plough Europe
Myocet®	Doxorubicin.HCl	Liposomal/ injection	Metastatic breast cancer (in combination with cyclophosphamide)	2000	Cephalon Europe
Visudyne®	Verteporfin	Liposomal/ injection	Age-related macular degeneration	2000	QLT Inc. /Novartis

Table 2. Current FDA or EMA-approved liposomal single drug formulations for different clinical applications. Source: official website of USA Food and Drug Administration (FDA) - http://www.fda.gov (2010) and European Medicines Agency (EMA) - http://www.ema.europa.eu (2010).

Formulation brand name	Therapeutic agent	Therapeutic indication	Company name	Status
Annamycin		Acute lymphocytic leukemia Acute myelogenous leukemia	Callisto Pharmaceuticals	Phase I/II
		Breast cancer	New York University School of Medicine	Phase I/II
Aroplatin	Platinum agent NDDP	Colorectal cancer	Aronex Pharmaceuticals	Phase II
Atragen	Tretinoin	Hodgkin's lymphoma	M.D. Anderson Cancer Center	Phase II
		Metastatic kidney cancer	Weill Medical College of Cornell University	Phase II
Cisplatin		Lung cancer	Transave	Phase II
LE-SN28	Irinotecan metabolite SN38	Advanced cancer	NeoPharm	Phase I
LEP-ETU	Paclitaxel	Advanced cancer	NeoPharm	Phase I
Marqibo®	Vincristine	Acute lymphoblastic leukemia Malignant melanoma	Hana Biosciences	Phase II Phase I/II
Mitoxantrone		Advanced cancer	NeoPharm	Phase I
Nystatin		Systemic fungal infection in patients with hematologic cancer	Aronex Pharmaceuticals	Phase III
OSI-211	Lurtotecan	Ovarian cancer Small cell lung carcinoma	OSI Pharmaceuticals	Phase II
SPI-77	Cisplatin	Ovarian cancer	New York University School of Medicine	Phase II
Stimuvax®	BLP25 vaccine	Non-small cell lung cancer	EMD Serono and Oncothyreon	Phase III
Topotecan		Small cell lung cancer Ovarian cancer Other solid tumors	Hana Biosciences, Inc	Phase I
Vinorelbine		Advanced solid tumors Non-Hodgkin's lymphoma Hodgkin's lymphoma	Hana Biosciences, Inc	Phase I

Table 3. Examples of emerging liposomal single drug formulations currently undergoing clinical evaluation for cancer treatment. Currently, some liposomal drugs have no brand name and, therefore, are identified by the drug name. Data was compiled from http://www.phrma.org (2009) and from literature references (Lammers et al., 2008; Dutta, 2007; Torchillin, 2007, 2005; Immordino et al., 2006; Hofheinz et al., 2005) with actualization of current clinical status after consult of http://clinicaltrials.gov/ (2010).

Currently, there are no approved liposomal drugs for treatment of urologic cancers. Nevertheless, some liposomal drug formulations listed in Table 4 are under clinical evaluation for prostate cancer treatment.

Formulation name	Treatment	Therapeutic indication	Company name	Status
Pegylated liposomal doxorubicin hydrochloride	Monotherapy	Prostate cancer (associated with hyperthermia treatment)	Celsion	Phase I
	Monotherapy	Hormone-refractory prostate cancer (HRPC)	Ireland Cancer Center	Phase II
Doxil®	In combination with estramustine		Ortho Biotech, Inc.	Phase I/II
Doxil®	In combination with thalidomide		Ortho Biotech, Inc.	Phase II
Doxil®	In combination with Taxotere®		James Graham Brown Cancer Center	Phase I/II

Table 4. Liposomal single drug formulations currently under clinical evaluation for prostate cancer treatment. Data was compiled after consult of http://clinicaltrials.gov/ (2010).

4.2.6 Liposomal formulations of anticancer drug combinations

4.2.6.1 General considerations

The use of drug combinations has been standard of care for the treatment of cancer over the last decades. Nevertheless, the application of liposomes as carriers for anticancer drug combinations has been described in literature only in the last few years (Tardi et al., 2009; Harasym et al., 2007; Tardi et al., 2007; Mayer et al, 2006). To our knowledge, there are no liposomal drug combinations approved for clinical application. As previously mentioned in section 3.1 drug combinations can act synergistically, additively or antagonistically depending on the ratio of the agents being combined (Chou, 2006). While this relationship can be readily evaluated in vitro, where drug ratios can be controlled, the translation of those ratios to the clinical setting is complex due to the independent pharmacokinetics, biodistribution and/or metabolism of the individual drugs intravenously administered as aqueous-based free drug cocktail (Mayer et al., 2006; Lee, 2006). Therefore, the referred uncoordinated pharmacokinetics results in exposure of tumor cells to drug concentrations below therapeutic threshold level or to antagonistic drug ratios with concomitant loss of therapeutic activity (Mayer & Janoff, 2007; Harasym et al, 2007). The inability to control drug ratios in systemic circulation, and mainly in tumor tissue, may partly explain the short outcome in clinical efficacy seen for conventional free drug combinations (Mayer & Janoff, 2007).

Drug delivery systems, such as liposomes, can control the release of drug combinations such that fixed drug ratios are maintained after systemic administration. This tight control provides significant improvements in efficacy as compared to free drug cocktail and to individual liposomal drugs (Tardi et al., 2009, Mayer & Janoff, 2007; Harasym et al., 2007; Mayer et al., 2006; Lee, 2006). In 2006, Mayer and colleagues were the first to investigate the importance of maintaining an optimal drug combination ratio in vivo through drug encapsulation in liposomes (Mayer et al., 2006). Further studies (Tardi et al., 2009; Harasym et al., 2007) have demonstrated that in vitro drug interaction effects can be translated in vivo since liposomes can synchronize pharmacokinetics and biodistribution of drug combinations and deliver them to tumor tissue at a specific drug ratio (Fig.7, lower panel).

This "ratiometric" dosing approach has the potential to be applied to other diseases besides cancer in which multiple interacting mechanisms are responsible for disease progression or response to therapeutic interventions (Mayer & Janoff, 2007). In contrast, the combination injected as a free drug cocktail rapidly distributes into healthy and tumor tissues at drug ratios that differ from the administered one (Fig.7, upper panel).

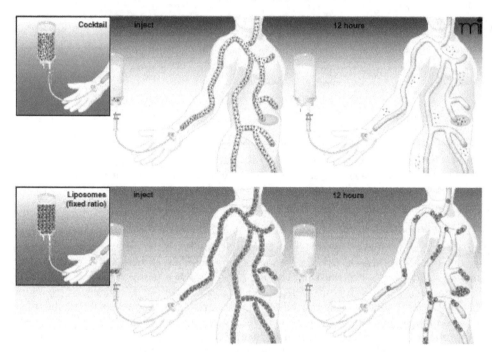

Fig. 7. Description of how clinical application of drug–drug synergy depends on controlled delivery of the desired drug ratio to the in vivo target. Upper panel - a drug cocktail is prepared at the desired ratio but biodistribution, metabolism and excretion processes will act differentially on the two drugs and cause the ratio to vary after intravenous injection. The two drugs distribute extensively into tissues shortly after injection and the ratio that reaches the tumor has been displaced 5-fold from the initially injected 1:1 ratio. Lower panel - liposomes that contain the synergistic 1:1 ratio maintain and selectively deliver this drug ratio to the tumor. The appropriately designed drug delivery vehicle maintains the drugs in the blood at higher concentrations for extended periods of time and, most importantly, at the effective synergistic ratio. Reproduced from reference (Mayer & Janoff, 2007).

Therefore, it can be concluded that liposome nanotechnology constitutes a valuable tool for preclinical assessment of drug combinations for clinical development (Lee, 2006). Advantages of liposomal drug combination delivery are summarized in Table 5.
Celator Pharmaceuticals were pioneers in liposomal drug combination design and have some products under clinical development and preclinical programs, which are summarized in Table 6. Currently, CPX-351 and CPX-1 are the only liposomal drug combinations under testing in clinical trials (http://clinicaltrials.gov (2010)) but none of them is intended for prostate cancer therapy.

1. Injection of multiple drugs simultaneously

2. Identical pharmacokinetic profile for multiple drugs reflecting the profile of the lipid carrier

3. Tight control of drug concentration at the target sites by changing the drug combined ratio in the liposome

4. Maximal combination effects can be achieved by synergistic action of multiple drugs after cellular uptake

5. Versatile design of the loading methods and membrane lipid composition to control drug release

6. Improvement of patient compliance and quality of life due to reduced number of injections and of side effects while increasing efficacy

Table 5. Advantages of liposomal drug combination delivery. Adapted from reference (Bae et al., 2007)

Product name	Liposomal drug combination	Therapeutic indication	Status
CPX-351	Cytarabine : daunorubicin	Acute myeloid leukemia	Phase II
CPX-1	Irinotecan HCl : floxuridine	Colorectal neoplasms	Phase II
CPX-571	Irinotecan HCl : cisplatin	Small cell lung cancer	Preclinical
CPX-8XY	Unknown	Unknown	Research

Table 6. Liposomal drug combinations developed by Celator Pharmaceuticals. Source: Celator Pharmaceuticals (http://www.celatorpharma.com (2010)).

4.2.6.2 Design of liposomal formulations for drug combination delivery

The concept of combining drugs, with dissimilar physicochemical properties, into a single vehicle, that efficiently encapsulates both drugs and releases them at the same rate after administration in vivo, represents a major scientific and technical challenge. Presently, liposomal encapsulation represents a new paradigm for formulating anticancer drug combinations. Although this approach has emerged as a promising strategy for cancer treatment, there are a limited number of research studies reporting successful drug co-loading in the same carrier (Tardi et al., 2009; Zhao et al., 2008; Harasym et al., 2007; Mayer et al., 2006). This is likely the result of technical difficulties associated with the efficient and stable encapsulation of two drugs inside a single carrier as well as challenges in controlling the drug leakage rate and still maintaining the entrapped drug:drug ratio after systemic administration (Harasym et al., 2007; Tardi et al., 2007).

There are three different approaches to formulate a drug combination involving liposomal design: i) combination of a liposomal drug with a free drug; ii) encapsulation of two drugs in individual liposomal carriers that are subsequently combined at the desired ratio and iii) co-encapsulation of two drugs in the same carrier by means of a simultaneous or a sequential drug loading. The advantages and limitations of each strategy are discussed below in more detail and in the mentioned order:

i.   A liposomal drug formulation can be administered together with a free drug but unfavorable liposome-free drug interactions may occur, such as hydrophobic interactions or loading of the free drug into liposomes exhibiting a pH gradient

(Waterhouse et al., 2001; Mayer et al., 1999). Therefore, these interactions may induce changes in the pharmacokinetic parameters of the free and encapsulated drugs as well as of the lipid carrier, leading to decreased efficacy and/or increased toxicity (Waterhouse et al., 2001).

ii. Perhaps the most straightforward approach to coordinate the pharmacokinetics of a drug combination would be to encapsulate each drug independently into different liposomes that provide the required drug retention properties and, subsequently, to mix the liposomes in a single suspension at the desired drug:drug ratio. Nevertheless, this protocol of formulating drugs in individual liposomes and ultimately administrate to patients would be extremely expensive due to the high costs inherent to lipid constituents and to the manufacturing process of two separate formulations (Harasym et al., 2007).

iii. Co-encapsulation of two drugs in the same liposomal carrier seems to be a preferable solution as compared to administration of individual liposomal drugs since it reduces cost production, minimizes lipid load to the patient, which has been associated to infusion-related side effects, and eliminates the potential interference that each liposome population may exert in the pharmacokinetic profile of the other (Harasym et al., 2007; Tardi et al., 2007). Furthermore, co-encapsulation overcomes potential uncertainties about drug biodistribution provided by the different liposome compositions. By encapsulating a drug combination into a single liposome, the two agents are no longer metabolized and eliminated independently but rather distributed as a unit, dictated by the characteristics of the carrier. However, this approach represents a technical challenge in order to develop a liposomal formulation that matches drug release kinetics for both drugs. To accomplish such purpose, experimental parameters and liposome features, such as drug loading methods and lipid composition, must be systematically optimized during formulation development (Harasym et al., 2007).

4.2.6.3 Development of a liposomal drug combination for prostate cancer: an example

In the last few years our group has performed an extensive and systematic preclinical study to evaluate the in vitro biologic activity of traditional and novel anticancer drugs and, ultimately, identify new drug combinations with therapeutic potential for the treatment of prostate cancer. Combinations were selected among different drugs (ciprofloxacin, docetaxel, doxorubicin, etoposide, imatinib, mitoxantrone and vinblastine) representative of distinct mechanisms of action. Several treatment schemes were evaluated by varying schedule, type of administration (simultaneous or sequential) and drug:drug molar ratio. The nature of antiproliferative combined effects (synergism, additivity or antagonism) against metastatic prostate cancer cell lines was quantitatively assessed by the median effect analysis method, whose main parameters are combination index (CI) and dose reduction index (DRI) (Pinto et al. 2011a, 2009).

Combination of two drugs tested simultaneously, comprising at least one topoisomerase II inhibitor, result in mild antagonistic effects against PC-3 and LNCaP cells. This antagonism of growth inhibition effects is translated by a CI superior to 1 and by a DRI inferior to twofold. In contrast, imatinib-mitoxantrone and ciprofloxacin-etoposide simultaneous combinations interact additively in inhibiting PC-3 cell growth, yielding CI values close to 1 and DRI values of 2.6 and 3.5-fold for mitoxantrone and etoposide, respectively (Pinto et al. 2011a, 2009).

The use of liposomes as drug delivery systems has been exploited in order to improve overall therapeutic index of anticancer drugs by increasing their antitumor activity and/or by reducing their toxicity profile. The main goal of our studies was to develop and characterize a novel liposomal formulation, for simultaneous co-loading and delivery of a drug combination previously identified in cytotoxicity screening studies performed in our laboratory, and to evaluate its in vitro and in vivo antitumor activity against HRPC preclinical models. The rationale for selecting imatinib-mitoxantrone combination was to investigate if co-loading of those two drugs into a liposome could translate the additive growth inhibition effects exerted on PC-3 cells when these drugs were combined simultaneously in the free form. Another selection criterion was that these drugs exhibit non-overlapping toxicity profiles and different mechanisms of action, so potential side effects and resistance phenomena could be minimized. Moreover, this combination is innovative for prostate cancer therapy since it conciliates a conventional antineoplastic drug (mitoxantrone), which is standard of care for palliative treatment of HRPC, with a molecular-targeted agent (imatinib), which has exhibited antitumor activity against in vitro and in vivo HRPC models.

Systematic development studies, by varying drug loading methods and incubation conditions, were carried out in order to design a liposomal imatinib-mitoxantrone (LIM) formulation that while being stable would exhibit adequate features for intravenous administration. Obtained results provide clear evidence that the two drugs can be simultaneously loaded, with high encapsulation efficiency (> 95%), in a single liposomal carrier using a transmembrane $(NH4)_2SO_4$ gradient-based procedure. According to literature, our study was the first to report an active loading method for imatinib (Pinto et al. 2011b).

In vitro studies performed on PC-3 cells showed that LIM formulation, at an optimized drug:drug molar ratio, exhibits enhanced tumor cell growth inhibition and promotes a 2.6-fold reduction of IC_{50} as compared to single liposomal mitoxantrone. This dose reduction is equivalent to the one found for mitoxantrone in free drug combination against the same cell line (Pinto et al. 2011a). Therefore, the therapeutic gain in mitoxantrone efficacy, mediated by imatinib and that result from free drug combination, is also attainable after liposomal encapsulation of the drugs at an optimized drug:drug ratio (Pinto et al. 2011b).

In vivo therapeutic activity of developed liposomal formulations, comprising different doses of single or imatinib-combined mitoxantrone, was evaluated in a nude mice bearing subcutaneous PC-3 xenograft model. Obtained results clearly demonstrate that intravenous administration of the liposomal formulation co-loading a low mitoxantrone dose (0.5 mg/kg) with imatinib (10 mg/kg) enables a tumor growth inhibition similar to the one yielded by single liposomal mitoxantrone (2.0 mg/kg), i.e. with a 4-fold inferior dose. This dose reduction could minimize the occurrence of side effects and hence increase therapeutic index of mitoxantrone (Pinto et al. 2011b).

Our results clearly emphasize the potential of incorporating clinically relevant drug combinations, at specific therapeutic ratios, within a lipid-based delivery system. Our research study is the first to provide a proof-of-principle for imatinib use in improving in vitro and in vivo antitumor efficacy of liposomal mitoxantrone. Overall, the developed LIM formulation constitutes a novel nanotechnology-based drug combined platform with improved therapeutic outcome against HRPC.

5. Conclusion

The up-to-date approach intended to develop novel chemotherapeutic drug combinations should be based on a rational selection of the drugs to be combined and on a systematic and quantitative screening of the ratio-dependent antiproliferative effects against human tumor cell lines. Drug combination studies on tumor cell lines, using a quantitative method to evaluate the nature of drug interactions, allow a more rational design of future chemotherapy protocols.

The translation of specific drug ratios, previously selected in vitro, to the clinical setting is complex due to the independent pharmacokinetics and biodistribution of individual drugs intravenously administered as aqueous-based free drug cocktail. The referred uncoordinated pharmacokinetics results in exposure of tumor cells to drug concentrations below therapeutic threshold level or to antagonistic drug ratios with concomitant loss of therapeutic activity. The inability to control drug ratios in systemic circulation, and mainly in tumor tissue, may partly explain the short outcome in clinical efficacy seen for conventional free drug combinations.

The extensive in vitro information on drug ratios can be used to formulate drug combinations in drug delivery systems. The use of liposomes as drug delivery systems has been successfully exploited in order to improve overall therapeutic index of anticancer drugs by increasing their antitumor activity and/or by reducing their toxicity profile. Successful clinical application of this rationally-designed approach to cancer therapy depends on the development of a liposomal formulation, with specific features, that delivers the drug combination in vivo so that the effective drug ratio is maintained after systemic administration and is ultimately exposed to tumors.

6. References

Abraham S.A., Waterhouse D.N., Mayer L.D., Cullis P.R., Madden T.D. & Bally M.B. (2005). The liposomal formulation of doxorubicin. *Methods Enzymol*, vol.391, (February 2005), pp. 71-97, ISNN 0076-6879

Alexis F., Rhee J.W., Richie J.P., Radovic-Moreno A.F., Langer R. & Farokhzad O.C. (2008). New frontiers in nanotechnology for cancer treatment. *Urol Oncol*, vol.26, No.1, (January 2008), pp. 74-85, ISNN 1078-1439

Allen T.M. (1998). Liposomal drug formulations. Rationale for development and what we can expect for the future. *Drugs*, vol.56, No.5, (November 1998), pp. 747-756, ISNN 0012-6667

Allen T.M. (1997). Liposomes. Opportunities in drug delivery. *Drugs*, vol.54, No.4, (January 1997), pp. 8-14, ISNN 0012-6667

Allen T.M. (1994). Long-circulating (sterically stabilized) liposomes for targeted drug delivery. *Trends Pharmacol Sc*, vol.15, No.7, (July 1994), pp. 215-220, ISNN 0165-6147

Andresen T.L., Jensen S.S. & Jorgensen K. (2005). Advanced strategies in liposomal cancer therapy: problems and prospects of active and tumor specific drug release. *Prog Lipid Res*, vol.44, No.1, (March 2005), pp. 68-97, ISNN 0163-7827

Armstrong A.J. & Carducci M.A. (2006). New drugs in prostate cancer. *Curr Opin Urol*, vol.16, No.3, (May 2006), pp. 138-145, ISNN 0963-0643

Bae Y., Diezi T.A., Zhao A. & Kwon G.S. (2007). Mixed polymeric micelles for combination cancer chemotherapy through the concurrent delivery of multiple chemotherapeutic agents. *J Control Release*, vol.122, No.3, (August 2007), pp. 324-330, ISNN 1873-4995

Bangham A.D., Standish M.M. & Watkins J.C. (1965). Diffusion of univalent ions across the lamellae of swollen phospholipids. *J Mol Biol*, vol.13, No.1, (August 1965), pp. 238-252, ISSN 0022-2836

Budman D.R., Calabro A. & Kreis W. (2002). Synergistic and antagonistic combinations of drugs in human prostate cancer cell lines in vitro. *Anticancer Drugs*, vol.13, No.10, (November 2002), pp. 1011-1016, ISSN 0959-4973

Cattel L., Ceruti M. & Dosio F. (2003). From conventional to stealth liposomes: a new frontier in cancer chemotherapy. *Tumori*, vol.89, No.3, (August 2003), pp. 237-249, ISSN 0300-8916

Charrois G.J. & Allen T.M. (2004). Drug release rate influences the pharmacokinetics, biodistribution, therapeutic activity, and toxicity of pegylated liposomal doxorubicin formulations in murine breast cancer. *Biochim Biophys Acta*, vol.1663, No.1-2, (January 2004), pp. 167-177, ISSN 0006-3002

Charrois G.J. & Allen T.M. (2003). Rate of biodistribution of STEALTH liposomes to tumor and skin: influence of liposome diameter and implications for toxicity and therapeutic activity. *Biochim Biophys Acta*, vol.1609, No.1, (January 2003), pp. 102-108, ISSN 0006-3002

Cho K., Wang X., Nie S., Chen Z.G. & Shin D.M. (2008). Therapeutic nanoparticles for drug delivery in cancer. *Clin Cancer Res*, vol.14, No.5, (March 2008), pp. 1310-1316, ISSN 1078-0432

Chonn A., Semple S.C. & Cullis P.R. (1992). Association of blood proteins with large unilamellar liposomes in vivo. Relation to circulation lifetimes. *J Biol Chem*, vol.267, No.26, (September 1992), pp. 18759-18765, ISSN 0021-9258

Chou T.C. & Talalay P. (1984). Quantitative analysis of dose-effect relationships: the combined effects of multiple drugs or enzyme inhibitors. *Adv Enzyme Regul*, vol.22, (January 1984), pp. 27-55, ISSN 0065-2571

Chou T.C., Motzer R.J., Tong Y. & Bosl G.J. (1994). Computerized quantitation of synergism and antagonism of taxol, topotecan, and cisplatin against human teratocarcinoma cell growth: a rational approach to clinical protocol design. *J Natl Cancer Inst*, vol.86, No.20, (October 1994), pp. 1517-1524, ISSN 0027-8874

Chou T.C. (2010). Drug combination studies and their synergy quantification using the Chou-Talalay method. *Cancer Res*, vol. 70, No.2, (January 2010), pp. 440-446, ISSN 1538-7445

Chou T.C. (2006). Theoretical basis, experimental design, and computerized simulation of synergism and antagonism in drug combination studies. *Pharmacol Rev*, vol.58, No.3, (September 2006), pp. 621-681, ISSN 0031-6997

Chou T.C. (1998). Drug combinations: from laboratory to practice. J Lab Clin Med 132, No.1, (July 1998), pp. 6-8, ISSN 0022-2143

Chou T.C. (1994). Assessment of synergistic and antagonistic effects of chemotherapeutic agents in vitro. *Contrib Gynecol Obstet*, vol.19, (January 1994), pp. 91-107, ISSN 0304-4246

Chou T.C. (1976). Derivation and properties of Michaelis-Menten type and Hill type equations for reference ligands. *J Theor Biol*, vol.59, No.2, (july 1976), pp. 253-276, ISSN 0022-5193

De La Taille A., Vacherot F., Salomon L., Druel C., Gil Diez De Medina S., Abbou C., Buttyan R. & Chopin D. (2001). Hormone-refractory prostate cancer: a multi-step and multi-event process. *Prostate Cancer Prostatic Dis*, vol.4, No.4, (December 2001), pp. 204-212, ISSN 1476-5608

Devalapally H., Chakilam A. & Amiji M.M. (2007). Role of nanotechnology in pharmaceutical product development. *J Pharm Sci*, vol.96, No.10, (August 2007), pp. 2547-2565, ISNN 0022-3549

Dong J.T. (2006). Prevalent mutations in prostate cancer. *J Cell Biochem* 97, No.3, (November 2005), pp. 433-447, ISNN 0730-2312

Drummond D.C., Meyer O., Hong K., Kirpotin D.B. & Papahadjopoulos D. (1999). Optimizing liposomes for delivery of chemotherapeutic agents to solid tumors. *Pharmacol Rev*, vol.51, No.4, (December 1999), pp. 691-743, ISNN 0031-6997

Dutta R.C. (2007). Drug carriers in pharmaceutical design: promises and progress. *Curr Pharm Des*, vol.13, No.7, (March 2007), pp. 761-769, ISNN 1873-4286

Fenske D.B., Chonn A. & Cullis P.R. (2008). Liposomal nanomedicines: an emerging field. *Toxicol Pathol*, vol.36, No.1, (March 2008), pp. 21-29, ISNN 1533-1601

Fenske D.B. & Cullis P.R. (2005). Entrapment of small molecules and nucleic acid-based drugs in liposomes. *Methods Enzymol*, vol.391, (February 2005), pp. 7-40, ISNN 0076-6879

Gabizon A.A., Shmeeda H. & Zalipsky S. (2006). Pros and cons of the liposome platform in cancer drug targeting. *J Liposome Res*, vol.16, No.3, (September 2006), pp. 175-183, ISNN 0898-2104

Gabizon A.A. (1992). Selective tumor localization and improved therapeutic index of anthracyclines encapsulated in long-circulating liposomes. *Cancer Res*, vol.52, No.4, (February 1992), pp. 891-896, ISNN 0008-5472

Gabizon A., Shmeeda H. & Barenholz Y. (2003). Pharmacokinetics of pegylated liposomal Doxorubicin: review of animal and human studies. *Clin Pharmacokinet*, vol.42, No.5, (may 2003), pp. 419-436, ISNN 0312-5963

Gabizon A. & Papahadjopoulos D. (1988). Liposome formulations with prolonged circulation time in blood and enhanced uptake by tumors. *Proc Natl Acad Sci USA*, vol.85, No.18, (September 1988), pp. 6949-6953, ISNN 0027-8424

Gabizon A., Goren D., Cohen R. & Barenholz Y. (1998). Development of liposomal anthracyclines: from basics to clinical applications. *J Control Release*, vol.53, No.1-3, (September 1998), pp. 275-279, ISNN 0168-3659

Goldie J.H. (2001). Drug resistance in cancer: a perspective. *Cancer Metastasis Rev*, vol.20, No.1-2, (February 2002), pp. 63-68, ISNN 0167-7659

Gregoriadis G. & Florence A.T. (1993). Liposomes in drug delivery. Clinical, diagnostic and ophthalmic potential. *Drugs*, vol.45, No.1, (January 1993), pp. 15-28, ISNN 0012-6667

Haley B. & Frenkel E. (2008). Nanoparticles for drug delivery in cancer treatment. *Urol Oncol*, vol.26, No.1, (January 2008), pp. 57-64, ISNN 1078-1439

Hanahan D. & Weinberg R.A. (2000). The hallmarks of cancer. *Cell*, vol.100, No.1, (January 2000), pp. 57-70, ISNN 0092-8674

Harasym T.O., Tardi P.G., Harasym N.L., Harvie P., Johnstone S.A. & Mayer L.D. (2007). Increased preclinical efficacy of irinotecan and floxuridine coencapsulated inside liposomes is associated with tumor delivery of synergistic drug ratios. *Oncol Res*, vol.16, No.8, (October 2007), pp. 361-374, ISNN 0965-0407

Harrington K.J., Syrigos K.N. & Vile R.G. (2002). Liposomally targeted cytotoxic drugs for the treatment of cancer. *J Pharm Pharmacol*, vol.54, No.12, (January 2003), pp. 1573-1600, ISNN 0022-3573

Hofheinz R.D., Gnad-Vogt S.U., Beyer U. & Hochhaus A. (2005). Liposomal encapsulated anti-cancer drugs. *Anticancer Drugs*, vol.16, No.7, (July 2005), pp. 691-707, ISNN 0959-4973

Immordino M.L., Dosio F. & Cattel L. (2006). Stealth liposomes: review of the basic science, rationale, and clinical applications, existing and potential. *Int J Nanomedicine*, vol.1, No.3, (August 2007), pp. 297-315, ISNN 1176-9114

Ismael G.F., Rosa D.D., Mano M.S. & Awada A. (2008). Novel cytotoxic drugs: old challenges, new solutions. *Cancer Treat Rev*, vol.34, No.1, (October 2007), pp. 81-91, ISNN 0305-7372

Kreis W., Budman D.R. & Calabro A. (2001). A reexamination of PSC 833 (Valspodar) as a cytotoxic agent and in combination with anticancer agents. *Cancer Chemother Pharmacol*, vol.47, No.1, (February 2001), pp. 78-82, ISNN 0344-5704

Lammers T., Hennink W.E. & Storm G. (2008). Tumour-targeted nanomedicines: principles and practice. *Br J Cancer*, vol.99, No.3, (July 2008), pp. 392-397, ISNN 1532-1827

Lasic D.D., Vallner J.J. & Working P.K. (1999). Sterically stabilized liposomes in cancer therapy and gene delivery. *Curr Opin Mol Ther*, vol.1, No.2, (November 2001), pp. 177-185, ISNN 1464-8431

Lee R.J. (2006). Liposomal delivery as a mechanism to enhance synergism between anticancer drugs. *Mol Cancer Ther*, vol.5, No.7, (August 2006), pp. 1639-1640, ISNN 1535-7163

Maeda H., Wu J., Sawa T., Matsumura Y. & Hori K. (2000). Tumor vascular permeability and the EPR effect in macromolecular therapeutics: a review. *J Control Release*, vol.65, No.1-2, (March 2000), pp. 271-284, ISNN 0168-3659

Mayer L.D., Harasym T.O., Tardi P.G., Harasym N.L., Shew C.R., Johnstone S.A., Ramsay E.C., Bally M.B. & Janoff A.S. (2006). Ratiometric dosing of anticancer drug combinations: controlling drug ratios after systemic administration regulates therapeutic activity in tumor-bearing mice. *Mol Cancer Ther*, vol.5, No.7, (Augusr 2006), pp. 1854-1863, ISNN 1535-7163

Mayer L.D. & Janoff A.S. (2007). Optimizing combination chemotherapy by controlling drug ratios. *Mol Interv*, vol.7, No.4, (Sptember 2007), pp. 216-223, ISNN 1534-0384

Mayer L.D., Reamer J. & Bally M.B. (1999). Intravenous pretreatment with empty pH gradient liposomes alters the pharmacokinetics and toxicity of doxorubicin through in vivo active drug encapsulation. *J Pharm Sci*, vol.88, No.8, (January 1999), pp. 96-102, ISNN 0022-3549

Mayer L.D., Tai L.C., Ko D.S., Masin D., Ginsberg R.S., Cullis P.R. & Bally M.B. (1989). Influence of vesicle size, lipid composition, and drug-to-lipid ratio on the biological activity of liposomal doxorubicin in mice. *Cancer Res*, vol.49, No.21, (November 1989), pp. 5922-5930, ISNN 0008-5472

Merlin J.L. (1994). Concepts of synergism and antagonism. *Anticancer Res*, vol.14, No.6A, (November 1994), pp. 2315-2319, ISNN 0250-7005

Mitchell S., Abel P., Ware M., Stamp G. & Lalani E. (2000). Phenotypic and genotypic characterization of commonly used human prostatic cell lines. *BJU Int*, vol.85, No.7, (May 2000), pp. 932-944, ISNN 1464-4096

Nagayasu A., Uchiyama K. & Kiwada H. (1999). The size of liposomes: a factor which affects their targeting efficiency to tumors and therapeutic activity of liposomal antitumor drugs. *Adv Drug Deliv Rev*, vol.40, No.1-2, (June 1999), pp.75-87, ISNN 1872-8294

Papahadjopoulos D., Allen T.M., Gabizon A., Mayhew E., Matthay K., Huang S.K., Lee K.D., Woodle M.C., Lasic D.D. & Redemann C. (1991). Sterically stabilized liposomes: improvements in pharmacokinetics and antitumor therapeutic efficacy. *Proc Natl Acad Sci USA*, vol.88, No.24, (December 1991), pp. 11460-11464, ISNN 0027-8424

Peer D., Karp J.M., Hong S., Farokhzad O.C., Margalit R. & Langer R. (2007). Nanocarriers as an emerging platform for cancer therapy. *Nat Nanotechnol*, vol.2, No.12, (July 2008), pp. 751-760, ISNN 1748-3395

Pinto A., Moreira J., Simões S. (2009). Ciprofloxacin sensitizes hormone-refractory prostate cancer cell lines to doxorubicin and docetaxel treatment on a schedule-dependent manner. *Cancer Chemother Pharmacol*, vol.64, No.3, (December 2008), pp. 445-454, ISNN 1432-0843

Pinto A., Ângelo S., Moreira J., Simões S. (2011a). Schedule treatment design and quantitative in vitro evaluation of chemotherapeutic combinations for metastatic prostate cancer therapy. *Cancer Chemother Pharmacol*, vol.67, No.2, (October 2010), pp. 275-284, ISNN 1432-0843

Pinto A., Moreira J., Simões S. (2011b). Liposomal imatinib-mitoxantrone combination: formulation development and therapeutic evaluation in an animal model of prostate cancer. *Prostate*, vol.71, No.1, (July 2010), pp.81-90, ISNN 1097-0045

Ramsay E.C., Dos Santos N., Dragowska W.H., Laskin J.J. & Bally M.B. (2005). The formulation of lipid-based nanotechnologies for the delivery of fixed dose anticancer drug combinations. *Curr Drug Deliv*, vol.2, No.4, (nvember 2005), pp. 341-351, ISNN 1567-2018

Song H., Zhang J., Han Z., Zhang X., Li Z., Zhang L., Fu M., Lin C. & Ma J. (2006). Pharmacokinetic and cytotoxic studies of pegylated liposomal daunorubicin. *Cancer Chemother Pharmacol*, vol.57, No.5, (September 2005), pp.591-598, ISNN 0344-5704

Suggitt M. & Bibby M.C. (2005). 50 years of preclinical anticancer drug screening: empirical to target-driven approaches. *Clin Cancer Res*, vol.11, No.3, (February 2005), pp.971-981, ISNN 078-0432

Tardi P., Johnstone S., Harasym N., Xie S., Harasym T., Zisman N., Harvie P., Bermudes D. & Mayer L. (2009). In vivo maintenance of synergistic cytarabine:daunorubicin ratios greatly enhances therapeutic efficacy. *Leuk Res*, vol.33, No.1, (August 2008), pp.129-139, ISNN 0145-2126

Tardi P.G., Gallagher R.C., Johnstone S., Harasym N., Webb M., Bally M.B. & Mayer L.D. (2007). Coencapsulation of irinotecan and floxuridine into low cholesterol-containing liposomes that coordinate drug release in vivo. *Biochim Biophys Acta*, vol.1768, No.3, (January 2007), pp.678-687, ISNN 0006-3002

Torchilin V.P. (2007). Targeted pharmaceutical nanocarriers for cancer therapy and imaging. *Aaps J*, vol.9, No.2, (July 2007), pp. E128-147, ISNN 1550-7416

Torchilin V.P. (2005). Recent advances with liposomes as pharmaceutical carriers. *Nat Rev Drug Discov*, vol.4, No.2, (February 2005), pp. 145-160, ISNN 1474-1776

Waterhouse D.N., Dos Santos N., Mayer L.D. & Bally M.B. (2001). Drug-drug interactions arising from the use of liposomal vincristine in combination with other anticancer drugs. *Pharm Res*, vol.18, No.9, (October 2001), pp.1331-1335, ISNN 0724-8741

Yuan F., Dellian M., Fukumura D., Leunig M., Berk D.A., Torchilin V.P. & Jain R.K. (1995). Vascular permeability in a human tumor xenograft: molecular size dependence and cutoff size. *Cancer Res*, vol.55, No.17, (September 1995), pp. 3752-3756, ISNN 0008-5472

Zhao X., Wu J., Muthusamy N., Byrd J.C. & Lee R.J. (2008). Liposomal coencapsulated fludarabine and mitoxantrone for lymphoproliferative disorder treatment. *J Pharm Sci*, vol.97, No.4, (August 2007), pp.1508-1518, ISNN 0022-3549

Zoli W., Ricotti L., Tesei A., Barzanti F. & Amadori D. (2001). In vitro preclinical models for a rational design of chemotherapy combinations in human tumors. *Crit Rev Oncol Hematol*, vol.37, No.1, (February 2001), pp.69-82, ISNN 1040-8428

3

Cytotoxic Plants: Potential Uses in Prevention and Treatment of Cancer

Zahra Tayarani-Najaran[1] and Seyed Ahmad Emami[2,*]
¹Department of Pharmacology and Pharmacological Research Centre of Medicinal Plants,
School of Medicine, Mashhad, University of Medical Sciences, Mashhad,
²Department of Pharmacognosy, School of Pharmacy, Mashhad,
University of Medical Sciences, Mashhad,
Iran

1. Introduction

Cancer is a leading cause of death worldwide and accounted for 7.6 million deaths (around 13% of all deaths) in 2008. Deaths from cancer worldwide are projected to continue to rise to over 11 million in 2030. [(2011) World health statistics]. Heredity and environmental changes affect the susceptibility to cancer affection. More than 30% of cancer could be prevented by modifying or avoiding key risk factors, including: tobacco use, being overweight or obese, low fruit and vegetable intake, physical inactivity, alcohol use, sexually transmitted HPV-infection, urban air pollution, indoor smoke from household use of solid fuels.

Plants have been used as a major source of remedies from the ancient time. The modern drug discovery and development is also dependent of medicinal plants (Saklani & Kutty, 2008). Using plants in the treatment of cancer has long history and dates back to ancient time. There are strong evidences about cancer preventing properties of various kinds of herbs used as food, fruit, spices, and vegetables (Dossus, 2008; Kruk, 2007; Moyad, 2004; Montesano, 2001; Lyman, 1992).

Dietary habits especially those involving fruits and vegetables have served the great interest in developing various preventive measures that influence cancer risk (Wu, 2009; Kurahashi, 2009). Phytochemicals of varied chemical structures from fruits and vegetables have already been studied extensively for their potential anticancer or chemopreventive efficacy (Ramos, 2008). Being the rich sources of vitamins, minerals, and fiber without posing "any side effects" made fruits and vegetables the best choice to lowering cancer risk and also in maintaining good general health.

The important role of plant derived compounds is undeniable. Paclitaxel (Wani et al., 1971), camptothecin (Wall, 1998), combrestatin (Cirla & Mann, 2003), epipodophyllotoxin (Canel et al., 2000) and Vinca alkaloids (vinblastine, vincristine) (Johnson et al., 1963) are some examples of herbal originated cancer treatments. These are also many other plant-derived compounds that are in clinical trials for cancers (Saklani & K. Kutty, 2008).

---

*Corresponding Author

Herbs and spices can defy the DNA damage which is the fundamental cause of cancer and can occur as a result of aging, genetic susceptibility, and exposure to an assortment of carcinogens.

Free radicals and different toxins have the important role in cancer development and progression through interaction with DNA. Numerous phytonutrients found in fruits, herbs and spices act as potent preventive agents against cancer by preventing the overproduction of toxic chemicals within the body, improving the body's detoxification processes.

Herbs and spices not only reduce the risks of developing cancer, but also act as efficient treatments for cancer. Herbs and spices are traditional cancer treatments of radiotherapy and chemotherapy enhancers, reducing the negative side effects of these therapies.

Edible vegetables, fruits, spices and whole grains contain significant amounts of bioactive phytochemicals, which are warrented health benefits beyond basic nutrition to reduce the risk of chronic disease and the process of carcinogenesis [Liu, 2004)

The National Cancer Institute (NCI) of the United States has introduced several plant-based foods that exert cancer-preventive properties, including garlic, soybeans, ginger, onion, turmeric, tomatoes and cruciferous vegetables (for example, broccoli, cabbage, cauliflower and Brussels sprouts). (Surh, 2003). Iridoids, phenols, phenolics, carotenoids, alkaloids, organosulfur compounds, and terpenoids are main class of phytochemicals.

Plants with cytotoxic effects respect to their sub family, species, phytochemical, and the stage of which they are in progress for cancer treatment are classified in table 1 to 38.

Each table is representive of phytochemical of a selected family. Each row illustrates the selected phytochemical of representative plant bioactives that have been shown to induce cytotoxic effects.

Anacardiaceae R.Brown

A family of 69 genera and 850 species mainly subtropical trees, shrubs, lianas or rarely perennial herbs with vertical resine – ducts in bark. The family contains dyeing and tanning materials and phenolic compounds (Evans 2009; Judd et al., 2008; Mabberley 2008).

Species	Compound	Class of Compound	Effect	Status	Ref.
Rhus verniciflua Stokes	total extract	not stated	metastatic colorectal cancer (mCRC)	clinical trial	Lee et al, 2009

Table 1. Anacardiaceae Cytotoxic Phytochemicals

Apiaceae Lindley

(Umbelliferae A.L. de Jussieu)

The plant family consists of 434 genera and 3780 species most members are herbs with furrowed stems and hollow internodes, some are annuals, some biennials, and some perennials. The three subfamilies are as follows: 1) Hydrocotyoideae 2) Saniculoideae and 3) Apioioideae.

Constituents of the family include essential oils, coumarins, furocumarins, chromonocoumarins, monoterpenes, sesquiterpenes, triterpenoid saponins, resins and acetylenic compounds. Alkaloids occur but are rare (Evans 2009; Judd et al., 2008; Mabberley 2008).

Species	Compound	Class of Compound	Effect	Status	Ref.
Angelica sinensis (Oliv.) Diels	citronellol	terpenoids	improve their immune function, improving their ability to fight off the cancer	randomized, double-blind, placebo-controlled study	Zhuang et al., 2009
Cuminum cyminum L.	apigenin and luteolin	flavonoids	cancer chemopreventive activities	cell culture, animal study	Aggarwal et al., 2008; Patel et al., 2007; Manju & Nalini, 2007
Foeniculum vulgare Mill.	anethole, [1-methoxy-4-(1-propenyl) benzene], anethole dithiolethione	phenylpropanoid	chemopreventive activities as indicated by suppression of the incidence and multiplicity of both invasive and non-invasive adenocarcinomas	cancer cells cell culture	Aggarwal et al., 2008

Table 2. Apiaceae Cytotoxic Phytochemicals

Apocynaceae A.L. de Jussieu

This family contains 380 genera and 4700 species
mostly in tropical and subtropical but also in few temperate regions. The members are trees, shrubs, lianas, vines, sometimes sscculent and cactuslike.
Constituents of the family are some types of alkaloids, cardioactive glycosides, cyanogenic glycosides leucoanthyocyanins, saponins, tannins, coumarins, phenolic acids, cyclitols and triterpenoids (Evans 2009; Judd et al., 2008; Mabberley 2008).

Species	Compound	Class of Compound	Effect	Status	Ref.
Catharanthus roseus (L.) G.Don	methyl jasmonate	cyclopentanone derivatives	induces apoptosis	A549 human lung adenocarcinoma cells, myeloid leukemia cells	Balbi & Devoto, 2007
Rhazya stricta Decne.	didemethoxycarbonyl-tetrahydrosecamine, sewarine, tetrahydrosecamine, tetrahydrosecaminediol diacetate vallesiachotamine DL-1-(oxo-3,4-thero-3,4,5-trihydroxy-1-pentyl)-β-carboline, 16-epi-Z-isositsirkine	alkaloids	cytotoxic	cell culture	Gilani et al., 2007

Table 3. Apocynaceae Cytotoxic Phytochemicals

Araliaceae A.L. de Jussieu

A family of 39 genera and 1425 species mainly tropical shrubs, lianas or trees to occasionally herbs, aromatic with secretary canals containing volatile oils and resins. other constituents include saponins, a few alkaloids, acetylenic compounds, coumarins, diterpenoids and triterpenoids (Evans 2009; Judd et al., 2008; Mabberley 2008).

Species	Compound	Class of Compound	Effect	Status	Ref.
Panax ginseng C.A.Mey.	ginsenosides	saponins	anticancer effects: regulation of cell cycle, Induction of apoptosis, Inhibition of angiogenesis	*in vitro* and *in vivo*	Qi et al., 2010
Panax ginseng C.A.Mey.	ginsenosides	saponins	Re and Rg1 enhance angiogenesis, whereas Rb1, Rg3 and Rh2 inhibit it. Rh2, an antitumor agent,, P quinquefolium has better anticancer effects	*in vitro* and *in vivo*	Chen et al., 2008
Panax ginseng C.A.Mey.	total extract	not stated	anticancer antitumor	cell culture	Xiang et al., 2008
Panax ginseng C.A.Mey.	ginsenosides	saponins	the risk of cancer was shown to be lower in those who used ginseng	prospective cohort study	Yun et al., 1998; Kiefer et al., 2003
Panax ginseng C. A. Mey.	ginsenosides	saponins	antitumor/cytotoxicity activities	*in vitro* and *in vivo* against a wide variety of cancer cell lines or *in vivo* neoplasms	Chang et al., 2003

Table 4. Araliaceae Cytotoxic Phytochemicals

Asteraceae Bercht. & J. Presl

(Compositae Giseke)
The family is the largest family of flowering plants and contains about 1590 genera and 23600 species that comprise of herbs, shrubs or trees. Asteraceae divided into 3 subfamilies: 1) Baradosioideae 2) Cichorioideae and 3) Asteroideae.
The Asteraceae contains a wide variety of chemical constituents. Some of the essential oils found in the family contain acetylenic compounds. sesquiterpenes known as azulenes. mono sesquiterpene lactones occur. Alkaloids of the pyridine, pyrrolizidine, quinoline and diterpenoid types also occur in the family, other constituents include triterpenoid saponins, cyclitols, coumarins and flavonols (Evans 2009; Judd et al., 2008; Mabberley 2008).

Species	Compound	Class of Compound	Effect	Status	Ref.
Artemisia annua L.	different fractions	not stated	antiproliferative effect	cancer cell lines	Rabe et al., 2011

Artemisia annua L.	artemisinin	sesquiterpenoids	colon cancer	*in vitro*	McGovern et al., 2010
Artemisia annua L.	artemisinin	sesquiterpenoids	anticancer effects, cell cycle arrest, apoptosis, inhibition of angiogenesis, disruption of cell migration, and modulation of nuclear receptor responsiveness	in a variety of human cancer cell model systems	Firestone et al., 2009
Artemisia annua L.	different fractions	not stated	cytotoxic and pro-apoptotic	variety of cancer cell lines	Emami et al., 2009b
Artemisia annua L.	artemisinins	sesquiterpenoids	anticancer properties	in cell lines and animal models	Krishna et al., 2008
Artemisia annua L.	artemisinin	sesquiterpenoids	regulation of proliferation (BUB3, cyclins, CDC25A), angiogenesis (vascular endothelial growth factor and its receptor, matrix metalloproteinase-9, angiostatin, thrombospondin-1) or apoptosis (BCL-2, BAX, NF-kappaB). p53-dependent and -independent apoptosis	tumor cells	Efferth et al., 2007
Artemisia annua L.	total extract	not stated	cytotoxic activity	human Caucasian hepatocyte carcinoma (HepG-2) and human Caucasian larynx carcinoma (Hep-2)	Vahdati-Mashhadian et al., 2009
Artemisia argyi H.Lév. & Vaniot	isoscopoletin	coumarins	lung cancer	*in vitro*	McGovern et al., 2010

Artemisia biennis Willd.	different fractions	not stated	antiproliferative effect		Rabe et al., 2011
Artemisia campestris L.	total extract	not stated	cytotoxic activity	human Caucasian hepatocyte carcinoma (HepG-2) and human Caucasian larynx carcinoma (Hep-2)	Vahdati-Mashhadian et al., 2009
Artemisia chamaemelifolia Vill.	total extract	not stated	cytotoxic activity	human Caucasian hepatocyte carcinoma (HepG-2) and human Caucasian larynx carcinoma (Hep-2)	Vahdati-Mashhadian et al., 2009
Artemisia ciniformis Krasch. & Popov ex Poljak.	different fractions	not stated	antiproliferative effect	cancer cell lines	Rabe et al., 2011
Artemisia diffusa Krasch. ex Poljakov	different fractions	not stated	antiproliferative effect	cancer cell lines	Rabe et al., 2011
Artemisia diffusa Krasch. ex Poljakov	total extract	not stated	cytotoxic activity	human Caucasian hepatocyte carcinoma (HepG-2) and human Caucasian larynx carcinoma (Hep-2)	Emami et al., 2009a
Artemisia fragrans Willd.	total extract	not stated	cytotoxic activity	human Caucasian hepatocyte carcinoma (HepG-2) and human Caucasian larynx carcinoma (Hep-2)	Vahdati-Mashhadian et al., 2009
Artemisia incana Druce	total extract	not stated	cytotoxic activity	human Caucasian	Vahdati-Mashhadian

				hepatocyte carcinoma (HepG-2) and human Caucasian larynx carcinoma (Hep-2)	et al., 2009
Artemisia khorassanica Podlech	different fractions	not stated	cytotoxic activity	variety of cancer cell lines	Mahmoudi et al., 2009
Artemisia kulbadica Boiss. & Buhse	total extract	not stated	cytotoxic activity	human Caucasian hepatocyte carcinoma (HepG-2) and human Caucasian larynx carcinoma (Hep-2)	Emami et al., 2009a
Artemisia persica Boiss.	different fractions	not stated	antiproliferative effect	cancer cell lines	Rabe et al., 2011
Artemisia persica Boiss.	total extract	not stated	cytotoxic activity	human Caucasian hepatocyte carcinoma (HepG-2) and human Caucasian larynx carcinoma (Hep-2)	Vahdati-Mashhadian et al., 2009
Artemisia santolina Schrenk	different fractions	not stated		cancer cell lines	Rabe et al., 2011
Artemisia santolina Schrenk	total extract	not stated	cytotoxic activity	human Caucasian hepatocyte carcinoma (HepG-2) and human Caucasian larynx carcinoma (Hep-2)	Emami et al., 2009a
Artemisia sieberi Besser	total extract	not stated	cytotoxic activity	human Caucasian hepatocyte carcinoma (HepG-2) and human	Emami et al., 2009a

				Caucasian larynx carcinoma (Hep-2)	
Artemisia turanica Krasch.	total extract	not stated	cytotoxic activity	human Caucasian hepatocyte carcinoma (HepG-2) and human Caucasian larynx carcinoma (Hep-2)	Emami et al., 2009a
Artemisia vulgaris L.	different fractions	not stated	antiproliferative effect	cancer cell lines	Rabe et al., 2011
Artemisia vulgaris L.	total extract	not stated	cytotoxic activity	human Caucasian hepatocyte carcinoma (HepG-2) and human Caucasian larynx carcinoma (Hep-2)	Vahdati-Mashhadian et al., 2009
Inula britannica M.Bieb.	1-O-acetylbritannilactone	sesquiterpene lactones	cytotoxic, apopotic	cell culture	Khan et al., 2010
Inula britannica M.Bieb.	1,6-*O,O*-diacetylbritannilactone	sesquiterpene lactones	cytotoxic, apopotic	cell culture	Khan et al., 2010
Inula britannica M.Bieb.	6α-O-(2-methylbutyryl)-britannilactone	sesquiterpene lactones	cytotoxic, apopotic, inflammation	cell culture	Khan et al., 2010
Inula britannica M.Bieb.	neobritannilactone A	sesquiterpenes lactones	cytotoxic, apopotic, inflammation	cell culture	Khan et al., 2010
Inula britannica M.Bieb.	neobritannilactone B	sesquiterpene lactones	cytotoxic, apopotic, inflammation	cell culture	Khan et al., 2010
Inula britannica M.Bieb.	quercetin, spinacetin, diosmetin	flavonoids	antioxidant, cytotoxic	cell culture	Khan et al., 2010
Saussurea costus (Falc.) Lipsch.	C17 polyene alcohol	polyenes	anticancer, antitumor, moderate cytotoxicity	against the human tumor cell lines A549, SK-OV3, SK-MEL-2, XF 498, and	Wang et al., 2010

				HCT 15	
Saussurea costus (Falc.) Lipsch.	lappadilactone, dehydrocostuslactone, and costunolide	sesquiterpene lactones	most potent cytotoxicities	HepG2, OVCAR-3, and HeLa cell lines	Wang et al., 2010
Saussurea costus (Falc.) Lipsch.	total extract	not stated	cytostatic effects, inducer of apoptosis	AGS gastric cancer cell line	Wang et al., 2010
Saussurea costus (Falc.) Lipsch.= *Saussurea lappa* C.B.Clarke	costunolide	sesquiterpene lactones	Anticancer, induction of apoptosis	in HL-60 human leukemia cells	Pandey et al., 2007
Saussurea costus (Falc.) Lipsch.= *Saussurea lappa* C.B.Clarke	total extract	not stated	induced apoptotic cell death	AGS gastric cancer cell line	Pandey et al., 2007
Saussurea costus (Falc.) Lipsch.= *Saussurea lappa* C.B.Clarke	lappadilactone, dehydrocostuslactone and costunolide	sesquiterpene lactones	cytotoxic	HepG2, OVCAR-3 and HeLa cell lines	Pandey et al., 2007
Saussurea costus (Falc.) Lipsch.= *Saussurea lappa* C.B.Clarke	dehydrocostus lactone	sesquiterpene lactone	induced apoptosis	human leukemia HL-60 cells	Pandey et al., 2007
Saussurea costus (Falc.) Lipsch.= *Saussurea lappa* C.B.Clarke	cynaropicrin	sesquiterpene lactones	pro-apoptotic activity	leukocyte cancer cell lines, such as U937, Eol-1 and Jurkat T cells	Pandey et al., 2007
Saussurea costus (Falc.) Lipsch.= *Saussurea lappa* C.B.Clarke	costunolide	sesquiterpene lactones	anti-angiogenic effect	vascular endothelial growth factor (VEGF)	Pandey et al., 2007
Saussurea costus (Falc.) Lipsch.= *Saussurea lappa* C.B.Clarke	C-17 polyene alcohol	polyenes	moderate cytotoxicities	human tumor cell lines A549, SK-OV3, SK-MEL-2, XF 498 and HCT 15	Pandey et al., 2007
Saussurea medusa Maxim.	arctiin and arctigenin	lignans	remarkable antitumorpromoting effect on two-stage carcinogenesis test	mouse-skin tumors, mouse pulmonary tumors	Wang et al., 2010

Saussurea spp.	costunolide	sesquiterpene lactones	inducer of apoptosis	HL-60 human leukemia cells	Wang et al., 2010
Saussurea spp.	arctigenin		inhibition of TNF-a induction		Wang et al., 2010
Saussurea spp.	dehydrocostuslactone	sesquiterpene lactones	induced apoptosis	human leukemia HL-60 cells	Wang et al., 2010
Saussurea spp.	cynaropicrin	sesquiterpene lactones	inhibited the proliferation, potential anticancer agent against some leukocyte cancer cells	leukocyte cancer cell lines, such as U937, Eol-1, and Jurkat T cells	Wang et al., 2010
Saussurea spp.	costunolide	sesquiterpene lactones	anti-angiogenic effect	human umbilical vein endothelial cells (HUVECs)	Wang et al., 2010
Silybum marianum (L.) Gaertn	total extract	not stated	prevention or treatment of liver dysfunction in patients undergoing anticancer therapy	patients with cancer	Ladas & Kelly, 2003
Silybum marianum (L.) Gaertn	silibinin, silymarin	flavonolignans	Prostate cancer, anticancer effects, inhibition of mitogenic and cell survival signaling	in different cancer cells, animal models	Singh et al., 2004
Silybum marianum (L.) Gaertn.	silibinin	flavonolignans	inhibition of multiple cancer cell signaling pathways, including growth inhibition, inhibition of angiogenesis, chemosensitization, and inhibition of invasion and metastasis	in animals and humans	Li et al., 2010
Silybum marianum (L.) Gaertn.	silybin, isosilybin, silychristin, silydianin and taxifoline	flavonolignans	suppression of the proliferation of a variety of tumor cells (e.g., prostate, breast,	cell culture, animal study and clinical trials	Agarwal et al., 2006

			ovary, colon, lung, bladder), angiogenesis (VEGF) and metastasis, as a chemopreventive agent, apoptosis induction, antitumor activity		
Silybum marianum (L.) Gaertn.	silybin and silymarin	flavonolignans	anticancer and canceroprotective	not stated	Kren et al., 2005
Silybum marianum (L.) Gaertn.	silymarin	flavonolignans	cancer prevention, adjuvant cancer treatment, and reduction of iatrogenic toxicity	clinical trials	Sagar et al., 2007
Silybum marianum (L.) Gaertn.	total extract	not stated	protective effect in certain types of cancer	clinical trials	Tamayo et al., 2007

Table 5. Asteraceae Cytotoxic Phytochemicals

Brassicaceae Burnett

(Cruciferae A.L. de Jussieu)
A family of 321 genera and about 3400 species of herbs and a few undershrubs. Many members of the family contain glucosinolates. Cardiac glycosides occur in some genera and the seeds usually contain mucilage and fixed oil (Evans 2009; Judd et al., 2008; Mabberley 2008).

Species	Compound	Class of Compound	Effect	Status	Ref.
Arabidopsis thaliana (L.) Heynh.	jasmonate	cyclopentanone derivatives	induces cell death and suppresses cell proliferation	in animals, several human cancer cell lines	Balbi & Devoto, 2007
Brassica spp.	indole-3-carbinol	glucosinolates	breast cancer, prostate cancer, endometrial cancer, colon cancer, and leukemic, induce G1/S arrest of the cell cycle, and induce apoptosis	*in vitro* and *in vivo*, clinical trials	Aggarwal & Ichikawa, 2005

Table 6. Brassicaceae Cytotoxic Phytochemicals

Campannlaceae A.L. de Juessieu

The family contains 79 genera and around 1900 species mostly herbs but some shrubs and pachycaul trees with a network of lacticifers in phloem. The members of the family contain phenolic compounds, tannins and triterpenoid glycosides (Evans 2009; Judd et al., 2008; Mabberley 2008).

Species	Compound	Class of Compound	Effect	Status	Ref.
Codonopsis pilosula Nannf.	a mixture of citronellol and extracts of *Ganoderma lucidum, Codonopsis pilosula* and *Angelicae sinensis*	not stated	Improvement of immune function, improving the ability to fight off the cancer, as well as any secondary infections that could compromise the treatment and the health	randomized, double-blind, placebo-controlled study	Zhuang et al., 2009

Table 7. Campannlaceae Cytotoxic Phytochemicals

Cannabaceae Martynov

A family of 10 genera and 80 species usually trees or shrubs but also herbs or vines. Widely distributed in tropical to temperate regions (Evans 2009; Judd et al., 2008; Mabberley 2008).

Species	Compound	Class of Compound	Effect	Status	Ref.
Humulus lupulus L.	hop acids	sesquiterpenoids	inhibiting cell proliferation and angiogenesis, by inducing apoptosis	*in vitro* and *in vivo*	Van Cleemput et al., 2009

Table 8. Cannabaceae Cytotoxic Phytochemicals

Clusiaceae Lindley

(**Guttiferae** A.L. de Jussieu)
The Clusiaceae contains about 30 genera and 1150 tropical species. They are trees shrubs or lianas with colored exudate in secretory canals or cavities. Constituents of the family include resins, volatile oils, alkaloids, xanthones and seed oil (Evans 2009; Judd et al., 2008; Mabberley 2008).

Species	Compound	Class of Compound	Effect	Status	Ref.
Garcinia cantleyana Whitmore	cantleyanones, 7-hydroxyforbesione, and deoxygaudichaudione A from	xanthones	cytotoxic effect	variety of cancer cell lines	Han et al., 2009
Garcinia gaudichaudii Planch. & Triana	gaudichaudiones, gaudichaudic acids, gaudichaudione H xanthones	xanthones	potent antitumor activity	variety of cancer cell lines	Han et al., 2009
Garcinia indica Choisy	gambogic acid (gamboges or kokum)	pigments	cytotoxic, apoptotic, antiangiogenesis and anticancer	*in vitro* and *in vivo*	Aggarwal et al., 2008

Garcinia spp.	gaudichaudione A	xanthones	induced the apoptosis	human leukemic cells	Han et al., 2009
Garcinia spp.	gambogic acid	pigments	induce apoptosis, can overcome the drug resistance, In vitro and in vivo studies	*in vitro* and *in vivo*	Han et al., 2009

Table 9. Clusiaceae Cytotoxic Phytochemicals

Combretaceae R. Brown

A family of 17 genera and 525 species, tropical and subtropical trees, shrubs or lianas, sometimes with erect monopodial trnnk supporting a series of horizontal, sympodial branches. Members of the family usually rich in tannin (Evans 2009; Judd et al., 2008; Mabberley 2008).

Species	Compound	Class of Compound	Effect	Status	Ref.
Combretum caffrum Kuntze	combretastatin A-4	phenolic compounds	potent antimitotic agent	cancer cells cell culture	Nam et al., 2003

Table 10. Combretaceae Cytotoxic Phytochemicals

Cornaceae Bercht. & Presl

A family of 2 genera and 80 species. Trees, shrubs or rarely rhizomatous herbs usually with iridoids, widespread; specially common in north temperate regions, rare in tropical and south temperate regions (Evans 2009; Judd et al., 2008; Mabberley 2008).

Species	Compound	Class of Compound	Effect	Status	Ref.
Camptotheca acuminata Decne.	camptothecin and its derivatives	alkaloids	anticancer drugs	cancer treatment in patients	Sirikantaramas et al., 2007

Table 11. Cornaceae Cytotoxic Phytochemicals

Crassulaceae J. St. Hilaire

The Crassulaceae contains 92 genera and around 1380 species almost cosmopolitan especially south Africa, rare in Australia and wcst Pacific. succulent herbs to shrubs; often with cortical or medullary vascular bundles; with crassulacean acid metabolism (CAM), tannins present, often with alkaloids, sometimes cyanogenic (Evans 2009; Judd et al., 2008; Mabberley 2008).

Species	Compound	Class of Compound	Effect	Status	Ref.
Rhodiola rosea L.	total extract	not stated	anticancer, decreased metastasis to the liver, and extended survival times	in animal experiments	Kelly et al., 2001

Table 12. Crassulaceae Cytotoxic Phytochemicals

Cupressaceae Gray

A family of 30 genera and 130 species. The family is subcosmopolitan of warm to cold temperate climate. Monoecious or dioecious resinous trees or shrubs. Leaves descussate or in whorls of 3 or 4, in young plants needle – like, usually small and scale – like in mature plants. Flowers, small, solitary, axillary or terminal on short shoots, cones terminals, woody, leathery or berry – like, cone – scales opposite or in whorls of 3, ovules usually several per scale. Seeds winged or not. Constituents of the family include essential oils, monoterpenes, sesquiterpenes diterpenes, tannins and flavomoids (Evans 2009; Judd et al., 2008; Mabberley 2008).

Species	Compound	Class of Compound	Effect	Status	Ref.
Cupressus sempervirens L. var. horizentalis (Mill.) Gordon	total extract	not stated	cytotoxic effect	cell culture	Emami et al., 2005
Juniperus excelsa M.Bieb. subsp. excelsa	total extract	not stated	cytotoxic effect	cell culture	Sadeghi-aliabadi et al., 2009a
Juniperus excelsa M.Bieb. subsp. polycarpos (K. Koch) Takhtajan	total extract	not stated	cytotoxic effect	cell culture	Sadeghi-aliabadi et al., 2009a
Juniperus foetidissima Willd.	total extract	not stated	cytotoxic effect	cell culture	Sadeghi-aliabadi et al., 2009b
Juniperus sabina L.	total extract	not stated	cytotoxic effect	cell culture	Sadeghi-aliabadi et al., 2009b
Platycladus orientalis (L.) Franco	total extract	not stated	cytotoxic effect	not stated	Emami et al., 2005

Table 13. Cupressaceae Cytotoxic Phytochemicals

Ericaceae A.L. de Jussieu

They Ericaceae contains 117 genera and 3850 species cosmopolitan except deserts usually montane in tropical regions. Trees, shrubs, lianas or subherbaceous, sometimes epiphytic, occasionally mycoparasitic herbs lacking chlorophyll, strongly associated with micorrhizal fungi. The family produces phenolic acids, phenolic glycosides aucubin glycosides, diterpenoids, triterpenoids, cyclitols and leucoanthecyanins. A few species are cyanogenic; saponins are absent (Evans 2009; Judd et al., 2008; Mabberley 2008).

Species	Compound	Class of Compound	Effect	Status	Ref.
Vaccinium macrocarpon Aiton	not stated	not stated	induction of apoptosis in tumor cells, reduced ornithine decarboxylase activity, decreased expression of matrix	in vitro tumor models	Neto et al., 2008

| Vaccinium macrocarpon Aiton | polyphenolic extracts flavonols, proanthocyanidin oligomers, and triterpenoids isolated from the fruit. | flavonoids | inhibit the growth and proliferation of breast, colon, prostate, lung, and other tumors, induction of apoptosis in tumor cells, reduced ornithine decarboxylase activity, decreased expression of matrix metalloproteinases associated with prostate tumor metastasis, and antiinflammatory activities including inhibition of cyclooxygenases | *in vitro* studies using a variety of tumor models | Neto et al., 2007 |

Table 14. Ericaceae Cytotoxic Phytochemicals

Fabaceae Lindley

(**Leguminosae** A.L. de Jussieu)

This is the second – largest family of flowering plants and contains 720 genera and 19500 cosmopolitan species. Herbs, shrubs, trees or vines / lianas climbing by twining or tendrils; with a high nitrogen metabolism and unusual aminoacids, often with root nodules containing nitrogen – fixing bacteria, sometimes with secretory canals or cavities, tannins usually present, often with alkaloids; sometimes cyanogenic, sieve cell plastids with protein crystals and usually also starch grains.

The family is divided into three subfamilies: 1) Papilionoideae; 2) Mimosoideae and 3) Caesalpinoideae (Evans 2009; Judd et al., 2008; Mabberley 2008).

Species	Compound	Class of Compound	Effect	Status	Ref.
Glycine max (L.) Merr.	soy saponins	saponins	cancer protective effects	epidemiological studies	Kerwin et al., 2004
Glycyrrhiza inflata Batalin	licochalcone E,	flavonoids	potent cytotoxic effect	in tumor cells	Asl & Hosseinzadeh, 2008
Glycyrrhiza spp.	total extract	not stated	inhibits angiogenesis, induced apoptosis	*in vivo* and *in vitro*	Asl & Hosseinzadeh, 2008
Glycyrrhiza spp.	glycyrrhetinic acid	triterpenoids	trigger the proapoptotic pathway	in tumor cells	Asl & Hosseinzadeh, 2008
Glycyrrhiza spp.	isoliquiritigenin (ILG)	triterpenoids	antiproliferative activity, trigger the proapoptotic pathway	in tumor cells	Asl & Hosseinzadeh, 2008
Glycyrrhiza spp.	glabridin dibenzoylmethane	triterpenoids	antiproliferative activity, trigger	in tumor cells	Asl & Hosseinzadeh,

	(DBM)		the proapoptotic pathway		2008
Trigonella foenum graecum	diosgenin	saponins	suppress proliferation, invasion inhibition, cytotoxic, apoptotic, anti-cancer activity	cell culture, animal study	Aggarwal et al., 2008

Table 15. Fabaceae Cytotoxic Phytochemicals

Ginkgoaceae Engler

A family contains only a monotypic genus, limited to remote mountain valleys of China; possibly extinct in the wild. From among the many groups of compounds isolated from *Ginkgo biloba* it is diterpenelactons and flavonoids which have been shown to possess therapeutic activity (Evans 2009; Judd et al., 2008; Mabberley 2008).

Species	Compound	Class of Compound	Effect	Status	Ref.
Ginkgo biloba L.	total extract	not stated	chemopreventive action at various levels with antioxidant, antiangiogenic properties, reduce angiogenesis	cell culture, cancer model	Mahadevan et al., 2008
Ginkgo biloba L.	total extract	not stated	anticancer (chemopreventive) properties are related to its antioxidant, antiangiogenic and gene-regulatory actions	cell culture	Dubey et al., 2004
Ginkgo biloba L.	ginkgolide B	sesquiterpenoids	anticancer (chemopreventive) properties that are related to their antioxidant, anti-angiogenic and gene-regulatory actions	molecular, cellular and whole animal models	DeFeudis et al., 2003
Ginkgo biloba L.	not stated	flavonoids	anticancer (chemopreventive) properties that are related to their antioxidant, anti-angiogenic and gene-regulatory actions	molecular, cellular and whole animal models	DeFeudis et al., 2003

Table 16. Ginkgoaceae Cytotoxic Phytochemicals

Hypericaceae A. L. de Jussieu

The Hypericaceae consists of 9 genera and 540 species. Members of this family are trees, shrubs or herbs with clear or block resinous sap in secretory cavities (Evans 2009; Judd et al., 2008; Mabberley 2008).

Species	Compound	Class of Compound	Effect	Status	Ref.
Hypericum perforatum L.	hypericin	naphthodianthrones	antineoplastic activity upon irradiation, photosensitizer can induce both apoptosis and necrosis	*in vivo* and *in vitro*, potential clinical anticancer agent	Agostinis et al., 2002

Table 17. Hypericaceae Cytotoxic Phytochemicals

Iridaceae A. L. de Jussieu

A family of 70 genera nd 2000 species. The species are widely distributed usually geophytic herbs with rhizomes, corms or bulbs, less often evergreen or even shrubby, rarely annuals or achlorophyllous mycotroph. Constituents include quinones, aromatic ketones, carotenoid pigments, terpenoids, and flavonoids (Evans 2009; Judd et al., 2008; Mabberley 2008).

Species	Compound	Class of Compound	Effect	Status	Ref.
Crocus sativus L.	total extract	not stated	antitumor and cancer preventive activities of saffron and its main ingredients	experimental *in vitro* and *in vivo* investigations	Abdullaev & Espinosa-Aguirre, 2004
Crocus sativus L.	total extract	not stated	apoptosis induction in MCF-7 and MDA-MB-231 breast cancer cells	*in vitro*	Mousavi et al., 2009; Chryssanthi et al., 2007

Table 18. Iridaceae Cytotoxic Phytochemicals

Lamiaceae Martynov

(Labiatae A. L. de Jussieu)
A family of 238 genera and 6500 species. Trees, shrubs, annual or perennial herbs, rarely lianas.Young stems often 4 – angleded. Leaves opposite and simple. Flower are bisexuals, usually bracteolate and in cymes, thyrse or verticillasters or single. The family divided into 7 subfamilies.The Lamiaceae contains many species that are economically important either for their volatile oils or for use as spices. Among the constituents found in the family are essential oils, saponins, tannins, quinones, irodoids: alkaloids appear to be rare (Evans 2009; Judd et al., 2008; Mabberley 2008).

Species	Compound	Class of Compound	Effect	Status	Ref.
Ocimum sanctum L.	ursolic acid	triterpenoids	antitumor	not stated	Prakash & Gupta, 2005

Phlomis armeniaca Willd.	Phenyl propanoid caffeic acid, phenylethyl alcohol and phenylethylalcohol glycosides	phenolic compounds	anticancer activity	several kinds of cancer cells	Limem-Ben Amor et al., 2009
Phlomis brunneogaleata Hub.-Mor.	verbascoside, isoverbascoside, forsythoside B and 3-O-caffeoylquinic acid methyl ester	phenolic compounds	cytotoxic activity	L6 cell lines	Limem-Ben Amor et al., 2009
*Rosmarinus officinalis*L.	ursolic acid (3β-hydroxy-urs-12-en-28-oic acid)	triterpenoids	suppress tumorigenesis, inhibit tumor promotion, and suppress angiogenesis, inhibited proliferation, induced apoptosis	*in vitro* and *in vivo*	Aggarwal et al., 2008
Salvia chamelaeagnea P.J.Bergius,	total extract	not stated	cyotoxic	animals and humans	Kamatou et al., 2008
Salvia namaensis Schinz	total extract	not stated	cyotoxic	animals and humans	Kamatou et al., 2008
Salvia runcinata L.f.	total extract	not stated	cyotoxic	animals and humans	Kamatou et al., 2008
*Salvia africana–caerulea*L.	total extract	not stated	cytotoxic effects on cancer cells	human cancer cell lines	Kamatou et al., 2008
Salvia chamelaeagnea P.J.Bergius	total extract	not stated	cytotoxic effects on cancer cells	human cancer cell lines	Kamatou et al., 2008
Salvia dolomitica Codd	total extract	not stated	cytotoxic effects on cancer cells	human cancer cell lines	Kamatou et al., 2008
Salvia gariepensis E.Mey.	total extract	not stated	cytotoxic effects on cancer cells	human cancer cell lines	Kamatou et al., 2008
Salvia hypargeia Fisch. & Mey.	total extract	not stated	cytotoxic effects on cancer cells	human cancer cell lines	Kamatou et al., 2008
Salvia lanceolata Lam.	total extract	not stated	cytotoxic effects on cancer cells	human cancer cell lines	Kamatou et al., 2008
Salvia miltiorrhiza Bunge	in mixture with *coriolus versicolor* in capsules	not stated	could be beneficial for promoting immunological function in post-treatment of breast cancer patients	clinical trial	Wong et al., 2005
Salvia muirii L.Bolus	total extract	not stated	cytotoxic effects on cancer cells	human cancer cell lines	Kamatou et al., 2008
Salvia namaensis Schinz	total extract	not stated	cytotoxic effects on cancer cells	human cancer cell lines	Kamatou et al., 2008

Salvia radula Benth.	total extract	not stated	cytotoxic effects on cancer cells	human cancer cell lines	Kamatou et al., 2008
Salvia repens Burch. ex Benth.	total extract	not stated	cytotoxic effects on cancer cells	human cancer cell lines	Kamatou et al.,2008
Salvia runcinata L.f.	total extract	not stated	cytotoxic effects on cancer cells	human cancer cell lines	Kamatou et al., 2008
Salvia verbenaca L.	total extract	not stated	cytotoxic effects on cancer cells	human cancer cell lines	Kamatou et al., 2008
Scutellaria barbata D.Don	aqueous extract	not stated	anticancer activity in women with metastatic breast cancer (MBC)	the trial was an open-label, phase 1B, multicenter, dose escalation study	Perez et al., 2010
Scutellaria spp.	Wogonin, Baicalein and Baicalin	flavones	potent anticancer activities, scavenge oxidative radicals, to attenuate NF-kappaB activity, to inhibit several genes important for regulation of the cell cycle, to suppress COX-2 gene expression and to prevent viral infections	*in vitro* and *in vivo*	Li-Weber 2009
Scutellaria lindbergii Rech. f.	different fractions	not stated	cytotoxic effects in different cancer cell lines in which apoptosis plays an important role, potential chemotherapeutic agent	cancer cell lines	Tayarani-Najaran et al., 2009
Scutellaria litwinowii Bornm. & Sint. ex Bornm	different fractions	not stated	cytotoxic effects in different cancer cell lines in which apoptosis plays an important role, potential chemotherapeutic agent	cancer cell lines	Tayarani-Najaran et al., 2011

Table 19. Lamiaceae Cytotoxic Phytochemicals

Liliaceae A. L. de Jussieu

A widely distributed family of 16 genera and about 600 species of perennials with bulbs or rhizomes; aerial stem unbranched. Leaves oval to filiform, usually parallel – veined.

Inflorescences usually raceme sometimes umbel, thyrse or 1 – flowered. Many members of the family contain alkaloids, which are of the steroidal, isoquinoline or purine types, other steroidal substances include sterols, cardenolides bufadienolides and steroidal saponins. Other constituents include quinones, flavonoids, the gamma – pyrone chelidonic acid, cyanogenic substances and fructosan – type carbohydrates. Some volatile oils of the family have antimicrobial properties (Evans 2009; Judd et al., 2008; Mabberley 2008).

Species	Compound	Class of Compound	Effect	Status	Ref.
Allium sativum L.	ajoene	thiosulfinates	anticancer activity, activation of the mitochondrial-dependent caspase cascade	*in vitro*	Kaschula et al., 2010
Allium sativum L.	not stated	not stated	garlic rich diet decreases risk of some cancers	epidemiological studies	Iciek et al., 2009
Allium sativum L.	not stated	not stated	Mortality in stomach cancer patients from the region where people have consumed high-garlic diet (about 20 g a day) was three times lower than in the second region in which consumption of plats of the family Allium was very low	trials carried out in China compared two big human populations living	Iciek et al., 2009
Allium sativum L.	not stated	not stated	negatively correlated with colon cancer, reduced risk of prostate cancer, reduced risk of breast cancer	epidemiological analysis,	Iciek et al., 2009
Allium sativum L.	DATS (diallyl trisulfide)	not stated	protection against gastric cancer	double-blind intervention study	Iciek et al., 2009
Allium sativum L.	alk (en)yl sulfides	thiosulfinates	anticancer effect	human colon cancer cells	Seki et al., 2008
Allium sativum L.	organosulfur compounds (OSCs)	thiosulfinates	inhibition of DNA adduct formation, upregulation of antioxidant defences and DNA repair systems, and suppression of cell proliferation by blocking cell cycle	epidemiological studies as well as laboratory data	Nagini et al., 2008

			progression and/or inducing apoptosis		
Allium sativum L.	diallylsulfides	thiosulfinates	not stated	not stated	Münchberg et al., 2007
Allium sativum L.	allicin and diallyltrisulfide	thiosulfinates	anticancer agents	cell culture	Münchberg et al., 2007
Allium sativum L.	allicin, methyl allyl trisulfide, and diallyl trisulfide	thiosulfinates	not stated	not stated	Ariga et al., 2006
Allium sativum L.	organosulfur compounds	thiosulfinates	anticarcinogenic and antitumorigenic	preclinical	Milner, 2006
Allium sativum L.	thiosulfinates such as allicin	thiosulfinates	anticancer and chemopreventive activities	not stated	Amagase, 2006
Allium sativum L.	organic allyl sulfur components	thiosulfinates	inhibitors of the cancer process, depression in nitrosamine formation and a reduction in carcinogen bioactivation	not stated	Milner et al., 2001
Allium sativum L.	thiosulfinates, allicin, S-allylcysteine, S-allylmercaptocysteine, N (alpha)-fructosyl arginine	thiosulfinates	not stated	not stated	Amagase et al., 2001
Aloe arborescens Mill.	in combination with pineal indole melatonin	not stated	stabilization of disease and survival, in patients with advanced solid tumors	a randomized study of chemotherapy versus biochemotherapy	Lissoni et al., 2009
Aloe vera L.	barbaloin,octapeptide, aloesin, aloe-emodin	antheraquinones	prolongation of the life span of tumor-transplanted animals, cytotoxicity, apoptosis	*in vitro* (acute myeloid leukemia (AML) and acute lymphocytes leukemia (ALL) cancerous cells) and *in vivo*	El-Shemy et al., 2010
Aloe vera L.	acemannan	polysaccharides	anti-tumour activity	*in vitro* models as well as in different animal species	Hamman et al., 2008
Aloe vera L.	gel	not stated	reduced tumour burden, tumour shrinkage, tumour necrosis and prolonged survival rates,	*in vitro* models as well as in different animal species	Hamman et al., 2008

			chemopreventative and anti-genotoxic effects on benzo[a]pyrene-DNA adducts		
Aloe vera L.	not stated	glycoproteins (lectins) and polysaccharides	anti-cancer effects, stimulation of the immune response	*in vitro* models as well as in different animal species	Hamman et al., 2008

Table 20. Liliaceae Cytotoxic Phytochemicals

Linaceae A. P. de Candolle ex Perleb.

A family of 10 genera and 280 species.
Lianas, shrubs and herbs sometimes cyanogenic. Leaves are spirals to opposites, simple, entire. Flowers bisexuals usually regulars and 5 – merous in cymose or racemose inflorescence. Constituents of the family in clued cyanogenaic glycosides, fixed oils, mucilage, diterpenes and triterpenes (Evans 2009; Judd et al., 2008; Mabberley 2008).
Family Linaceae

Species	Compound	Class of Compound	Effect	Status	Ref.
Linum usitatissimum L.	secoisolariciresinol	lignans	inhibited the invasion, inhibitory effect on breast and colon carcinoma, potent cytotoxic effect on human promyleocytic leukemia HL-60 cells, DNA damage and apoptosis, anticancer, antiapoptotic	cell culture	Sok et al., 2009
Linum usitatissimum L.	lariciresinol and pinoresinol	lignans	anticancer, antiapoptotic	cell culture	Sok et al., 2009
Linum usitatissimum L.	secoisolariciresinol diglucoside	lignans	anticancer, antiapoptotic	cell culture	Sok et al., 2009
Linum usitatissimum L.	hydroxymatairesinol, matairesinol	lignans	antitumor activity, anticarcinogenic effects	cell culture, animal experiment	Sok et al., 2009
Linum usitatissimum L.	enterolactone and enterodiol	Lignans	potential anticancer effects	randomized crossover study	Coulman et al., 2005

Table 21. Linaceae Cytotoxic Phytochemicals

Loranthaceae A. L. de Jussieu

A family of 84 genera and 950 species. Pantropical but no single genus spans both Old and New Worlds.

Typically brittle shroblets on tree – branches; less often trrestrial shrubs, lianas or even trees. The family contains glycoproteins, polypeptides, lignans, flavonoids, etc. (Evans 2009; Judd et al., 2008; Mabberley 2008).

Species	Compound	Class of Compound	Effect	Status	Ref.
Viscum album L.	total extracts	not stated	the evidence from RCTs to support the view that the application of mistletoe extracts has impact on survival or leads to an improved ability to fight cancer or to withstand anticancer treatments is weak.	randomized clinical trials (RCTs) and controlled clinical trials	Horneber et al., 2008
Viscum album L.	lectins	proteins	anti-metastatic effect, inhibition of tumour-induced angiogenesis, and in part due to an induction of apoptosis, suppress tumour growth	different tumour cell lines, in vivo	Pryme et al., 2006
Viscum album L.	aqueous extract (Isorel)	not stated	Isorel can improve immune competence and the overall health status of cancer patients undergoing surgery	clinical trial	Enesel et al., 2005
Viscum album L.	mistletoe lectins I, II, and III	proteins	improvement of quality of life in cancer patients	several preclinical studies, randomised phase III study	Stauder & Kreuser, 2002
Viscum album L.	total extract (Isorel)	not stated	benefit in terms of survival from combined postoperative chemotherapy and Isorel biotherapy, either adjuvant or palliative	Randomized and controlled study, patients with colorectal cancer stages Dukes C and D	Cazacu et al., 2003

Table 22. Loranthaceae Cytotoxic Phytochemicals

Lythraceae J. St. – Hilaire

A family contains 31 genera and 600 tropical with few temperate species. Herbs, less often sub shrubs or trees. Leaves are opposite and simple. Flowers are bisexuals, often heterostylons, solitary, fascicled in axils or terminal racemes, regular or not, with conspicuous hypanthium.

Constituents of the family include quinones, alkaloids and tannins (Evans 2009; Judd et al., 2008; Mabberley 2008).

Species	Compound	Class of Compound	Effect	Status	Ref.
Punica granatum L.	total exract	not stated	potential chemopreventive and anticancer agent	*in vitro* and *in vivo* animal models	Syed et al., 2007
Punica granatum L.	total exract	not stated	cancer chemoprevention, anticancer activities, interference with tumor cell proliferation, cell cycle, invasion and angiogenesis	mouse mammary organ culture, *in vitro* and *in vivo*, open-label, singlearm, 2-year, phase-2, Simon two-stage clinical trial	Lansky et al., 2007

Table 23. Lythraceae Cytotoxic Phytochemicals

Malvaceae A. L. de Jussieu

The Malvaceae consists of 113 genera and 5000 cosmopolitan species. Trees, shrubs, lianas and herbs, rarely scandent, usually with tufted or stellate hairs and parenchyma typically with scattered mucilage cell, mucilage cavities or mucilage canals. The family divided into 9 subfamilies. Constituents of the family include alkaloids, cardiac glycosides, saponins, tannins, pbenolic acids and mucilage (Evans 2009; Judd et al., 2008; Mabberley 2008).

Species	Compound	Class of Compound	Effect	Status	Ref.
Gossypium spp.	gossypol	polyphenols	anticancer	not stated	Wang et al., 2009

Table 24. Malvaceae Cytotoxic Phytochemicals

Melanthiaceae Batsch ex Borkh.

A family of 16 genera and about 120 species distributed in temperate and/or montane habitats. Members of this family perennial herbs sometimes pachycaul, with rhizomes and spirals of or distichous leaves. Inflorescence are spikes or racemes of usually bisexual flowers, steroidal saponins and various tonic alkaloids often present (Evans 2009; Judd et al., 2008; Mabberley 2008).

Species	Compound	Class of Compound	Effect	Status	Ref.
Veratrum grandiflorum O.Loes	resveratrol, trans-3,5,4'-trihydroxystilbene	stilbenoids	growth-inhibitory effects, suppression of angiogenesis, potentiate the	wide variety of tumor cells, including lymphoid and	Aggarwal et al., 2004

			apoptotic effects of cytokines (e.g., TRAIL), chemotherapeutic agents and gamma-radiation, chemopreventive effects, therapeutic effects against cancer	myeloid cancers; multiple myeloma; cancers of the breast, prostate, stomach, colon, pancreas, and thyroid; melanoma; head and neck squamous cell carcinoma; ovarian carcinoma; and cervical carcinoma	

Table 24. Melanthiaceae Cytotoxic Phytochemicals

Meliaceae A. L. de Jussieu

The Meliaceae contains 50 genera and 650 tropical and subtropical species. Trees, often pachycaul, rarely subshrubs or suckering shrublets, dioecious polygamous, monoecious or with only bisexual flowers, bark bitter and astringent. Leaves pinnate to bipinnate,unifolioate or simple, in spirals with usually entire leaflets and basally swollen petiole sometimes spiny. Flowers if unisexual often with rudiments of opposite sex, in spikes to thyrses, axillary to snpra – axillary. The family divided into two subfamilies. Significant constituents of the family are triterperoids and limonoids (Evans 2009; Judd et al., 2008; Mabberley 2008).
Family Meliaceae

Species	Compound	Class of Compound	Effect	Status	Ref.
Aglaia elliptifolia Merr.	rocaglamide	cyclopenta[b]benzofurans	antiproliferative activity, induce apoptosis in different human cancer cell lines	in a murine *in vivo* model, human cancer cell lines	Kim et al., 2006

Table 25. Meliaceae Cytotoxic Phytochemicals

Moraceae Gaudich.

A family of 38 genera and 1150 species of tropical and warm monoecious or dioecious trees, shrubs, lianas or rarely herbs, usually with laticifers with milky latex dis tribnted in all parenchy matous tissues. The family divided into 5 tribes. Constituents of the family include cardenolides and pyridine alkaloids (Evans 2009; Judd et al., 2008; Mabberley 2008).

Species	Compound	Class of Compound	Effect	Status	Ref.
Ficus spp.	6-O-acyl-d-glucosyl-sitosterol isoforms	latex	anti-proliferative activity, inhibited the growth of hepatic carcinoma xenografts by approximately 49%	in several tumor cell lines, *in vitro* in mice	Lansky et al., 2008

Ficus spp.	apigenin, carpachromene, and norartocarpetin	flavonoids	cytotoxic	In several cancer cell lines	Lansky et al., 2008
Ficus spp.	C-28 carboxylic acid functional groups	triterpenoids, phenanthroindolizidine alkaloids	cytotoxic	human cancer cell lines	Lansky et al., 2008
Ficus septica Burm. f.,	ficuseptine-A (6), (+)-tylophorine (19), and a mixture of (+)-antofine (1) and (+)-isotylocrebrine (12)	alkaloids	cytotoxic activity	in several cancer cell lines	Lansky et al., 2008
Ficus hispida L.f.	O-methyltylophorinidine	alkaloids	cytotoxic activity	in several cancer cell lines	Lansky EP 2008

Table 26. Moraceae Cytotoxic Phytochemicals

Oleaceae Hoffmannsegg & Link.

A family of 24 genera and 800 species of trees and shrubs, sometimes lianoid, usually with peltate secretory hairs. Sclereids often present, usually with phenolic glycosides. Other constituents of the family are saponins, tannins, coumarins and iridoid glycosides. Alkaloids are rare (Evans 2009; Judd et al., 2008; Mabberley 2008).

Species	Compound	Class of Compound	Effect	Status	Ref.
Olea europaea L.	not stated	Phenolic compounds	inhibit colon cancer development	in large intestinal cancer cell models, animals, and humans	Corona et al., 2009
Olea europaea L.	oleic acid	fatty acids	induces apoptosis and cell differentiation, colorectal chemoprotection	*in vitro* and *in vivo* studies	Waterman et al., 2007
Olea europaea L.	squalene	triterpenoids	chemoprotective effect, lower incidence of skin cancer, inhibitory action on chemically-induced skin carcinomas.	epidemiological data, animal studies	Waterman et al., 2007
Olea europaea L.	monounsaturated fatty acids, squalene, tocopherols, and phenolic compounds	Phenolic compounds	associated with low incidence and prevalence of cancer, including colorectal cancer	epidemiologic, *in vitro*, cellular, and animal studies	Hashim et al., 2005

Olea europaea L.	squalene and terpenoids acteosides, hydroxytyrosol, ????tyrosol and phenyl propionic acids hydroxytyrosol and tyrosol secoiridoids and lignans	phenolic antioxidants and squalene???	scavenging singlet oxygen generated by UV light, chemopreventive effects against colorectal cancer, potential as chemopreventive agents	animal, cellular and metabolic studie	Owen et al., 2004

Table 27. Oleaceae Cytotoxic Phytochemicals

Papaveraceae A. L. de Jussieu

The Papaveracea contains 430 genera and 770 species widely distributed in mainly temperate regions; specially diverse in the Northern Hemisphere, but also in southern Africa and eastern Australia. Herbs to soft – wooded shrubs; stem with vascular bundles sometimes in several rings with laticifers present and plants with white, cream, yellow, orange, or red sap, or with specialized elongated secretory cells and sap then mucilaginous, clear, sap with various alkaloids. The family is rich in alkaloids (Evans 2009; Judd et al., 2008; Mabberley 2008).

Species	Compound	Class of Compound	Effect	Status	Ref.
Chelidonium majus L.	total extract	not stated	has curative effects on a range of cancers	randomised clinical trials	Ernst & Schmidt, 2005

Table 28. Papaveraceae Cytotoxic Phytochemicals

Sapindaceae A. L. de Jussieu

The Sapindaceae is a family of 131 genera and 1450 species.
This family is divided into 3 subfamilies: 1) Hippocastanideae 2) Dodonaeoideae and 3) Sapindoideae. Mainly tropical and subtropical with a few genera most diverse in temperate regions. Trees, shrubs or lianas and herbaceous climbers. Constituents of the family inclued saponins, cyanogenic glycosides, cyclitols and coumarins.Alkaloids have been reported in a few species (Evans 2009; Judd et al., 2008; Mabberley 2008).

Species	Compound	Class of Compound	Effect	Status	Ref.
Litchi chinensis Sonn.	epicatechin, procyanidin B2, procyanidin B4	flavonoids	inhibition of proliferation and induction of apoptosis in cancer cells through upregulation and down-regulation of multiple genes, anti-breast cancer	cell culture	Li et al., 2007

Table 29. Sapindaceae Cytotoxic Phytochemicals

Solanaceae A. L. de Jussieu

The family comprise of 91 genera and 2450 species. Subcosmopolitan especially in tropical America. Shrubs, trees, lianas and herbs with branched hairs and often prickles; internal phloem around pith; some dioecious. Leaves simple, or lobed to pinnate or 3 – foliate, usually in spirals. Flowers solitary or in appearent basically cymose inflorescence. The Solanaceae is divided into two subfamilies: 1) Solanoideae and 2) Browallioideae.

The family contains a wide range of alkaloids which are great taxonomic interest. Types of alkaloid recorded are tropane, alkaloidal amine, indole, isoquinoline, purine, pyrazole, pyridine, pyrrolidine, quinolizidine, stroid alkaloids and glycoalkaloids. Other constituents include stroidal saponins, withanolides, coumarins, cyclitols, pungent principles, flavones, caretenoids and anthra quinons (Evans 2009; Judd et al., 2008; Mabberley 2008).

Species	Compound	Class of Compound	Effect	Status	Ref.
Capsicum annuum L.	capsanthin and capsorubin	carotenoids	potent P-gp inhibitors	cell culture	Molnár et al., 2010
Capsicum chinense Jacq.	capsaicin	capsaicinoids.	apoptosis inducer	cell culture	Meghvansi et al., 2010
Capsicum spp.	capsaicin (trans-8-methyl-N-vanillyl-6-nonenamide)	alkaloids	blocks the translocation of nuclear factor kappa B (NF-kB), activator protein 1 (AP-1), and signal transducer and activator of transcription (STAT3) signaling pathway	cell culture	Oyagbemi et al., 2010
Capsicum spp.	capsaicin (trans-8-methyl-N-vanillyl-6-nonenamide)	alkaloids	anticancer effects	cell culture, in animal models	Aggarwal et al., 2008
Lycopersicon esculentum Mill.	lycopene	carotenoids	prostate cancer	cell culture, animal, epidemiologic and case-control studies	Ansari & Ansari, 2005
Lycopersicon esculentum Mill.	lycopene	carotenoids	several types of cancer, including prostate cancer	*in vitro* and *in vivo* studies	Hwang et al., 2002
Lycopersicon esculentum Mill.	lycopene	carotenoids	cancer chemopreventive effects	animal models	Cohen et al., 2002
Nicotiana tabacum L.	alpha- and beta-2,7,11-cembratriene-4,6-diols	diterpenoids	anticancer activity	cell culture, mice, mouse, rats	El Sayed et al., 2007
Solanum incanum L.	diosgenin	saponins	suppress proliferation, invasion inhibition,	cell culture, animal study	Aggarwal et al., 2008

			Cytotoxic, apoptotic, anti-cancer activity		
Solanum xanthocarpum Schrad. & Wendl	diosgenin	saponins	suppress proliferation, invasion inhibition, Cytotoxic, apoptotic, anti-cancer activity	cell culture, animal study	Aggarwal et al., 2008

Table 30. Solanaceae Cytotoxic Phytochemicals

Ranunculaceae A. L. de Jussieu

A family of 56 genera and 2100 species. Widespread, but especially characteristic of temperate boreal regions of the Northern Hemisphere. Herbs, shrubs or occasionally vines. Leaves usually alternate and spiral, occasionally opposite, simples sometimes lobed or dissected, to compound, usually serrate, or crenate, with pinnate to occasionally palmate venation. Inflorescences determinate, sometimes appearing in de terminate or reduced to a single flower, terminal. Flowers usually bisexual. The family has diverse chemical constituents and is of considerable phytochemical and chemotaxonmic interest (Evans 2009; Judd et al., 2008; Mabberley 2008).

Species	Compound	Class of Compound	Effect	Status	Ref.
Nigella sativa L.	Thymoquinone	not stated	suppress proliferation, invasion inhibition, Cytotoxic, apoptotic, anti-cancer activity, anti angiogenic	cell culture, animal study, *in vitro* and *in vivo*	Aggarwal et al., 2008

Table 31. Ranunculaceae Cytotoxic Phytochemicals

Rosaceae A. L. de Jussieu

A family of 85 genera and around 3000 species. The family is subcosmopolitan and most abundant in the northern Hemisphere. Herbs, shrubs, or trees, often rhizomatous, in frequently climbing; thorns sometimes present. This family is divided into 3 subfamilies and 17 tribes. Constituents of the Rosaceae include cyanogenic glycosides, saponins, tannins, sugar alcohols, cyclitols, terpenoids and mucilage; alkaloids and coumarins are rare (Evans 2009; Judd et al., 2008; Mabberley 2008).

Species	Compound	Class of Compound	Effect	Status	Ref.
Aronia arbutifolia (L.) Pers.	not stated	anthocyanins and procyanidins	anticancer	*in vitro* and in *in vivo* studies	Kokotkiewicz et al., 2010
Aronia melanocarpa (Michx.) Elliott	not stated	anthocyanins and procyanidins	anticancer	*in vitro* and *in vivo* studies	Kokotkiewicz et al., 2010

Fragaria × *ananassa* (Weston) Duchesne ex Rozier	ellagic acid, and certain flavonoids: anthocyanin, catechin, quercetin and kaempferol	flavonoids	anticancer activity, blocking initiation of carcinogenesis, and suppressing progression and proliferation of tumors	in several different experimental systems	Hannum et al., 2004

Table 32. Rosaceae Cytotoxic Phytochemicals

Rubiaceae A. L. de Jussieu

The Rubiaceae consists of 563 genera and 10900 species. Members of the family are cosmopolitan, but most diverse in tropical and subtropical regions. The Rubiaceae divided into 4 subfamilies. In the family, alkaloids of indole, oxindole, quinoline and purine types are common; anthraquinones occur in some genera of the Rubiaceae. Other constituents of the family inclued anthocyanins, cyclitols, coumarins, diterpenoids, triterpenoids and iridoid glycosids.

Species	Compound	Class of Compound	Effect	Status	Ref.
Morinda citrifolia L.	total extract	not stated	potential anticancer activity, immunomodulatory activity	cell culture, phase I clinical study	McClatchey et al., 2002

Table 33. Rubiaceae Cytotoxic Phytochemicals

Rutaceae A. L. de Jussieu

A family of 158 genera and 1900 species. Nearly cosmopolitan, but mainly tropical and sub tropical. Usually trees or shrubs, sometimes with thorns, spines, or prickles. The Rutaceae is divided into 5 subfamilies.

Constituents of this family include a wide variety of alkaloids, volatile oils, rhamno – glucosides, coumarins and terpenoids. Alkaloids include alkaloidal amines, imidazole, indole isoquinoline, pyridine, pyrrolidine, quinazoline types. Many of the fruits are rich in citric and other acids and in vitamin c (Evans 2009; Judd et al., 2008; Mabberley 2008).

Species	Compound	Class of Compound	Effect	Status	Ref.
Citrus spp.	limonoids	triterpenoids	chemopreventive agents for cancer, Reduction of skin tumours	animal studies	Silalahi et al., 2002
Citrus spp.	nomilin	triterpenoids	inhibitor of carcinogenesis	animal studies for forestomach tumours	Silalahi, 2002
Citrus spp.	nobiletin and tangeretin dietary fibre	flavonoids	anticancer activity	*in vivo* and *in vitro*	Silalahi et al., 2002
Citrus spp.	β-carotene	not stated	pro-tumorigenic properties	not stated	Silalahi et al., 2002

Citrus spp.	ascorbic acid	not stated	prevents oxidation of specific chemicals to their active carcinogenic forms, protects against in vivo oxidation of lipids and DNA	in vivo, in humans	Silalahi et al., 2002
Citrus spp.	dietary fibre and pectin	polysaccharides	influence colon cancer by physical dilution of colon content, absorption of bile acids and carcinogens, decreased transit time, altered bile acid metabolism and the effects of fermentation, namely, the production of short-chain fatty acids, lowering of pH and stimulation of bacterial growth, absorbing carcinogens in the gastrointestinal tract, reducing the risk of bowel cancer,	in human	Silalahi et al., 2002
Citrus spp.	flavanone and flavone O- and C-glycosides and methoxylated flavones???	flavonoids	anti-inflammatory and anticancer actions	in vitro and in vivo	Manthey et al., 2001

Table 34. Rutaceae Cytotoxic Phytochemicals

Taxaceae Bercht. & J. Presl

A family of 6 genera and 28 species. Small or moderately sized dioecious trees or shrubs, usually not resinous or only slightly resinous, fragrant or not. Wood without resin canals, leaves simple, persistent for several years, shed singly, spirals, often twisted so as to appear 2 – ranked, linear, flattned, entire, acute at apex, with 0 – 1 resin canals. Some species of Taxus investigated for taxane alkaloids (Evans 2009; Judd et al., 2008; Mabberley 2008).

Species	Compound	Class of Compound	Effect	Status	Ref.
Taxus baccata L.	total extract	not stated	cytotoxic effect	Cell culture	Emami et al., 2005

Table 35. Taxaceae Cytotoxic Phytochemicals

Theaceae Mirbel

A family of 7 genera and about 240 species. Usually evergreen trees and shrubs. Leaves simple, entire to toothed usually in spirals and coriaceous, often withering red. Flowers usually large and bisexual, hypogynous to epigynous, solitary and axillary. Among the constituents are purine alkaloids, saponins, tannins and fixed oil (Evans 2009; Judd et al., 2008; Mabberley 2008).

Species	Compound	Class of Compound	Effect	Status	Ref.
Camellia sinensis (L.) Kuntze	(-)-epigallocatechin gallate (EGCG)	polyphenols	synergists with anticancer drugs	cell culture	Suganuma et al., 2011
Camellia sinensis (L.) Kuntze	catechins (specifically EGCG)	polyphenols	targeting of lipid rafts by EGCG	cell culture	Patra et al., 2008
Camellia sinensis (L.) Kuntze	catechins (specifically EGCG)	polyphenols	growth factor-mediated pathway, the mitogen-activated protein (MAP) kinase-dependent pathway, and ubiquitin/proteasome degradation pathways	phase I and II clinical trials	Chen et al., 2008
Camellia sinensis (L.) Kuntze	catechin, (-)-epigallocatechin	polyphenols	antioxidant, antiangiogenesis, and antiproliferative	review to summarize recent findings on the anticancer and medicinal properties of green tea	Cooper et al., 2005 b
Camellia sinensis (L.) Kuntze	epigallocatechin gallate (EGCg)	polyphenols	antioxidant, anti-angiogenesis, and antiproliferative	review to summarize recent findings on the anticancer and medicinal properties of green tea	Cooper et al., 2005 a
Camellia sinensis (L.) Kuntze	catechin EGCG	polyphenols	antioxidant properties of the catechins with anticancer effects	preclinical research	Moyers et al., 2004
Camellia sinensis (L.) Kuntze	catechins and polyphenols	polyphenols	both cytostatic and cytotoxic activity towards cancer cells	in vitro and in vivo research	Colic & Pavelic, 2000

Table 36. Theaceae Cytotoxic Phytochemicals

Zingiberaceae Martynov

The Zingiberaceae family of 50 genera and 1500 species widespread in tropical regions; chiefly in shaded to semi – shaded forest understory habitats; occasionally in wetlands. Small to large, spicy – aromatic herbs, scattered secretory cells containing ethereal oils, various terpenes, and phenyl – propanoid compounds. The family is divided into two subfamilies: 1) Costoideae and 2) Zingiberoideae.

Volatile oils and pungent principles are a feature of the family. Other constituents include the colouring matters known as curcominoids, tannins, phenolic acids, leucoantheyanins,flavonoids, ketones and terpenoids. Only a few isolated of alkaloids have been reported (Evans 2009; Judd et al., 2008; Mabberley 2008).

Species	Compound	Class of Compound	Effect	Status	Ref.
Curcuma longa L.	curcumin, difluorocurcumin analogs	polyphenols	prevention of tumor progression and/or treatments of human malignancies	promising leads for conducting first in-depth animal studies and subsequently clinical trials	Padhye et al., 2010
Curcuma longa L.	curcumin	polyphenols	anticancer activities	not stated	Agarwal et al., 2007
Curcuma longa L.	curcumin	polyphenols	cancer chemoprevention, antitumor	cell epidemiological studies, Preclinical studies	Thangapazham et al., 2006
Curcuma longa L.	curcumin	polyphenols	cancer prevention	human clinical trials	Aggarwal et al., 2008
Curcuma longa L.	curcumin, demethoxycurcumin and bisdemethoxycurcumin	polyphenols	Anti-cancer activity	progress clinical trials	Jurenka et al., 2009
Curcuma longa L.	turmerone, atlantone, and zingiberone	sesquiterpenoids	anti-cancer activity	progress clinical trials	Jurenka et al., 2009
Zingiber officinale Roscoe	[6]-gingerol	phenolic compounds	cytotoxic, apoptotic, anti-cancer activity	cell culture, animal study	Aggarwal et al., 2008
Zingiber officinale Roscoe	pungent vallinoids, viz. [6]-gingerol and [6]-paradol, shogaols, zingerene	phenolic compounds	cancer preventive activity	in experimental carcinogenesis	Shukla et al., 2007
Zingiber zerumbet Smith.	zerumbone [2,6,9,9-tetramethyl-(2E,6E,10E)-cycloundeca-2,6,10-trien-1-one]	phenolic compounds	cytotoxic, apoptotic, anti-cancer activity	cell culture, animal study	Aggarwal et al., 2008

Table 37. Zingiberaceae Cytotoxic Phytochemicals

Zygophyllaceae R. Brown

A family of 26 genera and 280 tropical species. Small trees, shrubs to herbs with stems often sympodial and jointed at the nodes, xylem with vessels, tracheids, and fibers arranged in horizon tally aligned tiers; usually producing steroidal or teriterponoid saponins, sesquiterpenes and alkaloids (Evans 2009; Judd et al., 2008; Mabberley 2008).

Species	Compound	Class of Compound	Effect	Status	Ref.
Larrea divaricata Cav.	nordihydroguaiaretic acid	phenolic compounds	anticancer, antioxidant, antimicrobial, anti-inflammatory and immunosuppressive activities	phase I/II clinical trials as an anticancer agent	Chen et al., 2009

Table 38. Zygophyllaceae Cytotoxic Phytochemicals

2. References

http://www.who.int/mediacentre/factsheets/fs297/en/

Abdullaev FI, Espinosa-Aguirre JJ. Biomedical properties of saffron and its potential use in cancer therapy and chemoprevention trials. Cancer Detect Prev. 2004;28 (6):426-32.

Agarwal R, Agarwal C, Ichikawa H, Singh RP, Aggarwal BB. Anticancer potential of silymarin: from bench to bed side. Anticancer Res. 2006 Nov-Dec;26 (6B):4457-98.

Aggarwal BB, Bhardwaj A, Aggarwal RS, Seeram NP, Shishodia S, Takada Y. Role of resveratrol in prevention and therapy of cancer: preclinical and clinical studies. Anticancer Res. 2004 Sep-Oct;24 (5A):2783-840.

Aggarwal BB, Ichikawa H. Molecular targets and anticancer potential of indole-3-carbinol and its derivatives. Cell Cycle. 2005 Sep;4 (9):1201-15. Epub 2005 Sep 6.

Aggarwal BB, Kunnumakkara AB, Harikumar KB, Tharakan ST, Sung B, Anand P. Potential of spice-derived phytochemicals for cancer prevention. Planta Med. 2008 Oct; 74 (13):1560-9. Epub 2008 Jul 8.

Aggarwal BB, Sundaram C, Malani N, Ichikawa H. Curcumin: the Indian solid gold. Adv Exp Med Biol. 2007;595:1-75.

Agostinis P, Vantieghem A, Merlevede W, de Witte PA. Hypericin in cancer treatment: more light on the way. Int J Biochem Cell Biol. 2002 Mar;34 (3):221-41.

Amagase H, Petesch BL, Matsuura H, Kasuga S, Itakura Y. Intake of garlic and its bioactive components. J Nutr. 2001 Mar;131 (3s):955S-62S.

Amagase H. Clarifying the real bioactive constituents of garlic. J Nutr. 2006 Mar;136 (3 Suppl):716S-725S.

Ansari MS, Ansari S. Lycopene and prostate cancer. Future Oncol. 2005 Jun;1 (3):425-30.

Ariga T, Seki T. Antithrombotic and anticancer effects of garlic-derived sulfur compounds: a review. Biofactors. 2006;26 (2):93-103.

Asl MN, Hosseinzadeh H. Review of pharmacological effects of *Glycyrrhiza* sp. and its bioactive compounds. Phytother Res. 2008 Jun;22 (6):709-24.

Balbi V, Devoto A. Jasmonate signalling network in *Arabidopsis thaliana*: crucial regulatory nodes and new physiological scenarios. New Phytol. 2008;177 (2):301-18. Epub 2007 Nov 27.

Canel C, Moraes R M., Dayan F E., Ferreira D, (2000) Podophyllotoxin. Phytochemistry 54, 115–120

Cazacu M, Oniu T, Lungoci C, Mihailov A, Cipak A, Klinger R, Weiss T, Zarkovic N. The influence of isorel on the advanced colorectal cancer. Cancer Biother Radiopharm. 2003 Feb;18 (1):27-34.

Chang YS, Seo EK, Gyllenhaal C, Block KI. *Panax ginseng*: a role in cancer therapy? Integr Cancer Ther. 2003 Mar;2 (1):13-33.

Chen CF, Chiou WF, Zhang JT.Comparison of the pharmacological effects of *Panax ginseng* and *Panax quinquefolium*. Acta Pharmacol Sin. 2008 Sep;29 (9):1103-8.

Chen D, Milacic V, Chen MS, Wan SB, Lam WH, Huo C, Landis-Piwowar KR, Cui QC, Wali A, Chan TH, Dou QP. Tea polyphenols, their biological effects and potential molecular targets. Histol Histopathol. 2008 Apr;23 (4):487-96.

Chen Q. Nordihydroguaiaretic acid analogues: their chemical synthesis and biological activities. Curr Top Med Chem. 2009;9 (17):1636-59.

Chryssanthi DG, Lamari FN, Iatrou G, Pylara A, Karamanos NK, Cordopatis P. Inhibition of breast cancer cell proliferation by style constituents of different Crocus species. Anticancer Res. 2007 Jan-Feb;27(1A):357-62. PubMed PMID:17352254.

Cirla, A. and Mann, J. (2003) Combrestatins: from natural product to drug discovery. Nat. Prod. Rep. 20, 558–564

Cohen LA. A review of animal model studies of tomato carotenoids, lycopene, and cancer chemoprevention. Exp Biol Med (Maywood). 2002 Nov;227 (10):864-8.

Colic M, Pavelic K. Molecular mechanisms of anticancer activity of natural dietetic products. J Mol Med. 2000;78 (6):333-6.

Cooper R, Morré DJ, Morré DM. Medicinal benefits of green tea: part II. review of anticancer properties. J Altern Complement Med. 2005a Aug;11 (4):639-52.

Corona G, Spencer JP, Dessì MA. Extra virgin olive oil phenolics: absorption, metabolism, and biological activities in the GI tract. Toxicol Ind Health. 2009 May-Jun;25 (4-5):285-93.

Coulman KD, Liu Z, Hum WQ, Michaelides J, Thompson LU. Whole sesame seed is as rich a source of mammalian lignan precursors as whole flaxseed. Nutr Cancer. 2005;52 (2):156-65.

DeFeudis FV, Papadopoulos V, Drieu K. *Ginkgo biloba* extracts and cancer: a research area in its infancy. Fundam Clin Pharmacol. 2003 Aug;17 (4):405-17.

Dossus L, Kaaks R. Nutrition, metabolic factors and cancer risk. Best Pract Res Clin Endocrinol Metab. 2008;22:551-71.

Dubey AK, Shankar PR, Upadhyaya D, Deshpande VY. Ginkgo biloba--an appraisal. Kathmandu Univ Med J (KUMJ). 2004 Jul-Sep;2 (3):225-9.

El Sayed KA, Sylvester PW. Biocatalytic and semisynthetic studies of the anticancer tobacco cembranoids. Expert Opin Investig Drugs. 2007 Jun;16 (6):877-87.

El-Shemy HA, Aboul-Soud MA, Nassr-Allah AA, Aboul-Enein KM, Kabash A, Yagi A. Antitumor properties and modulation of antioxidant enzymes' activity by *Aloe vera* leaf active principles isolated via supercritical carbon dioxide extraction. Curr Med Chem. 2010;17 (2):129-38.

Emami A, Sadeghi-aliabadi H, Saidi M, and Jafarian A (2005). Cytotoxic evaluation of Iranian conifers on cancer cells. Pharm. Biol. 43 (4): 299-304.

Emami SA, Rabe SZT, Ahi A, Mahmoudi M, Tabasi N. Study the cytotoxic and pro-apoptotic activity of *Artemisia annua* extracts. Pharmacol. online 3: 1062-1069 (2009b).

Emami SA, Vahdati-Mashhadian N, Oghazian MB, Vosough R (2009a). The anticancer activity of five species of *Artemisia* on Hep2 and HepG2 cell lines. Pharmacol. online 3: 327-339.

Enesel MB, Acalovschi I, Grosu V, Sbarcea A, Rusu C, Dobre A, Weiss T, Zarkovic N. Perioperative application of the *Viscum album* extract Isorel in digestive tract cancer patients. Anticancer Res. 2005 Nov-Dec;25 (6C):4583-90.

Ernst E, Schmidt K. Ukrain - a new cancer cure? A systematic review of randomised clinical trials. BMC Cancer. 2005 Jul 1;5:69.

Evans W. C., Trease and Evans Pharmacognosy,16th edition pp. 22, 24, 25, 28-42, W.B. Saunders, (2009).

Firestone GL, Sundar SN. Anticancer activities of artemisinin and its bioactive derivatives. Expert Rev Mol Med. 2009 Oct 30;11:e32.

Gilani SA, Kikuchi A, Shinwari ZK, Khattak ZI, Watanabe KN. Phytochemical, pharmacological and ethnobotanical studies of *Rhazya stricta* Decne. Phytother Res. 2007 Apr;21 (4):301-7.

Hamman JH. Composition and applications of *Aloe vera* leaf gel. Molecules. 2008 Aug 8;13 (8):1599-616.

Han QB, Xu HX. Caged *Garcinia* xanthones: development since 1937. Curr Med Chem. 2009;16 (28):3775-96.

Hannum SM. Potential impact of strawberries on human health: a review of the science. Crit Rev Food Sci Nutr. 2004;44 (1):1-17.

Hashim YZ, Eng M, Gill CI, McGlynn H, Rowland IR. Components of olive oil and chemoprevention of colorectal cancer. Nutr Rev. 2005 Nov;63 (11):374-86.

Horneber MA, Bueschel G, Huber R, Linde K, Rostock M. Mistletoe therapy in oncology. Cochrane Database Syst Rev. 2008 Apr 16; (2):CD003297.

Hwang ES, Bowen PE. Can the consumption of tomatoes or lycopene reduce cancer risk? Integr Cancer Ther. 2002 Jun;1 (2):121-32; discussion 132.

Iciek M, Kwiecień I, Włodek L. Biological properties of garlic and garlic-derived organosulfur compounds. Environ Mol Mutagen. 2009 Apr;50 (3):247-65.

Johnson, I.S. et al., (1963) The *Vinca* alkaloids: a new class of oncolytic agents. Cancer Res. 23, 1390

Judd, W. S.; Campbell, C. S.; Kellogg, E. A.; Stevens, P. F. and Donoghue, M. J. Plant Systematics, A Phylogenetic Approach " Third Edition " PP.208,215-217, 219-221,257

- 258, 260 - 262, 272 - 273, 302 - 304, 309-312,314 - 316, 334, 336, 342, 350 - 351, 362 - 364, 371 - 376, 379 - 381, 391 - 393, 408 - 410, 412 - 414, 416, 420 - 427, 429 - 437, 438 - 440, 443 - 445, 452 - 455, 459 - 462, 469 - 475, 480 - 481, 492 - 501, 508 - 515, Sinauer Associates, Inc. Publisher, Sunderland, Massachusetts,USA (2008).

Kamatou GP, Makunga NP, Ramogola WP, Viljoen AM. South African Salvia species: a review of biological activities and phytochemistry. J Ethnopharmacol. 2008 Oct 28;119 (3):664-72. Epub 2008 Jul 2.

Kaschula CH, Hunter R, Parker MI. Garlic-derived anticancer agents: structure and biological activity of ajoene. Biofactors. 2010 Jan-Feb;36 (1):78-85.

Kelly GS. *Rhodiola rosea*: a possible plant adaptogen. Altern Med Rev. 2001 Jun;6 (3):293-302.

Kerwin SM. Soy saponins and the anticancer effects of soybeans and soy-based foods. Curr Med Chem Anticancer Agents. 2004 May;4 (3):263-72.

Khan AL, Hussain J, Hamayun M, Gilani SA, Ahmad S, Rehman G, Kim YH, Kang SM, Lee IJ. Secondary metabolites from Inula britannica L. and their biological activities. Molecules. 2010 Mar 10;15 (3):1562-77.

Kiefer D, Pantuso T. *Panax ginseng*. Am Fam Physician. 2003 Oct 15;68 (8):1539-42.

Kim S, Salim AA, Swanson SM, Kinghorn AD. Potential of cyclopenta[b]benzofurans from *Aglaia* species in cancer chemotherapy. Anticancer Agents Med Chem. 2006 Jul;6 (4):319-45.

Kokotkiewicz A, Jaremicz Z, Luczkiewicz M. *Aronia* plants: a review of traditional use, biological activities, and perspectives for modern medicine. J Med Food. 2010 Apr;13 (2):255-69.

Kren V, Walterová D. Silybin and silymarin--new effects and applications. Biomed Pap Med Fac Univ Palacky Olomouc Czech Repub. 2005 Jun;149 (1):29-41.

Krishna S, Bustamante L, Haynes RK, Staines HM. Artemisinins: their growing importance in medicine. Trends Pharmacol Sci. 2008 Oct;29 (10):520-7. Epub 2008 Aug 25.

Kruk J. Lifetime physical activity and the risk of breast cancer: a casecontrol study. Cancer Detect Prev. 2007;31:18-28.

Kurahashi N, Inoue M, Iwasaki M, Tanaka Y, Mizokami M, Tsugane S, JPHC Study Group. Vegetable, fruit and antioxidant nutrient consumption and subsequent risk of hepatocellular carcinoma: a prospective cohort study in Japan. Br J Cancer. 2009;100:181-4.

Ladas EJ, Kelly KM. Milk thistle: is there a role for its use as an adjunct therapy in patients with cancer? J Altern Complement Med. 2003 Jun;9 (3):411-6.

Lansky EP, Newman RA. *Punica granatum* (pomegranate) and its potential for prevention and treatment of inflammation and cancer. J Ethnopharmacol. 2007 Jan 19;109 (2):177-206. Epub 2006 Sep 10.

Lansky EP, Paavilainen HM, Pawlus AD, Newman RA. *Ficus* spp. (fig): ethnobotany and potential as anticancer and anti-inflammatory agents.J Ethnopharmacol. 2008 Sep 26;119 (2):195-213. Epub 2008 Jun 28.

Lee SH, Choi WC, Yoon SW. Impact of standardized Rhus verniciflua stokes extract as complementary therapy on metastatic colorectal cancer: a Korean single-center experience. Integr Cancer Ther. 2009 Jun;8 (2):148-52.

Li J, Jiang Y. Litchi flavonoids: isolation, identification and biological activity. Molecules. 2007 Apr 11;12 (4):745-58.

Li L, Zeng J, Gao Y, He D. Targeting silibinin in the antiproliferative pathway. Expert Opin Investig Drugs. 2010 Feb;19 (2):243-55.

Limem-Ben Amor I, Boubaker J, Ben Sgaier M, Skandrani I, Bhouri W, Neffati A, Kilani S, Bouhlel I, Ghedira K, Chekir-Ghedira L. Phytochemistry and biological activities of *Phlomis* species.J Ethnopharmacol. 2009 Sep 7;125 (2):183-202. Epub 2009 Jun 27.

Lissoni P, Rovelli F, Brivio F, Zago R, Colciago M, Messina G, Mora A, Porro G. A randomized study of chemotherapy versus biochemotherapy with chemotherapy plus *Aloe arborescens* in patients with metastatic cancer. *In vivo*. 2009 Jan-Feb;23 (1):171-5.

Liu R H, Potential synergy of phytochemicals in cancer prevention: Mechanism of action. J. Nutr. 2004, 134, 3479S–3485S.

Li-Weber M. New therapeutic aspects of flavones: the anticancer properties of Scutellaria and its main active constituents Wogonin, Baicalein and Baicalin.Cancer Treat Rev. 2009 Feb;35 (1):57-68.

Lyman GH. Risk factors for cancer. Prim Care. 1992;19:465–79.

Mabberley D. J., The Plant-Book, 3th edition pp. 41, 56-57, 61-62, 143-144, 147, 205, 207-211, 218, 225-226, 231-232, 313-314, 359, 380-381, 424, 433, 445, 460-461, 474-477, 489, 502, 508, 518-519, 533-534,557-558, 598-599, 628, 688-689, 747-748, 750-751, 755-756, 766, 803-804, 852,884-885, 923, 925 Cambridge University Press, (2008).

Mahadevan S, Park Y. Multifaceted therapeutic benefits of *Ginkgo biloba* L.: chemistry, efficacy, safety, and uses. J Food Sci. 2008 Jan;73 (1):R14-9.

Mahmoudi M, Rabe SZT, Ahi A, Emami SA. Evaluation of the cytotoxic activity of different *Artemisia khorassanica* samples on cancer cell lines. Pharmacologyonline 2: 778-786 (2009).

Manju V, Nalini N. Protective role of luteolin in 1,2-dimethylhydrazine induced experimental colon carcinogenesis. Cell Biochem Funct 2007; 25: 189–94

Manthey JA, Grohmann K, Guthrie N. Biological properties of citrus flavonoids pertaining to cancer and inflammation. Curr Med Chem. 2001 Feb;8 (2):135-53.

McClatchey W. From Polynesian healers to health food stores: changing perspectives of *Morinda citrifolia* (Rubiaceae). Integr Cancer Ther. 2002 Jun;1 (2):110-20; discussion 120.

McGovern PE, Christofidou-Solomidou M, Wang W, Dukes F, Davidson T, El-Deiry WS. Anticancer activity of botanical compounds in ancient fermented beverages (review). Int J Oncol. 2010 Jul;37 (1):5-14.

Meghvansi MK, Siddiqui S, Khan MH, Gupta VK, Vairale MG, Gogoi HK, Singh L.Naga chilli: a potential source of capsaicinoids with broad-spectrum ethnopharmacological applications.J Ethnopharmacol. 2010 Oct 28;132 (1):1-14. Epub 2010 Aug 20.

Milner JA. Mechanisms by which garlic and allyl sulfur compounds suppress carcinogen bioactivation. Garlic and carcinogenesis. Adv Exp Med Biol. 2001;492:69-81.

Milner JA. Preclinical perspectives on garlic and cancer.J Nutr. 2006 Mar;136 (3 Suppl):827S-831S.

Molnár J, Engi H, Hohmann J, Molnár P, Deli J, Wesolowska O, Michalak K, Wang Q. Reversal of multidrug resitance by natural substances from plants. Curr Top Med Chem. 2010;10 (17):1757-68.

Montesano R, Hall J. Environmental causes of human cancers. Eur J Cancer. 2001; 37:S67-87.

Mousavi SH, Tavakkol-Afshari J, Brook A, Jafari-Anarkooli I. Role of caspases and Bax protein in saffron-induced apoptosis in MCF-7 cells. Food Chem Toxicol. 2009 Aug;47(8):1909-13. Epub 2009 May 18. PubMed PMID: 19457443.

Moyad MA, Carroll PR. Lifestyle recommendations to prevent prostate cancer, part II: time to redirect our attention? Urol Clin North Am. 2004;31:301-11.

Moyers SB, Kumar NB. Green tea polyphenols and cancer chemoprevention: multiple mechanisms and endpoints for phase II trials. Nutr Rev. 2004 May;62 (5):204-11.

Münchberg U, Anwar A, Mecklenburg S, Jacob C. Polysulfides as biologically active ingredients of garlic.Org Biomol Chem. 2007 May 21;5 (10):1505-18. Epub 2007 Apr 17.

Nagini S. Cancer chemoprevention by garlic and its organosulfur compounds-panacea or promise? Anticancer Agents Med Chem. 2008 Apr;8 (3):313-21.

Nam NH. Combretastatin A-4 analogues as antimitotic antitumor agents. Curr Med Chem. 2003 Sep;10 (17):1697-722.

Neto CC, Amoroso JW, Liberty AM. Anticancer activities of cranberry phytochemicals: an update. Mol Nutr Food Res. 2008 Jun;52 Suppl 1:S18-27.

Owen RW, Haubner R, Würtele G, Hull E, Spiegelhalder B, Bartsch H. Olives and olive oil in cancer prevention. Eur J Cancer Prev. 2004 Aug;13 (4):319-26.

Oyagbemi AA, Saba AB, Azeez OI. Capsaicin: a novel chemopreventive molecule and its underlying molecular mechanisms of action. Indian J Cancer. 2010 Jan-Mar;47 (1):53-8.

Padhye S, Chavan D, Pandey S, Deshpande J, Swamy KV, Sarkar FH. Perspectives on chemopreventive and therapeutic potential of curcumin analogs in medicinal chemistry. Mini Rev Med Chem. 2010 May;10 (5):372-87.

Pandey MM, Rastogi S, Rawat AK. Saussurea costus: botanical, chemical and pharmacological review of an ayurvedic medicinal plant.J Ethnopharmacol. 2007 Apr 4;110 (3):379-90. Epub 2007 Jan 20.

Patel D, Shukla S, Gupta S. Apigenin and cancer chemoprevention: progress, potential and promise (review). Int J Oncol 2007; 30: 233–45

Patra SK, Rizzi F, Silva A, Rugina DO, Bettuzzi S. Molecular targets of (-)-epigallocatechin-3-gallate (EGCG): specificity and interaction with membrane lipid rafts. J Physiol Pharmacol. 2008 Dec;59 Suppl 9:217-35.

Perez AT, Arun B, Tripathy D, Tagliaferri MA, Shaw HS, Kimmick GG, Cohen I, Shtivelman E, Caygill KA, Grady D, Schactman M, Shapiro CL. A phase 1B dose escalation trial of Scutellaria barbata (BZL101) for patients with metastatic breast cancer.Breast Cancer Res Treat. 2010 Feb;120 (1):111-8.

Prakash P, Gupta N. Therapeutic uses of Ocimum sanctum Linn (Tulsi) with a note on eugenol and its pharmacological actions: a short review. Indian J Physiol Pharmacol. 2005 Apr;49 (2):125-31.

Pryme IF, Bardocz S, Pusztai A, Ewen SW. Suppression of growth of tumour cell lines *in vitro* and tumours *in vivo* by mistletoe lectins. Histol Histopathol. 2006 Mar;21 (3):285-99.

Qi LW, Wang CZ, Yuan CS. American ginseng: potential structure-function relationship in cancer chemoprevention. Biochem Pharmacol. 2010 Oct 1;80 (7):947-54. Epub 2010 Jun 25.

Rabe SZT, Mahmoudi M, Ahi A, Emami SA. Antiproliferative effects of extracts from Iranian *Artemisia* species on cancer cell lines. Pharm. Biol. 2011, 1-8, Early Online.

Ramos S. Cancer chemoprevention and chemotherapy: dietary polyphenols and signaling pathways. Mol Nutr Food Res. 2008;52:507–26.

Sadeghi-aliabadi H, Emami A, Sadeghi B and Jafarian A (2009a). *In vitro* cytotoxicity of two subspecies of *Juniperus excelsa* on cancer cells. Iranian Journal of Basic Medical Sciences 11 (4): 250-253.

Sadeghi-aliabadi H, Emami A, Saidi M, Sadeghi B and Jafarian A (2009b). Evaluation of *in vitro* cytotoxic effects of *Juniperus foetidissima* and *Juniperus sabina* extracts against a panel of cancer cells. IJPR 8 (4): 281-286.

Sagar SM. Future directions for research on Silybum marianum for cancer patients. Integr Cancer Ther. 2007 Jun;6 (2):166-73.

Saklani A, Kutty SK. Plant-derived compounds in clinical trials. Drug Discov Today. 2008 Feb;13 (3-4):161-71. Epub 2007 Nov 26.

Saklani A. and K. Kutty S. Plant-derived compounds in clinical trials Drug Discovery Today.Volume 13, Numbers 3/4, 2008

Seki T, Hosono T, Hosono-Fukao T, Inada K, Tanaka R, Ogihara J, Ariga T. Anticancer effects of diallyl trisulfide derived from garlic. Asia Pac J Clin Nutr. 2008;17 Suppl 1:249-52.

Silalahi J. Anticancer and health protective properties of citrus fruit components.Asia Pac J Clin Nutr. 2002;11 (1):79-84.

Singh RP, Agarwal R. A cancer chemopreventive agent silibinin, targets mitogenic and survival signaling in prostate cancer. Mutat Res. 2004 Nov 2;555 (1-2):21-32.

Sirikantaramas S, Asano T, Sudo H, Yamazaki M, Saito K. Camptothecin: therapeutic potential and biotechnology. Curr Pharm Biotechnol. 2007 Aug;8 (4):196-202.

Sok DE, Cui HS, Kim MR. Isolation and bioactivities of furfuran type lignan compounds from edible plants. Recent Pat Food Nutr Agric. 2009 Jan;1 (1):87-95.

Stauder H, Kreuser ED. Mistletoe extracts standardised in terms of mistletoe lectins (ML I) in oncology:current state of clinical research. Onkologie. 2002 Aug;25 (4):374-80.

Suganuma M, Saha A, Fujiki H. New cancer treatment strategy using combination of green tea catechins and anticancer drugs. Cancer Sci. 2011 Feb;102 (2):317-23.

Surh, Y. J., Cancer chemoprevention with dietary phytochemicals. Nat. Rev. Cancer 2003, 3, 768–780.

Syed DN, Afaq F, Mukhtar H. Pomegranate derived products for cancer chemoprevention. Semin Cancer Biol. 2007 Oct;17 (5):377-85. Epub 2007 May 29.

Tamayo C, Diamond S. Review of clinical trials evaluating safety and efficacy of milk thistle (*Silybum marianum* [L.] Gaertn.). Integr Cancer Ther. 2007 Jun;6 (2):146-57.

Tayarani-Najaran Z, Emami SA, Asili J, Mirzaei A, Mousavi SH. Analyzing cytotoxic and apoptogenic properties of *Scutellaria litwinowii* root extract on cancer cell lines. Evid Based Complement Alternat Med. 2011

Tayarani-Najaran Z, Mousavi SH, Asili J, Emami SA. Growth-inhibitory effect of *Scutellaria lindbergii* in human cancer cell lines. Food Chem Toxicol. 2010 Feb;48 (2):599-604. Epub 2009 Nov 22.

Thangapazham RL, Sharma A, Maheshwari RK. Multiple molecular targets in cancer chemoprevention by curcumin. AAPS J. 2006 Jul 7;8 (3):E443-9.

Vahdati-Mashhadian N, Emami SA, Oghazian MB, Vosough R (2009). The cytotoxity evaluation of seven species of *Artemisia* on human tumor cell lines. Pharmacoly online 3: 327-339.

Van Cleemput M, Cattoor K, De Bosscher K, Haegeman G, De Keukeleire D, Heyerick A. Hop (*Humulus lupulus*)-derived bitter acids as multipotent bioactive compounds. J Nat Prod. 2009 Jun;72 (6):1220-30.

Wall, M.E. (1998) Camptothecin and Taxol: discovery to clinic. Med. Res. Rev. 18, 299–314

Wang X, Howell CP, Chen F, Yin J, Jiang Y. Gossypol--a polyphenolic compound from cotton plant. Adv Food Nutr Res. 2009;58:215-63.

Wang YF, Ni ZY, Dong M, Cong B, Shi QW, Gu YC, Kiyota H. Secondary metabolites of plants from the genus Saussurea: chemistry and biological activity. Chem Biodivers. 2010 Nov;7 (11):2623-59.

Wani, M.C. et al., (1971) Plant antitumor agents. VI. The isolation and structure of Taxol, a novel antileukemic and antitumor agent from Taxus brevifolia. J. Am. Chem. Soc. 93, 2325–2327

Waterman E, Lockwood B. Active components and clinical applications of olive oil. Altern Med Rev. 2007 Dec;12 (4):331-42.

Wong CK, Bao YX, Wong EL, Leung PC, Fung KP, Lam CW. Immunomodulatory activities of Yunzhi and Danshen in post-treatment breast cancer patients. Am J Chin Med. 2005;33 (3):381-95.

World health statistics 2008. pp. 1–80, WHO (2008) (http://www.who.int/)

Wu H, Dai Q, Shrubsole MJ, Ness RM, Schlundt D, Smalley WE, Chen H, Li M, Shyr Y, et al., Fruit and vegetable intakes are associated with lower risk of colorectal adenomas. J Nutr. 2009;139:340–4.

Xiang YZ, Shang HC, Gao XM, Zhang BL. A comparison of the ancient use of ginseng in traditional Chinese medicine with modern pharmacological experiments and clinical trials. Phytother Res. 2008 Jul;22 (7):851-8.

Yun TK, Choi SY. Non-organ specific cancer prevention of ginseng: a prospective study in Korea. Int J Epidemiol 1998;27:359-64.

Zhuang SR, Chen SL, Tsai JH, Huang CC, Wu TC, Liu WS, Tseng HC, Lee HS, Huang MC, Shane GT, Yang CH, Shen YC, Yan YY, Wang CK. Effect of citronellol and the Chinese medical herb complex on cellular immunity of cancer patients receiving chemotherapy/radiotherapy.Phytother Res. 2009 Jun;23 (6):785-90.

4

Multimodal Therapies for Upper Gastrointestinal Cancers – Past, Now, and Future

Shouji Shimoyama
Gastrointestinal Unit, Settlement Clinic
Japan

1. Introduction

Gastric and esophageal cancers are one of the most aggressive malignancies worldwide. Complete surgical resection offers the only chance of cure but many cases are presented at advanced stages or recur even after R0 resections. In gastric cancer (GC), 5-year survival rates (SRs) of stages II and III after curative resection range respectively from 30%-49% and 10-20% in Western countries, and respectively 70-80% and 40-50% in Japan and Korea (Fujii et al., 1999; Hundahl et al., 2000; J.P.Kim et al., 1998; Shimada et al., 1999). With regard to esophageal cancer (EC), the 5-year SRs in older series were 14-20% in the United States (Daly et al., 1996; Ries et al., 2007) and ranging from 3 to 11% in European countries, with an average of 10% (Faivre et al., 1998) while they improved to 42% in a recent series (Rice et al., 2009; Ruol A et al., 2009), which is comparable to those (36-46%) after an esophagectomy in Japan (The Japan Esophageal Society). Even in Japan, however, T3 or stage III EC, the most frequently encountered tumor depth or tumor stage, has exhibited respectively lower 5-year SRs of 27-29% and 17-20% after esophagectomy (Ando et al., 2000; The Japan Esophageal Society). Although stage-specific survival rates differ between reports from Western and Asian institutions, the survival decline according to the stage progression suggests that recurrence does occur even for those who undergo curative resection. Furthermore, a more extended (>D2) lymph node dissection (LND) in GC unfortunately fails to improve survival outcomes (Sasako et al., 2008).

Such disappointing treatment results in GC and EC even in Japan -where aggressive LND has been performed- have reminded researchers a plateau effectiveness of, and little likelihood of further improvement by, surgical therapy only. These facts have encouraged physicians to establish more effective multimodal strategies to improve survival, including newly developed regimens incorporating molecular targeting agents as well as to determine candidate molecules or genes that could help establish individualized therapies. These multimodal therapies have mainly consisted of chemotherapy (CTx), radiotherapy (RTx), and chemoradiotherapy (CRTx) administered after curative resection (adjuvant settings), or for recurrent or inoperable diseases (advanced settings), or before surgical resection (neoadjuvant settings). Recently, CRTx has become a focus of research, because of the radiosensitizing properties of some chemotherapeutic agents that could potentiate the anticancer activities of both CTx and RTx (Kleinberg et al., 2007).

Table lists the theoretical advantages and disadvantages of adjuvant and neoadjuvant treatments (Rice et al., 2003). Adjuvant and neoadjuvant treatments require balancing advantages and disadvantages to maximize treatment effects. This chapter focuses on past, current, and potential future directions in the field of multimodal therapies in GC and EC.

	Advantages	Disadvantages
Adjuvant treatment	Prevention of potential recurrence from occult micrometastasis which would become overt postoperatively.	Inability to assess final treatment effects until diseases recur.
	Less consideration for increase in morbidity and mortality that would be sometimes harm in case of neoadjuvant treatment.	Destruction of vasculature that decreases delivery of drugs or oxygen compromising CTx and/or RTx effects.
	Treatment decision based on the full staging information, which can avoid unnecessary treatment in patients who may not otherwise require it, i.e., in patients with earlier stage of the disease than expected.	Preclusion of early commencement of therapy if patient recovery delays due to postoperative complications or reduced functional status. Requirement of longer period to recover from surgery allows tumor cells for further growth.
	Especially in EC, relief of tumor-associated complaints such as dysphagia or alimentary support by surgically-placed feeding tube, allowing for better tolerance of postoperative therapy.	In RTx, removal of target that make definition of radiation field more difficult.
Neoadjuvant treatment	Increased surgical R0 resection rate by downstaging which would otherwise have been regarded as incurable (R1/R2 resection).	Surgical delay due to toxicities that would cancel the potential survival benefit of responders.
	Early elimination of undetectable micrometastasis.	Loss of opportunity to undergo surgery by tumor growth during treatment period in nonresponders. No reliable methods available to predict tumor response that could discriminate responders and non-responders before treatment.
	Intact vasculature that maintains accessibility of drugs to the tumor bed and oxygenation, realizing more effective CTx and/or RTx.	
	Determination of tumor and patient specific chemo(radio)sensitivity that would be applicable to postoperative treatment.	Increased surgical complaints due to preoperative treatment-related toxicities.
	Possibility to administer a more intensive regimen because of the maintained physical and nutritional state. The same regimen would become more toxic if given postoperatively due to surgical-related complication.	Preclusion of effective regimen due to dysphagia or tumor related worse nutritional state, especially in EC.
		Possibility of overtreatment for early stage tumor because treatment is based on clinical stage that is not necessarily accurate.

Table 1. Advantages and disadvantages of adjuvant and neoadjuvant treatment [Rice TW, et al. 2003].

2. General considerations

In consideration of the establishment of multimodal therapies against GC and EC, one should bear in mind the difference in surgical treatment and pathology between Japan and the West. First, the scope of LND influences local tumor control rate and postoperative survival. A wider scope of LND has the theoretical potential to reduce local recurrence rates, which may improve postoperative survival. Second, it is also a fact that a wider scope of LND increases postoperative morbidity and mortality, which may cancel the anticipated survival benefit of LND. This phenomenon is especially observed in the West, providing one reason for the difference in the standard scope of LND between here and Japan. As a result, for GC, the standard scope of LND is a D2 (second-tier node dissection) in Japan but a D1 (first-tier node dissection) in the West, and for EC, the routinely performed node clearance encompasses three fields (cervical, thoracic, and abdominal) or at least any two of the three fields in Japan, while it encompasses a limited area in the West. Since the effect of hospital volume on a perioperative mortality hazard is larger than those on hazards for death at 5 years postoperatively (Bilimoria et al., 2008; Birkmeyer et al., 2002), the perioperative patient control reflects the subsequent overall survival; thus, LND by specialists is now an important issue. Third, a wider scope of LND results in a more accurate nodal staging than a narrower one. Therefore, under conditions of a limited extent of LND, judgement regarding R0 resection is not always accurate, and resections deemed R0 might sometimes be actually equivalent to R1 resection. For example, in a Dutch trial, 38% of GC patients classified as stage II on D1 dissection were reclassified as stage IIIA on D2 dissection (Bunt,1995). This discordance is reflected by the stage migration phenomenon which implies that a narrower scope of LND results in a significant risk of understaging. Therefore, results of clinical trials of multimodal therapies are undoubtedly influenced if they recruit such understaged patients. Fourth, the scope of LND depends on the pathological characteristics of the tumor. With regard to EC, adenocarcinoma is observed at a substantial ratio (43-56%) in the United States (Daly et al., 1996; Trivers et al., 2008), while squamous cell cancer comprises a majority in Japan (The Japan Esophageal Society), the incidences twice those of the United States (90% vs. 38%) (Trivers et al., 2008). Such histological differences reflect tumor location and surgical approach. In Japan, the incidences of middle and lower third thoracic EC were respectively 50% and 25% (The Japan Esophageal Society), whereas those in the United States were respectively 25% and 50% (Daly et al., 1996). Considering that upper thoracic or cervical nodal involvement occurs more frequently in the middle third than lower third thoracic EC, such histological and topographical differences also influence surgical approach and ultimately the scope of LND. In Japan, a right thoracotomy is a main approach while a transhiatal approach is considered in the West (Hulscher et al., 2001). Finally, the different stances in surgical therapy between Japan and the West reflect the different stances of multimodal therapies. Since a wider scope of LND is more effective in local tumor control than a limited one, CTx rather than CRTx has been developed in Japan for the purpose of preventing systemic relapse rather than local recurrence, whereas CRTx rather than CTx has been developed in the West for the purpose of preventing both local and systemic relapse.

3. Gastric cancer

3.1 Adjuvant setting

Many randomized controlled trials (RCTs) have been conducted to assess the advantage of adjuvant CTx on survival compared with surgery alone. However, they have shown mixed results and have been mostly disappointing. The difficulties in making definitive conclusions concerning the significance of adjuvant CTx are accounted for -at least in part- by the small size of the studies and suboptimal CTx regimens. Many trials recruited relatively small numbers of patients -usually less than 200- and were therefore inadequate to detect clinically significant survival differences between the CTx arm and surgery alone arm. In addition, many CTx regimens employed old types of drug with low response rates (RRs) and short durations of response. Therefore, the negative results of most previous clinical trials do not necessarily mean that the adjuvant CTx does not work.

Several meta-analyses of adjuvant trials have been published (Earle & Maroun, 1999; GASTRIC Group, 2010; Hermans et al., 1993; Hu et al., 2002; Janunger et al., 2002; Liu et al., 2008; Mari et al., 2000; Oba et al., 2006; Panzini et al., 2002; Zhao & Fang, 2008) in order to overcome the drawbacks of small patient accrual and to assess any potential benefit by adjuvant therapy that may have been missed in the individual trials. Unfortunately, definitive evidence concerning benefits of adjuvant CTx is lacking, with results ranging from an odds ratio for death of 0.56-0.9 to no benefit. However, the first meta-analysis (Hermans et al., 1993), which failed to demonstrate a clear benefit of adjuvant CTx, was later updated by an inclusion of 318 patients who had been erroneously omitted from the initial analysis, resulting in a reduction of the odds ratio for death to a significant 0.82 (Hermans & Bonenkamp, 1994).

Nevertheless, criticism still persists as to the methodologies applied in these meta-analyses that make this interpretation too complicated. For example, there was a great heterogeneity among individual studies in terms of quality of surgery, adjuvant therapy regimens administered, clinical stage, and intervals between surgery and the commencement of CTx. Accordingly, patient recruitment was not uniform within each meta-analysis. Some meta-analyses included studies of palliative resections and curative resections, or studies of CTx, RTx, and immunotherapy together. The quality of surgery could not be evaluated because the scope of LND was not always clarified. Studies with old generation drug(s) and those with newer generation drug(s) were also included together. In addition, one meta-analysis (Hu et al., 2002) included a previous meta-analysis (Hermans et al., 1993).

The most recent meta-analysis (GASTRIC Group, 2010), which was the first patient-level analysis, was published in the year 2010. It demonstrated both mortality and relapse hazard reduction by 18% each by adjuvant CTx. This trend was also reproduced irrespective of the number of CTx drugs (monochemotherapy and polychemotherapies). Furthermore, a survival improvement of 6% by CTx at 5 years postoperatively was maintained during the ensuing 5 years. These consecutive results of the meta-analyses suggest that the benefit of adjuvant CTx change from 'none or inconclusive or borderline' to 'significant'.

Subset metaanalysis have demonstrated inconsistent results, however. When Asian and non-Asian adjuvant trials were grouped together or analyzed separately, survival benefits were seen only in the non-Asian studies (Earle & Maroun, 1999), or only in the Asian studies (Janunger et al., 2002), or in both (Zhao & Fang, 2008). The extant metaanalyses are therefore difficult to interpret due to significant heterogeneity. Interestingly, in the pivotal Japanese RCT for adjuvant CTx (JCOG9206-1) (Nashimoto et al., 2003), the total recurrence rate at 69 months was almost double in the surgery only arm than in the CTx arm (13.8% vs. 7.1%), indicating a possible role by CTx for the prevention of recurrence. Against these backgrounds, several large RCTs of postoperative or perioperative CTx have been conducted in Japan, the United States, and Europe, and each result has been recently published.

The ACTS-GC (Adjuvant Chemotherapy Trial of TS-1 for Gastric Cancer) trial is so far the largest adjuvant RCT conducted in Japan, in which oral S-1, a new generation of fluoropyrimidine derivative, was administered for 1 year as an adjuvant treatment (Sakuramoto et al., 2007). The survival benefit of S-1 at three years postoperatively has also been confirmed at 5 years (Sasako et al., 2010). The results are consistent with the previous metaanalysis demonstrating the survival advantage of oral fluoropyrimidine containing adjuvant regimen (Oba et al., 2006). Of note in this trial is that most of the recruited patients underwent D2 or a wider scope of LND, and even under such circumstances of qualified surgery, the oral fluoropyrimidine derivative alone was able to render benefits in an adjuvant setting. However, caution is required when these results are applied to clinical use. The subanalysis of the ACTS-GC trial revealed that survival benefit was maintained in stages II and IIIA GC but disappeared in stage IIIB. Such stage specific survival differences suggest that oral fluoropyrimidine alone lacks power to exhibit statistically meaningful survival advantages in more advanced stages.

The phase III intergroup-0116 trial (INT0116) is one of the most important adjuvant trials against adenocarcinoma of the stomach or esophagogastric junction ever conducted in North America (Macdonald et al., 2001). The adjuvant treatment in this study was a CRTx consisting of fluorouracil, leucovorin, and extra-beam radiation delivered to the tumor bed with 2cm beyond the proximal and distal margins of resection as well as to the areas of regional draining lymph nodes. Adjuvant CRTx yielded a significant prolongation of disease free survival (DFS) and overall survival (OS) at 3 years postoperatively (Macdonald et al., 2001). More than six years of median follow-up confirmed no deterioration of survival over time (Macdonald et al., 2004), making this regimen optimal as the standard of care in the United States. However, there has also been some criticism directed towards this study. First, the extent of surgery performed in this study has been a focus of much debate. The trial has been criticized for the surgical undertreatment of patients: 54% and 36% of the patients in the trial respectively underwent a D0 and a D1 LND despite a recommendation of a D2 LND in the trial protocol. Such noncompliance clearly undermined survival and led to a high relapse rate of 64% in the surgery only arm after a median follow-up of 5 years, the results contrasting sharply with those of the JCOG9206-1 trial (Nashimoto et al., 2003). Considering that more than two thirds and 85% of the recruited patients respectively had T3/T4 diseases and were node positive, the survival benefit by CRTx seen in this study seemed to be simply a compensation for the control residual disease left by the inadequately limited surgery (D0 or D1), which could otherwise be resected by a D2 LND. Second, usage of 5FU as a radiosensitizer and chemotherapy of 5FU and leucovorin seemed appropriate at the time when INT-0116 was designed (in the 1980's) and executed (in the 1990's); however, new generation agents with a superior antitumor activity and greater radiosensitizing effect continue to be developed (Rice et al., 2003).

As discussed in the General Considerations section, this context raises another important insight that outcomes of adjuvant therapy undoubtedly depend on the quality of surgery, in particular, on the scope of LND. The incidence of locoregional recurrence after curative resection has been higher in the West (Roviello et al., 2003) (45%) than in Japan (Maehara et al., 2000) (22%), suggesting a benefit from the routine performance of a D2 LND for local tumor control. Such a benefit is guaranteed by the safe performance of a D2 LND in Japan, with a 0-2.2% mortality rate (Fujii et al., 1999; Maruyama et al., 1987; Maruyama et al., 2006; Nashimoto et al., 2003; Sano et al., 2002). Indeed, in the JCOG9206-1 trial, 98% of the patients underwent a D2 or greater LND, with just one (0.8%) postoperative death in the surgery only arm. The number of patients with local recurrence was two (1.6%) in the surgery only arm and none in the adjuvant treatment arm, suggesting a remarkable local control rate by the Japanese style D2 LND. Therefore, convinced of the benefit of a D2 LND, Japanese investigators have always been reluctant to conduct any trial comparing D2 with D1 LND. In contrast, operative mortality remains high within Europe, ranging between 5-16% (Lepage et al., 2010). Under these circumstances, the initial phase III trials conducted in the West demonstrated that a D2 LND provided neither survival improvements nor decreased relapse rates, and that it was even harmful in terms of a 43-46% morbidity and 10-13% mortality (Bonenkamp et al., 1995; Bonenkamp et al., 1999; Cuschieri et al., 1996; Cuschieri A et al., 1999; Hartgrink et al., 2004a; Songun et al., 2010). Such higher D2-associated morbidity and mortality were initially considered to nullify its potential survival benefit by local control; however, a subsequent long-term 15-year follow up of a Dutch trial observed significantly higher local recurrence rates and cancer-related death rates in D1 than in D2 (Songun et al., 2010), leading the authors to conclude that a D2 LND has efficacy for local control and can be recommended for resectable GC, given that a safer, spleen-preserving D2 LND is available. Subsequent studies have supported this procedure-related safety. Several nonrandomized trials have also demonstrated no differences in morbidity and mortality between a D1 and a D2 or wider LND (Bösing et al., 2000; Edwards et al., 2004; Danielson et al., 2007; Zilberstein et al., 2004). The RCTs conducted in the dedicated centers in the West elucidated a safer performance with a D2 or wider LND, with morbidity and hospital mortality being 17-22% and <2%, respectively, if resection of the pancreas and/or spleen was performed for selected patients.

Considering that postoperative CRTx can be a substitution for a D2 LND, adjuvant CRTx constitutes an alternative option for countries where a D1 LND is the primary treatment or at institutions where surgeons are not keen on a D2, whereas its effect is questionable where a D2 dissection is both routine and safe -such as in Japan or in some Western specialized centers (Degiuli et al., 2004a; Degiuli et al., 2004b; Degiuli et al., 2010; Kulig et al., 2007; Sano et al., 2004; C.W.Wu et al., 2004; C.W.Wu et al., 2006). Interestingly, a Korean group (S.Kim et al., 2005) reported the superiority of adjuvant CRTx over surgery alone in gastric cancer patients undergoing a D2 dissection. Since the CRTx protocol in this study was identical to that of INT0116, the results, although observational, suggest that CRTx is promising even for patients undergoing a qualified LND.

Two RCTs assessing the benefits of perioperative chemotherapy have been conducted. The MAGIC trial (Medical Research Council Adjuvant Gastric Infusional Chemotherapy) (Cunningham et al., 2006) was a randomized perioperative CTx trial in United Kingdom for patients with stage II or higher resectable adenocarcinoma of the stomach, esophagogastric junction, or lower esophagus. In this trial, the perioperative CTx consisted of three preoperative and three postoperative cycles of epirubicin, cisplatin, and fluorouracil (ECF). The perioperative CTx significantly improved 5-year DFS and 5-year OS. Another was a French trial (FNCLCC94012-FFCD9703) comparing perioperative cisplatin and 5FU (CF). Again, however, there are several limitations and criticisms regarding these trials. The scope of LND in MAGIC trial was not standardized, with a D1 or a D2 LND being left to the discretion of the surgeons, resulting in only 41% of the patients undergoing a D2 LND. Curative resection rates in the surgery only arm accounted only for 66% (MAGIC trial) or 73% (FFCD trial) of the patients, suggesting that both were not purely adjuvant CTx trials and likely recruited extremely advanced cases. Perioperative CTx may be harsh because of the relatively higher rate (9%) of not completing the three planned cycles of ECF, and of low rates of commencement (55%) and completion (42%) of the postoperative ECF, predominantly due to toxic effects, early disease progression, patient request, and postoperative complications. In addition, the 30-day mortality rate in both arms of the MAGIC trial was approximately 6%, which is relatively higher than those of a D2 (0-5%) (Degiuli et al., 2004a; Degiuli et al., 2004b; Degiuli et al., 2010; Kulig et al., 2007; Nashimoto et al., 2003; Sano et al., 2004; C.W.Wu et al., 2004; C.W.Wu et al., 2006) or wider scope of LND (0.8-2%) (Kulig et al., 2007; Sano et al., 2004) in Japanese and Western specialized institutions. Pathological T1 disease patients comprised 8% of the surgery only arm, suggesting that preoperative staging was not necessarily accurate and such earlier stage patients received unnecessary CTx, which would be more harmful than beneficial. Finally, the continuous infusion of 5FU that requires an infusion pump and long term infusional access may be associated with a risk of catheter-related complications.

Taking these results concerning benefit and harm of LND into account, a D2 surgery is at least equal to an adjuvant CRTx with D0/D1 surgery, and an adjuvant S-1 improve survivals more than a D2 LND alone -at least in Japan. Encouraged by the positive results of INT0116 and MAGIC trials, a more combined multidisciplinary approach has been investigated in a CRITICS trial, in which adjuvant CRTx (investigational arm) after 3 preoperative cycles of ECC (epirubicine, cisplatin, capecitabine) and D1 surgery (clearance of >15 nodes) was compared with 3 adjuvant cycles of ECC (control arm) after the same preoperative ECC and the same quality of surgery (http://www.critics.nl).

3.2 Advanced setting

Evidence of benefits of CTx for patients with advanced or recurrent GC was obtained from the previous RCTs demonstrating a significantly improved survival by CTx as compared with the best supportive care (Glimelius et al., 1994; Murad et al., 1993; Pyrhönen et al., 1995). In Western countries, FAMTX (5FU, adriamycin, methotrexate) then became the standard regimen from the results of the EORTC randomized study, demonstrating the superiority of FAMTX over FAM (5FU, adriamycin, mitomycin C) with regard to median survival time (MST) (42 weeks vs. 29 weeks), RR (41% vs. 9%), and toxicity (Wils et al., 1991). Subsequently, a standard FAMTX regimen was compared with ECF. The RR and MST by ECF (46% and 8.7 months) were both found to be superior to FAMTX (21% and 6.1 months) (Waters et al., 1999). In addition, ECF was less toxic, afforded patients better quality of life, and was more favorable in cost effectiveness as compared with FAMTX (Webb et al., 1997), leading the investigators to propose an ECF regimen as a standard therapy. A recent systematic review revealed that the best survival results are achieved with a three-drug regimen containing 5FU, anthracycline, and cisplatin (Wagner et al., 2006).

In this century, docetaxel, one of the new generation agents, has become available and been recognized as a promising agent, being incorporated in several clinical trials. The non-overlapping toxicity profiles of docetaxel, cisplatin, and 5FU (DCF), as well as synergism among these agents in vitro (Maeda et al., 2004) in a schedule dependent manner or in human GC xenografts (Kodera et al., 2005), warrant this combination to be evaluated in treating GC. In Europe, a three-arm, randomized phase II study was conducted to compare DCF (docetaxel, cisplatin, 5FU), DC (docetaxel, cisplatin), and a standard reference regimen ECF (Roth et al., 2007). The RR and MST of the DCF (37% and 10.4 months) were superior to those of the DC (18% and 11.0 months) and ECF (25% and 8.3 months), leading to the recommendation of DCF as an investigational regimen for further clinical trials. Similarly, in the United States, a randomized phase II trial found that DCF and DC were both active while DCF produced higher RR (43%) than DC (26%) (Ajani et al., 2005b). The DCF was then further positioned as an investigational regimen in a subsequent phase III trial (Van Cutsem et al., 2006), in which DCF was found to be significantly superior to CF with regard to RR (37% vs. 25%, p=0.01) and MST (9.2 months vs. 8.6 months, p=0.02). In addition, DCF was able to maintain patient performance status longer. However, a higher incidence of grade 3/4 hematological toxicities (82% of neutropenia, 65% of leucopenia, and 29% of neutropenic fever) emphasized a need for a vigilant patient selection and careful patient management and monitoring, which might preclude its more widespread acceptance as a new treatment option.

The requirement for a balance between survival gains and experienced toxicities has prompted several modifications of the DCF regimen to improve tolerability. A weekly administration of DCF may yield an improved safety profile without compromising the efficacy. In lung, breast, and prostate cancers, toxicities were less with weekly taxane than with triweekly taxane, while OS did not significantly differ between the two schedules or was even better in weekly taxane (Bria et al., 2006; Engels & Verweij, 2005; Sparano et al., 2008). There are several trials of DCF modifications (C.P. Li, 2010; Lorenzen et al., 2007; Overman et al., 2010; Park et al., 2005; Sato et al., 2010; Tebbutt et al., 2010). Among these investigations, GASTRO-TAX-1 (Lorenzen et al., 2007) proved modified DCF to have a remarkably prolonged MST (17.9 months) and median time to progression (TTP) (9.4 months), with a reduced incidence of grade 3/4 neutropenia (22%) and febrile neutropenia (5%).

On the other hand, in Japan, JCOG conducted a randomized study comparing mitomycin C (MMC) plus tegafur with MMC plus UFT (uracil and tegafur) (UFT-M). Although MSTs were equivalent in both arms (6 months), significantly higher RR (25%) in the UFT-M arm than in the MMC plus tegafur arm (8%) (Kurihara et al., 1991) led the investigators to recommend UFT-M as a candidate regimen for further clinical trials. JCOG then conducted a three-arm RCT comparing UFT-M, CF, and a continuous infusion of 5FU (JCOG9205) (Ohtsu et al., 2003). In this trial, patient recruitment for the UFT-M arm was stopped due to poor survivals with significant toxicities, and the survival curves of the remaining two arms were overlapping. Taking efficacy and toxicity together into account, a continuous infusion of 5FU monotherapy with a MST of 7.1 months remained as a reference arm for further clinical trials.

At the end of the last century, when S-1 became available, JCOG conducted another three-arm RCT comparing the continuous infusion of 5FU monotherapy (reference regimen) with S-1, or irinotecan plus cisplatin (JCOG9912) (Boku et al., 2009). The investigators observed a noninferiority of S-1 to 5FU, and the convenience of oral administration lead to the conclusion that a continuous infusion of 5FU monotherapy could be replaced by S-1 for the first-line CTx.

Encouraged by these results, several randomized trials have been conducted by placing S-1 as a reference arm, and some trials have recently yielded results (Y.H. Kim et al., 2011; Koizumi et al., 2008; Narahara et al., 2011). Taking all these into account, a S-1 plus cisplatin combination (CS) is currently considered as a standard regimen in Japan for the treatment of advanced GC.

Globally, this combination has been investigated in a FLAGS study (First Line Advanced Gastric Cancer Study) (Ajani et al., 2010), in which 1053 patients were randomly assigned to either receive infusional CF or CS in non-Asian patients. Unfortunately, CS failed to prolong MST (8.6 months) as compared with CF (7.9 months). However, significant safety advantages of CS over CF suggested the possibility of the substitution of S-1 for infusional 5FU. The different results between the Japanese SPIRITS trial and Caucasian FLAGS trial are ascribed to the different recommended doses of S-1 between the two studies, presumably due to different metabolic profiles among races. Tegafur, a cytotoxic component of S-1, is converted to 5FU by cytochrome P450 2A6 (CYP2A6). Racial differences for gene polymorphism of CYP2A6 have been identified (Yoshida et al., 2003) (Daigo et al., 2002; M. Nakajima et al., 2006), and the variants are more frequent in Asians than in Caucasians (M. Nakajima et al., 2006). Since such polymorphism accounts for a lower enzymatic activity, Caucasians have a relatively higher enzymatic activity than Asians, leading to a faster conversion from FT to 5FU, more accumulation of 5FU, and consequently less tolerance to S-1. Accordingly, the recommended dose of S-1 in the FLAGS study (50mg/m2/day) was lower than that (80mg/m2/day) for Japanese (Ajani et al., 2005a). Another reason for the different results of the two trials may be the different ratio of patients receiving second-line therapies, which were respectively 74% and 75% in the CS and S-1 arms in the SPIRITS trial (Koizumi W et al., 2008), while they were respectively 30% and 33% in the CS and CF arms in the FLAGS trial (Ajani et al., 2010).

In China, a similar randomized study is now ongoing. In this study, the S-1 dose is the same (80mg/m2/day, twice daily) as that in Japan, but cisplatin is given in four administrations, each being 20mg/m2 (http://www.ClinicalTrial.gov. NCT 01198392).

Although the results of the FLAGS trial were unfortunately negative, an oral administration route is undoubtedly convenient; its advantages include the alleviation of the requirement for control of a central venous catheter implantation, which in turn may improve the patient's quality of life. Against these backgrounds, there have been attempts to replace intravenous chemotherapy agents with the oral chemotherapy. Two-by-two designed RCTs (REAL-2 trial) have evaluated whether capecitabine (oral fluoropyrimidine) could be an alternative to infusional 5FU (Cunningham et al., 2008) and also whether cisplatin could be replaced by the new platinum compound oxaliplatin. In the REAL-2 study, the incorporated agents were epirubicin (E), cisplatin (C), 5FU (F), capecitabine (X), and oxaliplatin (O). Some 1002 patients were randomly assigned to receive either one of triplet therapies such as ECF, EOF, ECX, and EOX. Interestingly, MST by EOX (11.2 months) was longer than that (9.9 months) of a current European standard regimen ECF. Toxicities of capecitabine and 5FU were similar. Cisplatin requires hydration while oxaliplatin does not. As compared with cisplatin, oxaliplatin was associated with lower incidences of grade 3/4 neutropenia, alopecia, renal toxicity, and thromboembolism, but with higher incidences of grade 3/4 diarrhea and neuropathy. These results, together with the results of the recent RCTs (Al-Batran et al., 2008; Y.K. Kang et al., 2009), suggest the feasibility of substituting 5FU with capecitabine, or cisplatin with oxaliplatin. Indeed, the superiority of capecitabine over 5FU has been confirmed by a recent meta-analysis (Okines et al., 2009)

Trends towards oral administration have prompted researchers to investigate whether 5FU can be replaced by oral fluoropyrimidine S-1 in the DCF regimen. Surprisingly, a combination of docetaxel, cisplatin, and S-1 (DCS) yielded remarkable RR (84%) and MST (23 months) (Sato et al., 2010). The optimal doses of docetaxel and/or cisplatin of this triplet therapy have been investigated in several phase I studies (Fushida et al., 2009; Hironaka et al., 2010; Nakayama et al., 2008). No requirement of hydration in oxaliplatin has prompted the substitution of cisplatin with oxaliplatin in the DCS regimen, forming a new triplet docetaxel, oxaliplatin, and S-1. However, it achieved modest MST (12 months) with 38% grade 3/4 neutropenia, despite high RR and CR rates (60% and 7.5%) (Zang et al., 2010). Since these studies are preliminary, the efficacy and safety of DCS should be confirmed by large-scale clinical trials. Finally, a multicenter phase II trial has very recently demonstrated that an S-1 and oxaliplatin combination (SOX) can be a substitution for a CS regimen; this has just been indicated as a standard regimen in Japan or a safer regimen than FP in the West. The SOX regimen yielded remarkable MST (16.5 months), while grade 3/4 neutropenia developed in 22% of the patients (Yamada et al., 2010).

Another important concern lies in the fact that the net survival time cannot necessarily be achieved by a single regimen. As discussed earlier, negative results of the FLAGS trial may be attributable to the relatively small number of patients receiving second-line therapies. One should bear in mind that most of the chemotherapy regimens introduced above could yield a median TTP of less than 7 months, suggesting the urgent need for the establishment of effective second-line regimens. The contribution of a second line treatment on survival has been also confirmed by the combined analysis of two large Japanese randomized trials (JCOG9205 and JCOG9912) (Takashima et al., 2010). Because the number of active drugs against GC is increasing, attempts to establish the best second or third line regimen(s) are important, as has been seen for colorectal cancer as well. Currently, several RCTs have been conducted or are now ongoing to provide one answer for this unresolved issue.

3.3 Neoadjuvant setting

Many RCTs for neoadjuvant CTx (NAC) trials have been performed, but the majority have failed to provide evidence concerning the superiority of NAC as compared with controls (Hartgrink et al., 2004b; Imano et al., 2010; Nio et al., 2004; Schuhmacher et al., 2010; Yonemura et al., 1993; C.W. Zhang et al., 2004). The negative results may be accounted for by the small number of recruited patients -usually less than 200, heterogeneous tumor stage- i.e., some studies recruited earlier T1/T2 tumors, heterogeneity in the scope of the LND or drug administration route, and allowance of additional postoperative adjuvant therapies. Therefore, the NAC value remains controversial because of a lack of well-powered trials, and the results of several meta-analyses are conflicting (H. Li et al., 2010; W. Li et al., 2010; A.W. Wu et al., 2007). Although the most recent two analyses revealed benefits of NAC in terms of OS, resection rate, and tumor down staging without increasing perioperative mortality (H. Li et al., 2010; W. Li et al., 2010), the effect of NAC alone on OS remains questionable since individual pure NAC trials, i.e., comparison between surgery alone and NAC without postoperative CTx, failed to demonstrate positive effects on survival (W. Li et al., 2010). Similarly, surgery plus postoperative CTx with or without NAC provided similar survival results (Nio et al., 2004).

As discussed in the General Considerations section, the selection of patients who receive the most benefit from NAC is an important concern (Table). The benefit of NAC was observed only in more advanced (T3/T4) cancers but not in earlier (T1/T2) cancers (W. Li et al., 2010), suggesting that any potential survival benefit may be confined to those patients at greatest risk of relapse (T3/T4). Whether early stage GC received the same benefit of NAC remains unclear since serosa-negative gastric cancer in Japan exhibited 83% DFS and 86% OS by a D2 LND without adjuvant CTx (JCOG9206-1) (Nashimoto et al., 2003). Similar favorable survival results by qualified surgery in earlier stage GC were also reported from the West (Roukos et al., 2001; Siewert et al., 1998), suggesting that patients with a low risk of recurrence can be cured with adequate surgery alone (Roukos, 2004). The benefit of NAC is also influenced by the quality of surgery. As discussed in the MAGIC trial, positive effects of NAC, if present when the combined surgery is a <D2 LND, can be attributable to a mere substitution for a LND rather than the effects of the NAC itself. When determining the NAC regimen, one providing the highest likelihood of tumor shrinkage is theoretically the best regimen for NAC because subsequent surgery can extirpate the residual disease of the NAC. In this sense, several NAC trials using CS, which provides currently the highest RR (74%) (Koizumi et al., 2003), are ongoing in Japan. First, JCOG0501 is a RCT comparing surgery alone with neoadjuvant CS for type 4 or large type 3 GC (http://www.ClinicalTrial.gov. NCT00252161). Second, JCOG0405 is a phase II study investigating the efficacy of neoadjuvant CS for GC with bulky second-tier nodes or positive paraaortic nodes (Kawashima et al., 2008). The third study is a comparison between surgery alone and neoadjuvant CS, both containing adjuvant S-1 for stage III GC (http://www.ClinicalTrial.gov. NCT00182611).

4. Esophageal cancer

4.1 Adjuvant setting
In the West, a number of RCTs have been conducted to investigate the efficacy of adjuvant CTx or adjuvant RTx. A subsequent meta-analysis, however, failed to find any survival benefit at three years by adjuvant CTx or at one year by adjuvant RTx (Malthaner et al., 2004). This conclusion concerning the efficacy of adjuvant CTx was, however, drawn from the pooled data of only 2 studies. So far, there have been no RCTs evaluating adjuvant CRTx versus surgery alone (Malthaner et al., 2004); however, several phase II trials have demonstrated that adjuvant CRTx appeared to prolong survival (Bédard et al., 2001; Rice et al., 2003).
In Japan, an earlier RCT of adjuvant CTx consisting of cisplatin plus vindesine conducted in the 1980s failed to exhibit a survival benefit over surgery alone (JCOG8806) (Ando et al., 1997). JCOG then conducted a RCT (JCOG9204) comparing adjuvant CF with surgery alone (Ando et al., 2003). Although 5-year SR did not differ between the two arms (p=0.13), adjuvant CF was able to yield significantly improved 5-year DFS (p=0.04), which was more evident in node positive patients. In Japan, no adequate RCTs have been conducted to assess adjuvant RTx or adjuvant CRTx as compared with surgery alone.

4.2 Neoadjuvant setting
Multimodal therapies as a neoadjuvant setting have been developed mostly in the West, but their efficacy is conflicting. The significance of survival prolongation by NAC has changed from inconclusive in earlier metaanalyses (mortality hazard=0.88, 95% CI=0.75-1.04) (Malthaner et al., 2004; Malthaner et al., 2006) to just reaching positive (mortality hazard=0.90, 95% CI=0.81-1.00, p=0.05) (Gebski et al., 2007). The significance was more evident in adenocarcinomas by subgroup analyses by histology (mortality hazard=0.78, CI=0.64-0.95, p=0.014) (Gebski et al., 2007). Fortunately, treatment morbidity and mortality did not differ between NAC and surgery alone (Malthaner et al., 2006; Urschel et al., 2002). However, the positive NAC effects on survival (Gebski et al., 2007) seem to be influenced by one MRC study (Medical Research Council Oesophageal Cancer Working Group 2002) with

the largest sample size (n=802), while most of the included RCTs in this meta-analysis in which the number of recruited patients was less than 100 showed no or marginal benefit for NAC. Although the survival benefit of the MRC study has been recently confirmed by a long-term follow-up study (Allum et al., 2009), the interpretation of this study requires caution, because the 5-year SR of the surgery only arm was only 17% despite half of the recruited EC being T3 or less (Medical Research Council Oesophageal Cancer Working Group 2002). This low SR contrasts with that (52%) of the surgery only arm in the JCOG9204 study, in which 65% and 55% of patients had T3/T4 and stage III/IV diseases, respectively. Conceivably, the advantage of neoadjuvant treatment is more likely to be demonstrated when SR in the control (surgery only) arm is lower. In addition, the survival benefit initially observed in adenocarcinoma in the MRC study disappeared in the later analysis (Allum et al., 2009). Finally, although NAC could enhance the chance of R0 resection, the pattern of the first recurrence was similar between the neoadjuvant CTx arm and surgery only arm (Allum et al., 2009), suggesting that NAC showed no clear trend toward fewer patients with distant metastasis as the first site of metastasis. These characteristics were also confirmed in the second largest study (RTOG8911) (Kelsen et al., 1998).

There are several systematic overviews concerning neoadjuvant RTx. These studies have consistently failed to reveal any improvement of survival by neoadjuvant RTx in patients with potentially resectable EC (Arnott et al., 2005; Ask et al., 2003; Malthaner et al., 2004).

In contrast, there are increasing expectations for neoadjuvant CRTx which are also supported by a recent RCT showing that neoadjuvant CRTx resulted in a significantly higher pathological CR rate compared with neoadjuvant CTx (Stahl et al., 2009). This could translate into a marginally significant (p=0.07) improvement in 3-year SR from 28% in neoadjuvant CTx to 47% in neoadjuvant CRTx in patients with locally advanced adenocarcinomas of the esophagogastric junction. Although some inconsistencies do exist (Luu et al., 2008), several neoadjuvant randomized CRTx trials have been conducted in the West and elucidated the rates of downstaging (Fiorica et al., 2004), R0 resection (Urschel & Vasan, 2003), and 3-year survival (Fiorica et al., 2004; Urschel & Vasan, 2003) in favor of neoadjuvant CRTx. Such survival benefits in favor of neoadjuvant CRTx were observed in both adenocarcinoma and squamous cell carcinoma (Gebski et al., 2007).

In Japan, the results of JCOG9204 have led to the subsequent RCT (JCOG9907) to determine which timing of the CTx administration is optimal, preoperatively or postoperatively. Preoperative CF was superior to postoperative CF both in progression free survival (PFS) (p=0.044) and OS (p=0.014), suggesting that neoadjuvant CF is superior to adjuvant CF or surgery alone. Whether the novel active regimen such as DCF or weekly DCF in GC can be extrapolated to EC has been investigated in a phase I/II trial (JCOG0807).

Comparing Japanese trials with Western ones, one should notice the dramatic difference in terms of postoperative mortality and survival outcomes. In Japan, surgery with at least 2-field LND yielded >50% 5-year SR with extremely low mortality, while Western studies demonstrated increased mortality (>5%) with lower 5-year SR. In addition, neoadjuvant CRTx resulted in increased postoperative in-hospital mortality than surgery alone (Fiorica et al., 2004), due to the three most frequent adverse events of respiratory complications, heart failure, and anastomotic leakage (Fiorica et al., 2004). As discussed in the General Considerations section, 3-field LND realizes local control, so that neoadjuvant CTx can afford a most impressive survival advantage and be regarded as a new standard regimen in stage II/III squamous cell carcinoma in Japan.

4.3 Definitive CRTx for resectable EC

CRTx only (definitive CRTx) undoubtedly represents an alternative treatment for patients with EC considered unsuitable for surgery on the basis of comorbidity, poor performance status, and locoregional diseases too extensive for curative resection. For respectable EC, although esophagectomy has still been designated as -at least a part of- a pivotal treatment modality, it is indeed a complex, highly invasive procedure. Operative morbidity and mortality undoubtedly depend on hospital volume; however, reports on this topic from the West, some of which were from high volume centers, documented a near 50% morbidity and 10% mortality (Bailey et al., 2003; Birkmeyer et al., 2002; Jamieson et al., 2004). Since CRTx does have a significant downstaging effect but increases postoperative mortality when combined with surgery, there is growing enthusiasm for the definitive CRTx to treat potentially resectable EC. The choice of CRTx as a definitive treatment option is based on the RTOG 8501 trial, which was instrumental in defining the superiority of definitive CRTx with a 50Gy radiation dose over definitive 64Gy RTx alone (Herskovic et al., 1992). A subsequent metaanalysis has confirmed its promise (Wong & Malthaner, 2006).

Two large RCTs examined whether surgery was necessary after CRTx. A German group demonstrated similar 2-year SR in the neoadjuvant CRTx to a total dose of 40Gy followed by surgery (40%), and in the definitive CRTx with at least 65Gy (35%) in locally advanced squamous cell cancer (Stahl et al., 2005). A subsequent French trial (FFCD9102) (Bedenne et al., 2007; Bonnetain et al., 2006) also confirmed no benefit for additional surgery after CRTx to the responding patients with locally advanced squamous cell cancer. In addition, a nonrandomized comparison revealed the same impact on survival between definitive CRTx and surgery only (without adjuvant treatment) (Hironaka et al., 2003). A single arm phase II study in Japan (JCOG9906) (K. Kato et al., 2010) demonstrated that definitive CRTx in stage II/III esophageal squamous cell cancer could yield a complete response rate of 62%, with 3-year and 5-year SR being 45% and 37%, respectively, comparable to those for esophagectomy (33-47% and 20-52%, respectively) (The Japan Esophageal Society). However, these findings are still inferior to those of the neoadjuvant CF arm in the JCOG 9907 trial. Accordingly, definitive CRTx is not regarded as a standard treatment for stage II/III esophageal squamous cell cancer in Japan.

Nevertheless, these encouraging reports have led to the further activation of several studies to assess the efficacy of definitive CRTx for patients with earlier stage squamous cell cancer. JCOG9708 trial (H. Kato et al., 2009) elucidated 2-year and 4-year SRs of 93% and 81%, respectively, which were comparable to those of the stage I SCC undergoing esophagectomy (The Japan Esophageal Society). Other investigators also reported a high complete response rate (88%) and 3-year SR (79%) in patients with stage I SCC by definitive CRTx (Minashi et al., 2006). However, definitive CRTx is accompanied by several problems.

First, and unfortunately, crude locoregional control rates remain poor, with a respective 23-65% and 13-67% of patients having persistent disease or relapse at the primary site (Coia et al., 2000; Cooper et al., 1999; Minsky et al., 2002; Murakami et al., 1998; Stahl et al., 2005; K.S. Wilson & J.T. Lim, 2000). Tumor recurrence among patients whose treatment results deemed CR is a problem with definitive CRTx because no perfect diagnostic methods currently exist for the evaluation of CR. In the JCOG 9708 trial, although the complete response rate was high (88%), half of the total patients relapsed. In another definitive CRTx trial (Minashi et al., 2006), locoregional diseases were discovered later in 14 (39%) of 36 complete response patients. Although surgery is not intended as part of the definitive CRTx, salvage surgery that could offer the only chance of cure for patients with recurrent or residual diseases after definitive CRTx should be considered. In addition, definitive CRTx-related local complications such as esophageal stenosis and perforation are also indications for salvage surgery. However, salvage surgery is a highly invasive and complex treatment leading to increased morbidity (50-79%) and in-hospital mortality (7-22%) as compared with those after neoadjuvant CRTx, due to the adverse events of predominantly respiratory complications and anastomotic leakage (Chao et al., 2009; Nakamura et al., 2004; M. Nishimura et al., 2007; Oki et al., 2007; Smithers et al., 2007; Swisher et al., 2002; Tachimori et al., 2009; Tomimaru et al., 2006). These hospital mortality rates are obviously higher than those for esophagectomy in Japan reported from specialized centers (2%) (Tachimori et al., 2009) or the nationwide registry (5%) (The Japan Esophageal Society). Second, definitive CRTx for resectable EC has the merit of preserving the esophagus, though it may increase late toxicity such as pericardial or pleural effusion (Ishikura et al., 2003; Kumekawa et al., 2006). Pericardial and pleural effusion developed in nearly 20% of complete response patients, leading to 10-12% of treatment-related deaths (Ishikura et al., 2003; Kumekawa et al., 2006). Even in the earlier stage squamous cell cancer, definitive CRTx-related mortality was observed in 8% of complete response patients (Minashi et al., 2006). These facts suggest that late toxicities are often progressive in severity and may compromise the long term health-related quality of life of a cancer survivor, leading to nullifying the anticipated treatment benefit from therapy. Since conventional toxicity reporting tends to present the more intensive treatments as less toxic than they really are (Trotti et al., 2007), one should bear in mind that the actual toxicities are likely to be underestimated.

These complications are accounted for by the radiation *per se* that renders risks of pulmonary complications, partly due to the fibrogenic response pathway (Bentzen, 2006), and the radiation induced injury in the thoracic cavity that makes surgical procedures technically more difficult and subsequently increases bleeding. In addition, the irradiated stomach, esophagus, and trachea become fragile with the impaired blood supply that eventually causes anastomotic leakage or conduit necrosis. The incidences of morbidity after salvage surgery were associated with radiation doses rather than clinical factors (Wang et al., 2006), suggesting that a dosimetric aspect should be taken into account in planning a definitive CRTx. On this basis, several attempts have been made to reduce the incidences of postoperative morbidity and mortality of salvage surgery. RTOG94-05/INT0123 elucidated the possibility of total radiation volume reduction (50.4Gy), which was equally effective as compared with higher doses (64.8Gy) (Minsky et al., 2002). A novel radiation technique has been developed to ensure an increased volume of lung unexposed to radiation to deliver large and uniform doses to the tumor while sparing nearby normal tissues (X. Zhang et al., 2008). In Japan, based on the phase I study results (T.E. Nakajima et al., 2009), a phase II study of definitive CRTx with a radiation dose of 50.4Gy for stage II/III esophageal squamous cell cancer is ongoing (JCOG0909). In planning a definitive CRTx, therefore, a higher radiation dose is not recommended because it does not improve survival but would presumably increase the risks of salvage surgery if needed.

Given the highly invasive and formidable procedures of salvage surgery, patient selection of those who would receive the most benefit or who would be unfit for surgery is a major concern in the clinical field. Several factors have been proposed for patient selection for salvage surgery. First, there is some evidence that patients with recurrence after CRTx had a significantly better survival after salvage surgery than those with persistent disease (Swisher et al., 2002). Salvage surgery could be avoided in complete response patients, but the diagnosis of complete response by imaging is not always reliable and is possible merely by resected specimen. Indeed, 10-13% of patients undergoing salvage surgery were proved to have pathologically complete response (Murakami et al., 1998; M Nishimura et al., 2007; Tachimori et al., 2009). Unfortunately, positron emission tomography using 2-[fluorine-18]-fluoro-2-deoxy-D-glucose (FDG-PET) (Klaeser et al., 2009) or its combination with other imaging modalities such as computed tomography and/or endoscopic ultrasonography (Swisher et al., 2004) failed to distinguish between patients with >10% viable cells and those with <10% viable cells, resulting in a false negative rate of 16-31% by each modality (Swisher et al., 2004). In this study, the accuracy rates decreased dramatically when an attempt was made to distinguish microscopic residual disease (1% to 10% viable cell) from the "true" pathological complete response (0% viable cells), implying that these modalities have limited value for response assessment for patients receiving preoperative treatment. Consequently, patients whose tumor response is deemed complete response after CRTx could have residual diseases and not be ascribed a reason to preclude further additional treatment. To solve these drawbacks, recent research has focused on the gene expression that can predict CRTx response (Eschrich et al., 2009; He et al., 2009; Maher et al., 2009). Second, multivariate analysis revealed that the most significant factor associated with long-term survival was a R0 resection (Chao et al., 2009; Tomimaru et al., 2006). No patients left with gross or microscopic residual tumors after salvage surgery (R1/R2 resections) survived more than 24 months in any series (Chao et al., 2009; Nakamura et al., 2004; Oki et al., 2007; Swisher et al., 2002; Tachimori et al., 2009; Tomimaru et al., 2006). However, the R1/R2 resection rate has been substantially high, ranging from 15-50% (Chao et al., 2009; Nakamura et al., 2004; Oki et al., 2007; Swisher et al., 2002; Tachimori et al., 2009; Tomimaru et al., 2006), and the resection status cannot be confidently predicted before surgery or even during surgery because of the indistinct planes between tumor and fibrotic masses within the irradiated mediastinum. Therefore, FDG-PET or other imaging modalities are used to select patients who are absolutely unfit for salvage surgery. There is an urgent need for the development of more reliable, accurate diagnostic tools for the assessment of response and resection status prediction.

5. Molecular targeting therapy

Despite the many challenges for establishment of more active multimodal therapy regimens, the mean average survival benefit remains only slight in GC and EC. The MST remains consistently around or less than 12 months in metastatic GC and EC (Ishida et al., 2004; Koizumi et al., 2008; Y. Nishimura et al., 2002; Ohtsu et al., 1999), underscoring a need for more active new agents and regimens. Against these backgrounds, a new generation of therapies designed to target epidermal growth factor receptor (EGFR) and subsequent cellular responses, or angiogenic processes, which both involve and promote tumor growth and survival, have been very recently introduced.

There are several approaches to target EGFR or angiogenic processes. First is monoclonal antibodies against EGFR, including cetuximab (a chimeric monoclonal immunoglobulin G1 antibody), panitumumab (a fully human monoclonal immunoglobulin G2 antibody), and trastuzumab (a monoclonal antibody against human epidermal growth factor receptor-2 (HER2)). Second is an inhibition of the tyrosine kinase (TK) domain and subsequent signal cascade; the molecules which play the role include gefitinib, erlotinib (both are inhibitors of EGFR-TK), lapatinib (a dual inhibitor of HER2-TK and EGFR-TK), sunitinib (inhibitor of TK of various kinds of proteins), and everolimus (RAD001) (inhibitor of mammalian target of rapamycin). Third is an inhibitor of tumor vascularization to anticipate the prevention of eventual tumor invasion and metastasis such as bevacizumab, a monoclonal antibody developed to target vascular endothelial growth factor (VEGF). There are several planned or ongoing RCTs incorporating molecular targeting therapies, and some trials have provided encouraging results.

5.1 Anti-EGFR antibody

A positive HER2 protein or amplified HER2 gene was observed in approximately 20% of GC patients (Jørgensen, 2010). An efficacy of trastuzumab for GC has been very recently demonstrated by a global RCT (ToGA trial; NCT01041404) which has revealed a significantly (p<0.005) prolonged MST (13.8 months) and RR (47%) by adding trastuzumab to 5FU (or capecitabine) and cisplatin as compared with those (11.1 months and 35%) without trastuzumab (Bang et al., 2010). However, it should be noted that the RR by adding trastuzumab to CTx was at best 50% even among the HER2 positive GC patients. Furthermore, the improvement of MST (13.8 months) was -although promising- only marginal as compared with those of a CS in SPIRITS trial (Koizumi et al., 2008). Furthermore, subanalysis by region revealing the efficacy of adding trastuzumab was observed in Europe and Central/South America but not in Asia. Considering that second-line treatment was performed more in Asia than in Europe or Central/South America, the power of second-line therapy in the control (without trastuzumab) arm may bring the treatment results of the two arms closer, leading to non-significant results in Asia.

5.2 Anti-VEGF antibody

The AVAGAST trial (NCT00548548) is the first RCT investigating the efficacy of bevacizumab, in which GC patients were randomized to 5-fluorouracil (or capecitabine) and cisplatin with or without bevacizumab (Y. Kang et al., 2010). Adding bevacizumab achieved a longer PFS (6.7 months vs. 5.3 months) and higher overall RR (38% vs. 30%); however, it failed to produce significant MST prolongation (12.1 months vs. 10.1 months). Several explanations are possible for these negative results. The results appeared to differ among subgroups according to geographic region. As was seen in the ToGA trial, adding bevacizumab proved to be effective in the pan-American region and in Europe but not in Asia, reflecting the role of a second-line treatment (van Cutsem et al., 2010). Alternatively, a potential disadvantage of the AVAGAST trial is a lack of a specific target that would allow for the optimal patient selection that was possible in the ToGA trial.

6. Future perspectives

While many regimens incorporating multimodal therapies have been investigated, it is also true that there is a great variability in tumor response and patient survival among regimens. In addition, even among patients receiving the same regimen, a given regimen may prove too active or too toxic for an individual. Unfortunately, however, it is difficult to predict perfectly the efficacy and toxicity prior to therapy. Therefore, there is a pressing need to explore the molecules and genes that could help explain the interindividual differences in drug response and toxic events. Such a discovery and validation of predictive biomarkers could allow us to develop a model for selecting the optimal therapy on an individual basis and reduce morbidity and reduce health care costs by avoiding potentially unnecessary or futile treatment, ultimately allowing treatment to be individualized (Shimoyama, 2009). One example is a predictive role of a biomarker in the usage of anti-EGFR therapy. Since mutant K-Ras or mutant B-Raf causes cells to escape from adequately controlled cell proliferation and consequently confers resistance to anti-EGFR therapies, K-Ras (Lièvre et al., 2008) or B-Raf (Tol et al., 2009) is considered a negative predictor for the efficacy of anti-EGFR therapy such as cetuximab and panitumumab in colorectal cancer (Allegra et al., 2009; Amado et al., 2008; Jiang et al., 2009). In contrast, incidences of K-Ras mutation were 3-21% in GC (Hongyo et al., 1995; I.J. Kim et al., 2003; Lee et al., 2003; Yoo et al., 2002; W. Zhao et al., 2004) and 0-9% in EC (Janmaat et al., 2006; Lorenzen et al., 2009), both relatively low as compared with those of colorectal cancer (Andreyev et al., 1998). In addition, the predictive value of the K-Ras mutation concerning the efficacy of anti-EGFR therapy has not been clearly established in esophagogastric cancer (Park et al., 2010). Furthermore, incidences of B-Raf mutation in GC were also low (2.2-3%). Therefore, whether mutations of K-Ras or B-Raf as negative predictors seen in colorectal cancer can be extrapolated into gastric and esophageal cancers requires further study. Actually, current phase III trials of cetuximab or panitumumab in GC and EC allow the inclusion of patients irrespective of K-Ras mutation status or EGFR immunohistochemical positivity. In addition, since racial difference does exist in some drug metabolizing enzymes (Shimoyama, 2010), the usefulness of predictive biomarkers may differ between Western and Eastern hemispheres as well as between tumor types.

Another perspective is the incorporating of molecular targeting therapy or other agents into conventional therapy. As discussed in the INT0116 trial, new generation agents with radiosensitizing effects should be continuously incorporated into future clinical trials. Accordingly, several promising results have been reported by the use of new generation agents in combination with molecular targeting therapy, or with radiation, or both (Gaast et al., 2010; Knox et al., 2010; Pinto et al., 2007; Safran et al., 2008; Spigel et al., 2010; Syrigos et al., 2008). Furthermore, non-cytotoxic agents such as statins are theoretical candidates for overcoming current problems of molecular targeting therapy (Shimoyama, 2011).

It is impossible to conduct RCTs for exhaustive drug combinations. There must be continuing efforts to obtain knowledge on specific drug interactions that could bypass clinical trials from one administration schedule to another or from one tumor type to another. This stance may most efficiently facilitate the establishment of the best multimodal therapies.

7. Conclusion

In GC, recent RCTs have elucidated the promising efficacy of multimodal therapies in an adjuvant and advanced settings, where S-1 plays a pivotal role in these settings. This is in agreement with the recent stance in which oral administration takes advantage over the intravenous administration. In EC, CRTx in neoadjuvant or definitive setting has gained the most intensive research topic; however, the latter setting is inevitably associated with highly morbid salvage surgery. Furthermore, researches in novel targeted therapies against growth signal transduction cascade have just begun and their efficacy has been anticipated.

For the treatment of GC and EC, we should say "good-by" for the surgery only treatment era while the "multimodal treatment era" is welcomed. It is hugely encouraged to consider multimodal therapies on the adjuvant, neoadjuvant, and advanced settings, as well as by the usage of conventional treatment (CTx, RTx, and CRTx) and targeted therapies, alone or in combination. Recent attempts have continuously clarified the molecular profiles or genetic events to stratify patients who receive the best benefit, which realizes maximization of the treatment effects instead of "one-regimen-fits-all" stance.

8. References

Ajani, J.A., Faust, J., Ikeda, K., Yao, J.C., Anbe, H., Carr, K.L., Houghton, M., & Urrea, P. (2005a). Phase I pharmacokinetic study of S-1 plus cisplatin in patients with advanced gastric carcinoma. *J Clin Oncol*. Vol.23, No.28, pp6957-6965.

Ajani, J.A., Fodor, M.B., Tjulandin, S.A., Moiseyenko, V.M., Chao, Y., Cabral Filho, S., Majlis, A., Assadourian, S., & Van Cutsem, E. (2005b). Phase II multi-institutional randomized trial of docetaxel plus cisplatin with or without fluorouracil in patients with untreated, advanced gastric, or gastroesophageal adenocarcinoma. *J Clin Oncol*. Vol.23, No.24, pp5660-5667.

Ajani, J.A., Rodriguez, W., Bodoky, G., Moiseyenko, V., Lichinitser, M., Gorbunova, V., Vynnychenko, I., Garin, A., Lang, I., & Falcon, S. (2010). Multicenter phase III comparison of cisplatin/S-1 with cisplatin/infusional fluorouracil in advanced gastric or gastroesophageal adenocarcinoma study: the FLAGS trial. *J Clin Oncol*. Vol.28, No.9, pp1547-1553.

Al-Batran, S.E., Hartmann, J.T., Probst, S., Schmalenberg, H., Hollerbach, S., Hofheinz, R., Rethwisch, V., Seipelt, G., Homann, N., Wilhelm, G., Schuch, G., Stoehlmacher, J., Derigs, H.G., Hegewisch-Becker, S., Grossmann, J., Pauligk, C., Atmaca, A., Bokemeyer, C., Knuth, A., & Jäger, E.; Arbeitsgemeinschaft Internistische Onkologie. (2008). Phase III trial in metastatic gastroesophageal adenocarcinoma with fluorouracil, leucovorin plus either oxaliplatin or cisplatin: a study of the Arbeitsgemeinschaft Internistische Onkologie. *J Clin Oncol*. Vol.26, No.9, pp1435-1442.

Allegra, C.J., Jessup, J.M., Somerfield, M.R., Hamilton, S.R., Hammond, E.H., Hayes, D.F., McAllister, P.K., Morton, R.F., & Schilsky, R.L. (2009). American Society of Clinical Oncology provisional clinical opinion: testing for KRAS gene mutations in patients with metastatic colorectal carcinoma to predict response to anti-epidermal growth factor receptor monoclonal antibody therapy. *J Clin Oncol*. Vol.27, No.12, pp2091-2096

Allum, W.H., Stenning, S.P., Bancewicz, J., Clark, P.I., & Langley, R.E. (2009). Long-term results of a randomized trial of surgery with or without preoperative chemotherapy in esophageal cancer. *J Clin Oncol*. Vol. 27, No.30, pp5062-5067.

Amado, R.G., Wolf, M., Peeters, M., Van Cutsem, E., Siena, S., Freeman, D.J., Juan, T., Sikorski ,R., Suggs, S., Radinsky, R., Patterson, S.D., & Chang, D.D. (2008). Wild-type KRAS is required for panitumumab efficacy in patients with metastatic colorectal cancer. *J Clin Oncol*. Vol.26, No.10, pp1626-1634.

Ando, N., Iizuka, T., Kakegawa, T., Isono, K., Watanabe, H., Ide, H., Tanaka, O., Shinoda, M., Takiyama, W., Arimori, M., Ishida, K., & Tsugane, S. (1997). A randomized trial of surgery with and without chemotherapy for localized squamous carcinoma of the thoracic esophagus: the Japan Clinical Oncology Group Study. *J Thorac Cardiovasc Surg*. Vol.114, No.2, pp205-209.

Ando, N., Ozawa, S., Kitagawa, Y., Shinozawa, Y., & Kitajima, M. (2000). Improvement in the results of surgical treatment of advanced squamous esophageal carcinoma during 15 consecutive years. *Ann Surg*. Vol.232, No.2, pp225-232.

Ando, N., Iizuka, T., Ide, H., Ishida, K., Shinoda, M., Nishimaki, T., Takiyama, W., Watanabe, H., Isono, K., Aoyama, N., Makuuchi, H., Tanaka, O., Yamana, H., Ikeuchi, S., Kabuto, T., Nagai, K., Shimada, Y., Kinjo, Y., & Fukuda, H.; Japan Clinical Oncology Group. (2003). Surgery plus chemotherapy compared with surgery alone for localized squamous cell carcinoma of the thoracic esophagus: a Japan Clinical Oncology Group Study--JCOG9204. *J Clin Oncol*. Vol.21, No.24, pp4592-4596.

Andreyev, H.J., Norman, A.R., Cunningham, D., Oates, J.R., & Clarke, P.A. (1998). Kirsten ras mutations in patients with colorectal cancer: the multicenter "RASCAL" study. *J Natl Cancer Inst*. Vol.90, No.9, pp675-684.

Arnott, S.J., Duncan, W., Gignoux, M., Hansen, H.S., Launois, B., Nygaard, K., Parmar, M.K., Rousell, A., Spilopoulos, G., Stewart, G., Tierney, J.F., Wang, M., & Rhugang, Z.; Oeosphageal Cancer Collaborative Group. (2005). Preoperative radiotherapy for esophageal carcinoma. Cochrane Database Syst Rev. Vol.19, No4, CD001799.

Ask, A., Albertsson, M., Järhult, J., & Cavallin-Ståhl, E. (2003). A systematic overview of radiation therapy effects in oesophageal cancer. *Acta Oncol*. Vol.42, No.5-6, pp462-475.

Bailey, S.H., Bull, D.A., Harpole, D.H., Rentz, J.J., Neumayer, L.A., Pappas, T.N., Daley, J., Henderson, W.G., Krasnicka, B., & Khuri, S.F. (2003). Outcomes after esophagectomy: a ten-year prospective cohort. *Ann Thorac Surg*. Vol.75, No.1, pp217-222.

Bang, Y.J., Van Cutsem, E., Feyereislova, A., Chung, H.C., Shen, L., Sawaki, A., Lordick, F., Ohtsu, A., Omuro, Y., Satoh, T., Aprile, G., Kulikov ,E., Hill, J., Lehle, M., Rüschoff, J., & Kang, Y.K.; ToGA Trial Investigators. (2010). Trastuzumab in combination with chemotherapy versus chemotherapy alone for treatment of HER2-positive advanced gastric or gastro-oesophageal junction cancer (ToGA): a phase 3, open-label, randomised controlled trial. *Lancet*. Vol.376, No.9742, pp687-697.

Bédard, E.L., Inculet, R.I., Malthaner, R.A., Brecevic, E., Vincent, M., & Dar, R. (2001). The role of surgery and postoperative chemoradiation therapy in patients with lymph node positive esophageal carcinoma. *Cancer*. Vol.91, No.12, pp2423-2430.

Bedenne, L., Michel, P., Bouché, O., Milan, C., Mariette, C., Conroy, T., Pezet, D., Roullet, B., Seitz, J.F., Herr, J.P., Paillot, B., Arveux, P., Bonnetain, F., & Binquet, C. (2007). Chemoradiation followed by surgery compared with chemoradiation alone in squamous cancer of the esophagus: FFCD 9102. *J Clin Oncol*. Vol.25, No.10, pp1160-1168.

Bentzen, S.M. (2006). Preventing or reducing late side effects of radiation therapy: radiobiology meets molecular pathology. *Nat Rev Cancer*. Vol.6, No.9, pp702-713.

Bilimoria, K.Y., Bentrem, D.J., Feinglass, J.M., Stewart, A.K., Winchester, D.P., Talamonti, M.S., & Ko, C.Y. (2008). Directing surgical quality improvement initiatives:

comparison of perioperative mortality and long-term survival for cancer surgery. *J Clin Oncol*. Vol.26, No.28, pp4626-4633

Birkmeyer, J.D., Siewers, A.E., Finlayson, E.V., Stukel, T.A., Lucas, F.L., Batista, I., Welch, H.G., & Wennberg, D.E. (2002). Hospital volume and surgical mortality in the United States. *N Engl J Med*. Vol.346, No.15, pp1128-1137.

Boige, V., Pignon, J.P., Saint-Aubert, B., Lasser, P., Conroy, T., Bouche, O., Segol, P., Bedenne, L., Rougier, P., & Ychou, M. (2007). Final results of a randomized trial comparing preoperative 5-fluorouracil (F)/cisplatin (P) to surgery alone in adenocarcinoma of stomach and lower esophagus (ASLE): FNLCC ACCORD 07-FFCD 9703 trial. *Proc ASCO*. Abs 4510.

Boku, N., Yamamoto, S., Fukuda, H., Shirao, K., Doi, T., Sawaki, A., Koizumi, W., Saito, H., Yamaguchi, K., Takiuchi, H., Nasu, J., & Ohtsu, A.; Gastrointestinal Oncology Study Group of the Japan Clinical Oncology Group. (2009). Fluorouracil versus combination of irinotecan plus cisplatin versus S-1 in metastatic gastric cancer: a randomised phase 3 study. *Lancet Oncol*. Vol.10, No.11, pp1063-1069.

42. Bonenkamp JJ, Songun I, Hermans J, Sasako M, Welvaart K, Plukker JT, van Elk P, Obertop H, Gouma DJ, Taat CW, van Lanschot, J., Meyer, S., De Graaf, P.W., von Meyenfeldt, M.F., Tilanus, H., & van de Velde, C.J.H. (1995). Randomised comparison of morbidity after D1 and D2 dissection for gastric cancer in 996 Dutch patients. *Lancet*. Vol.345, No.8952, pp745-748.

43. Bonenkamp, J.J., Hermans, J., Sasako, M., van de Velde, C.J., Welvaart, K., Songun, I., Meyer, S., Plukker, J.T., Van Elk, P., Obertop, H., Gouma, D.J., van Lanschot, J.J., Taat, C.W., de Graaf, P.W., von Meyenfeldt, M.F., & Tilanus, H.; Dutch Gastric Cancer Group. (1999). Extended lymph-node dissection for gastric cancer. *N Engl J Med*. Vol.340, No.12, pp908-914.

Bonnetain, F., Bouché, O., Michel, P., Mariette, C., Conroy, T., Pezet, D., Roullet, B., Seitz, J.F., Paillot, B., Arveux, P., Milan, C., & Bedenne, L. (2006). A comparative longitudinal quality of life study using the Spitzer quality of life index in a randomized multicenter phase III trial (FFCD 9102): chemoradiation followed by surgery compared with chemoradiation alone in locally advanced squamous resectable thoracic esophageal cancer. *Ann Oncol*. Vol.17, No.5, pp827-834.

Bösing, N.M., Goretzki, P.E., & Röher, H.D. (2000). Gastric cancer: which patients benefit from systematic lymphadenectomy? *Eur J Surg Oncol*. Vol.26, No.5, pp498-505.

Bria, E., Cuppone, F., Ciccarese, M., Nisticò, C., Facciolo, F., Milella, M., Izzo, F., Terzoli, E., Cognetti, F., & Giannarelli, D. (2006). Weekly docetaxel as second line chemotherapy for advanced non-small-cell lung cancer: meta-analysis of randomized trials. *Cancer Treat Rev*. Vol.32, No.8, pp583-587.

Bunt, A.M., Hermans, J., Smit, V.T., van de Velde, C.J., Fleuren, G.J., & Bruijn, J.A. (1995). Surgical/pathologic-stage migration confounds comparisons of gastric cancer survival rates between Japan and Western countries. *J Clin Oncol*. Vol.13, No.1, pp19-25.

Chao, Y.K., Chan, S.C., Chang, H.K., Liu, Y.H., Wu, Y.C., Hsieh, M.J., Tseng, C.K., & Liu, H.P. (2009). Salvage surgery after failed chemoradiotherapy in squamous cell carcinoma of the esophagus. *Eur J Surg Oncol*. Vol.35, No.3, pp289-294.

Coia, L.R., Minsky, B.D., Berkey, B.A., John, M.J., Haller, D., Landry, J., Pisansky, T.M., Willett, C.G., Hoffman, J.P., Owen, J.B., & Hanks, G.E. (2000). Outcome of patients receiving radiation for cancer of the esophagus: results of the 1992-1994 Patterns of Care Study. *J Clin Oncol*. Vol.18, No.3, pp455-462.

Cooper, J.S., Guo, M.D., Herskovic, A., Macdonald, J.S., Martenson, J.A. Jr, Al-Sarraf, M., Byhardt, R., Russell, A.H., Beitler, J.J., Spencer, S., Asbell, S.O., Graham, M.V., & Leichman, L.L. (1999). Chemoradiotherapy of locally advanced esophageal cancer: long-term follow-up of a prospective randomized trial (RTOG 85-01). Radiation Therapy Oncology Group. *JAMA*. Vol.281, No.17, pp1623-1627.

http://www.ClinicalTrial.gov. NCT 01198392, Accessed April, 2011

http://www.ClinicalTrial.gov. NCT00252161, Accessed April, 2011

http://www.ClinicalTrial.gov. NCT00182611, Accessed April, 2011

http://www.critics.nl, Accessed April, 2011

Cunningham, D., Allum, W.H., Stenning, S.P., Thompson, J.N., Van de Velde, C.J., Nicolson, M., Scarffe, J.H., Lofts, F.J., Falk, S.J., Iveson, T.J., Smith, D.B., Langley, R.E., Verma, M., Weeden, S., & Chua, Y.J., MAGIC Trial Participants. (2006). Perioperative chemotherapy versus surgery alone for resectable gastroesophageal cancer. *N Engl J Med*. Vol.355, No.1, pp11-20.

Cunningham, D., Starling, N., Rao, S., Iveson, T., Nicolson, M., Coxon, F., Middleton, G., Daniel, F., Oates, J., & Norman, A.R.; Upper Gastrointestinal Clinical Studies Group of the National Cancer Research Institute of the United Kingdom. (2008). Capecitabine and oxaliplatin for advanced esophagogastric cancer. *N Engl J Med*. Vol.358, No.1, pp36-46.

Cuschieri, A., Fayers, P., Fielding, J., Craven, J., Bancewicz, J., Joypaul, V., & Cook, P. (1996). Postoperative morbidity and mortality after D1 and D2 resections for gastric cancer: preliminary results of the MRC randomised controlled surgical trial. The Surgical Cooperative Group. *Lancet*. Vol.347, No.9007, pp995-999.

Cuschieri, A., Weeden, S., Fielding, J., Bancewicz, J., Craven, J., Joypaul, V., Sydes, M,, & Fayers, P. (1999). Patient survival after D1 and D2 resections for gastric cancer: long-term results of the MRC randomized surgical trial. Surgical Co-operative Group. *Br J Cancer*. Vol.79, No.9-10, pp1522-1530.

Daigo, S., Takahashi, Y., Fujieda, M., Ariyoshi, N., Yamazaki, H., Koizumi, W., Tanabe, S., Saigenji, K., Nagayama, S., Ikeda, K., Nishioka, Y., & Kamataki, T. (2002). A novel mutant allele of the CYP2A6 gene (CYP2A6*11) found in a cancer patient who showed poor metabolic phenotype towards tegafur. *Pharmacogenetics*. Vol.12, No.4, pp299-306.

Daly, J.M., Karnell, L.H., & Menck, H.R. (1996). National Cancer Data Base report on esophageal carcinoma. *Cancer*. Vol.78, No.8, pp1820-1828.

Danielson, H., Kokkola, A., Kiviluoto, T., Sirén, J., Louhimo, J., Kivilaakso, E., & Puolakkainen, P. (2007). Clinical outcome after D1 vs D2-3 gastrectomy for treatment of gastric cancer. *Scand J Surg*. Vol.96, No,1, pp35-40.

Degiuli, M., Sasako, M., Calgaro, M., Garino, M., Rebecchi, F., Mineccia, M., Scaglione, D., Andreone, D., Ponti, A., & Calvo, F.; Italian Gastric Cancer Study Group. (2004a). Morbidity and mortality after D1 and D2 gastrectomy for cancer: interim analysis of the Italian Gastric Cancer Study Group (IGCSG) randomised surgical trial. *Eur J Surg Oncol*. Vol.30, No.3, pp303-308.

Degiuli, M., Sasako, M., Ponti, A., & Calvo, F. (2004b). Survival results of a multicentre phase II study to evaluate D2 gastrectomy for gastric cancer. *Br J Cancer*. Vol.90, No.9, pp1727-1732.

Degiuli, M., Sasako, M., & Ponti, A.; Italian Gastric Cancer Study Group. (2010). Morbidity and mortality in the Italian Gastric Cancer Study Group randomized clinical trial of D1 versus D2 resection for gastric cancer. *Br J Surg*. Vol.97, No.5, pp643-649.

Earle, C.C. & Maroun, JA. (1999). Adjuvant chemotherapy after curative resection for gastric cancer in non-Asian patients: revisiting a meta-analysis of randomised trials. *Eur J Cancer*. Vol.35, No.7, pp1059-1064.

Edwards, P., Blackshaw, G.R., Lewis, W.G., Barry, J.D., Allison, M.C., & Jones, D.R. (2004). Prospective comparison of D1 vs modified D2 gastrectomy for carcinoma. *Br J Cancer*. Vol.90, No.10, pp1888-1892.

Engels, F.K. & Verweij, J. (2005). Docetaxel administration schedule: from fever to tears? A review of randomised studies. *Eur J Cancer*. Vol.41, No.8, pp1117-1126.

Eschrich, S.A., Pramana, J., Zhang, H., Zhao, H., Boulware, D., Lee, J.H., Bloom, G., Rocha-Lima, C., Kelley, S., Calvin, D.P., Yeatman, T.J., Begg, A.C., & Torres-Roca, J.F. (2009). A gene expression model of intrinsic tumor radiosensitivity: prediction of response and prognosis after chemoradiation. *Int J Radiat Oncol Biol Phys*. Vol.75, No.2, pp489-496.

Faivre, J., Forman, D., Estève, J., & Gatta, G. (1998). Survival of patients with oesophageal and gastric cancers in Europe. EUROCARE Working Group. *Eur J Cancer*. Vol.34, No.14, pp2167-2175.

Fiorica, F., Di Bona, D., Schepis, F., Licata, A., Shahied, L., Venturi, A., Falchi, A.M., Craxì, A., & Cammà, C. (2004). Preoperative chemoradiotherapy for oesophageal cancer: a systematic review and meta-analysis. *Gut*. Vol.53, No.7, pp925-930.

Fujii, M., Sasaki, J., & Nakajima, T. (1999). State of the art in the treatment of gastric cancer: from the 71st Japanese Gastric Cancer Congress. *Gastric Cancer*. Vol.2, No.3, pp151-157.

Fushida, S., Fujimura, T., Oyama, K., Yagi, Y., Kinoshita, J., & Ohta, T. (2009). Feasibility and efficacy of preoperative chemotherapy with docetaxel, cisplatin and S-1 in gastric cancer patients with para-aortic lymph node metastases. *Anticancer Drugs*. Vol.20, No.8, pp752-756.

Gaast, A.V., van Hagen, P., Hulshof, M., Richel, D., van Berge Henegouwen, M.I., Nieuwenhuijzen, G.A., Plukker, J.T., Bonenkamp, J.J., Steyerberg, E.W., & Tilanus, H.W., CROSS Study Group. (2010). Effect of preoperative concurrent chemoradiotherapy on survival of patients with resectable esophageal or esophagogastric junction cancer: Results from a multicenter randomized phase III study. *Proc ASCO*. Abs. 4004.

GASTRIC (Global Advanced/Adjuvant Stomach Tumor Research International Collaboration) Group. Paoletti, X., Oba, K., Burzykowski, T., Michiels, S., Ohashi, Y., Pignon, J.P., Rougier, P., Sakamoto, J., Sargent, D., Sasako, M., Van Cutsem, E., & Buyse, M. (2010). Benefit of adjuvant chemotherapy for resectable gastric cancer: a meta-analysis. *JAMA*. Vol.303, No.17, pp1729-1737.

Gebski, V., Burmeister, B., Smithers, B.M., Foo, K., Zalcberg, J., & Simes, J.; Australasian Gastro-Intestinal Trials Group. (2007). Survival benefits from neoadjuvant chemoradiotherapy or chemotherapy in oesophageal carcinoma: a meta-analysis. *Lancet Oncol.* Vol.8, No.3, pp226-324.

Glimelius, B., Hoffman, K., Haglund, U., Nyrén, O., & Sjödén, P.O. (1994). Initial or delayed chemotherapy with best supportive care in advanced gastric cancer. *Ann Oncol.* Vol.5, No.2, pp189-190.

Hartgrink, H.H., van de Velde, C.J., Putter, H., Bonenkamp, J.J., Klein Kranenbarg, E., Songun, I., Welvaart, K., van Krieken, J.H., Meijer, S., Plukker, J.T., van Elk, P.J., Obertop, H., Gouma, D.J., van Lanschot, J.J., Taat, C.W., de Graaf, P.W., von Meyenfeldt, M.F., Tilanus, H., & Sasako, M. (2004a). Extended lymph node dissection for gastric cancer: who may benefit? Final results of the randomized Dutch gastric cancer group trial. *J Clin Oncol.* Vol.22, No.11, pp2069-2077.

Hartgrink, H.H., van de Velde, C.J., Putter, H., Songun, I., Tesselaar, M.E., Kranenbarg, E.K., de Vries, J.E., Wils, J.A., van der Bijl, J., & van Krieken, J.H.; Cooperating Investigators of The Dutch Gastric Cancer Group. (2004b). Neo-adjuvant chemotherapy for operable gastric cancer: long term results of the Dutch randomised FAMTX trial. *Eur J Surg Oncol.* Vol.30, No.6, pp643-649.

He, L.R., Liu, M.Z., Li, B.K., Rao, H.L., Deng, H.X., Guan, X.Y., Zeng, Y.X., & Xie, D. (2009). Overexpression of AIB1 predicts resistance to chemoradiotherapy and poor prognosis in patients with primary esophageal squamous cell carcinoma. *Cancer Sci.* Vol.100, No.9, pp1591-1596.

Hermans, J., Bonenkamp, J.J., Boon, M.C., Bunt, A.M., Ohyama, S., Sasako, M., & Van de Velde, C.J. (1993). Adjuvant therapy after curative resection for gastric cancer: meta-analysis of randomized trials. *J Clin Oncol.* Vol.11, No.8, pp1441-1447.

Hermans, J. & Bonenkamp, H. (1994). In reply. *J Clin Oncol.* p879.

Herskovic, A., Martz, K., al-Sarraf, M., Leichman, L., Brindle, J., Vaitkevicius, V., Cooper, J., Byhardt, R., Davis, L., & Emami, B. (1992). Combined chemotherapy and radiotherapy compared with radiotherapy alone in patients with cancer of the esophagus. *N Engl J Med.* Vol.326, No.24, pp1593-1598.

Hironaka, S., Ohtsu, A., Boku, N., Muto, M., Nagashima, F., Saito, H., Yoshida, S., Nishimura, M., Haruno, M., Ishikura, S., Ogino, T., Yamamoto, S., & Ochiai, A. (2003). Nonrandomized comparison between definitive chemoradiotherapy and radical surgery in patients with T(2-3)N(any) M(0) squamous cell carcinoma of the esophagus. *Int J Radiat Oncol Biol Phys.* Vol.57, No.2, pp425-433.

Hironaka, S., Yamazaki, K., Taku, K., Yokota, T., Shitara, K., Kojima, T., Ueda, S., Machida, N., Muro, K., & Boku, N. (2010). Phase I study of docetaxel, cisplatin and S-1 in patients with advanced gastric cancer. *Jpn J Clin Oncol.* Vol.40, No.11, pp1014-1020.

Hongyo, T., Buzard, G.S., Palli, D., Weghorst, C.M., Amorosi, A., Galli, M., Caporaso, N.E., Fraumeni, J.F. Jr, & Rice, J.M. (1995). Mutations of the K-ras and p53 genes in gastric adenocarcinomas from a high-incidence region around Florence, Italy. *Cancer Res.* Vol.55, No.12, pp2665-2672.

Hu, J.K., Chen, Z.X., Zhou, Z.G., Zhang, B., Tian, J., Chen, J.P., Wang,L., Wang, C.H., Chen, H.Y., & Li, Y.P. (2002). Intravenous chemotherapy for resected gastric cancer: meta-analysis of randomized controlled trials. *World J Gastroenterol.* Vol.8, No.6, pp1023-1028.

Hulscher, J.B., Tijssen, J.G., Obertop, H., & van Lanschot, J.J. (2001). Transthoracic versus transhiatal resection for carcinoma of the esophagus: a meta-analysis. *Ann Thorac Surg.* Vol.72, No.1, pp306-313.

Hundahl, S.A., Phillips, J.L., & Menck, H.R. (2000). The National Cancer Data Base Report on poor survival of U.S. gastric carcinoma patients treated with gastrectomy: Fifth Edition American Joint Committee on Cancer staging, proximal disease, and the "different disease" hypothesis. *Cancer.* Vol.88, No.4, pp921-932.

Imano, M., Itoh, T., Satou, T., Sogo, Y., Hirai, H., Kato, H., Yasuda, A., Peng, Y.F., Shinkai, M., Yasuda, T., Imamoto, H., Okuno, K., Shiozaki, H., & Ohyanagi, H. (2010). Prospective randomized trial of short-term neoadjuvant chemotherapy for advanced gastric cancer. *Eur J Surg Oncol.* Vol.36, No.10, pp963-968.

Ishida, K., Ando, N., Yamamoto, S., Ide, H., & Shinoda, M. (2004). Phase II study of cisplatin and 5-fluorouracil with concurrent radiotherapy in advanced squamous cell carcinoma of the esophagus: a Japan Esophageal Oncology Group (JEOG)/Japan Clinical Oncology Group trial (JCOG9516). *Jpn J Clin Oncol.* Vol.34, No.10, pp615-619.

Ishikura, S., Nihei, K., Ohtsu, A., Boku, N., Hironaka, S., Mera, K., Muto, M., Ogino, T., & Yoshida, S. (2003). Long-term toxicity after definitive chemoradiotherapy for squamous cell carcinoma of the thoracic esophagus. *J Clin Oncol.* Vol.21, No.14, pp2697-2702.

Jamieson, G.G., Mathew, G., Ludemann, R., Wayman, J., Myers, J.C., & Devitt, P.G. (2004). Postoperative mortality following oesophagectomy and problems in reporting its rate. *Br J Surg.* Vol.91, No.8, pp943-947.

Janmaat, M.L., Gallegos-Ruiz, M.I., Rodriguez, J.A., Meijer, G.A., Vervenne, W.L., Richel, D.J., Van Groeningen, C., & Giaccone, G. (2006). Predictive factors for outcome in a phase II study of gefitinib in second-line treatment of advanced esophageal cancer patients. *J Clin Oncol.* Vol.24, No.10, pp1612-1619.

Janunger, K.G., Hafström, L., & Glimelius, B. (2002). Chemotherapy in gastric cancer: a review and updated meta-analysis. *Eur J Surg.* Vol.168, No.11, pp597-608.

Jiang, Y., Kimchi, E.T., Staveley-O'Carroll, K.F., Cheng, H., & Ajani, J.A. (2009). Assessment of K-ras mutation: a step toward personalized medicine for patients with colorectal cancer. *Cancer.* Vol.115, No.16, pp3609-3617.

Jørgensen, J.T. (2010). Targeted HER2 treatment in advanced gastric cancer. *Oncology.* Vol.78, No.1, pp26-33.

Kang, Y., Ohtsu, A., Van Cutsem, E., Rha, S.Y., Sawaki, A., Park, S., Lim, H., Wuk J., Langerk, B., & Shah, M.A. (2010). AVAGAST: A randomized, double-blind, placebo-controlled, phase III study of first-line capecitabine and cisplatin plus bevacizumab or placebo in patients with advanced gastric cancer (AGC). *Proc ASCO.* Abs. LBA 4007

Kang, Y.K., Kang, W.K., Shin, D.B., Chen, J., Xiong, J., Wang, J., Lichinitser, M., Guan, Z., Khasanov, R., Zheng, L., Philco-Salas, M., Suarez, T., Santamaria, J., Forster, G., & McCloud, P.I. (2009). Capecitabine/cisplatin versus 5-fluorouracil/cisplatin as first-line therapy in patients with advanced gastric cancer: a randomised phase III noninferiority trial. *Ann Oncol*. Vol.20, No.4, pp666-673.

Kato, H., Sato, A., Fukuda, H., Kagami, Y., Udagawa, H., Togo, A., Ando, N., Tanaka, O., Shinoda, M., Yamana, H., & Ishikura, S. (2009). A phase II trial of chemoradiotherapy for stage I esophageal squamous cell carcinoma: Japan Clinical Oncology Group Study (JCOG9708). *Jpn J Clin Oncol*. Vol.39, No.10, pp638-643.

Kato, K., Muro, K., Minashi, K., Ohtsu, A., Ishikura, S., Boku, N., Takiuchi, H., Komatsu, Y., Miyata, Y., & Fukuda, H.; Gastrointestinal Oncology Study Group of the Japan Clinical Oncology Group (JCOG). (2010). Phase II Study of Chemoradiotherapy with 5-Fluorouracil and Cisplatin for Stage II-III Esophageal Squamous Cell Carcinoma: JCOG Trial (JCOG 9906). *Int J Radiat Oncol Biol Phys*. 2010 Oct 5.

Kawashima, Y., Sasako, M., Tsuburaya, A., Sano, T., Tanaka, Y., Nashimoto, A., Fukushima, N., Iwasaki, Y., Yamamoto, S., & Fukuda, H. (2008). Phase study of preoperative neoadjuvant chemotherapy (CX) with S-1 plus cisplatin for gastric cancer (GC) with bulky and/or paraaortic lymph node metastasis: A Japan Clinical Oncology Group Study (JCOG0405). *ASCO Gastrointestinal Cancer Symposium*. Abs 118.

Kelsen, D.P., Ginsberg, R., Pajak, T.F., Sheahan, D.G., Gunderson, L., Mortimer, J., Estes, N., Haller, D.G., Ajani, J., Kocha, W., Minsky, B.D., & Roth, J.A. (1998). Chemotherapy followed by surgery compared with surgery alone for localized esophageal cancer. *N Engl J Med*. Vol.339, No.27, pp1979-1984.

Kim, I.J., Park, J.H., Kang, H.C., Shin, Y., Park, H.W., Park, H.R., Ku, J.L., Lim, S.B., & Park, J.G. (2003). Mutational analysis of BRAF and K-ras in gastric cancers: absence of BRAF mutations in gastric cancers. *Hum Genet*. Vol.114, No.1, pp118-120.

Kim, J.P., Lee, J.H., Kim, S.J., Yu, H.J., & Yang, H.K. (1998). Clinicopathologic characteristics and prognostic factors in 10 783 patients with gastric cancer. *Gastric Cancer*. Vol.1, No.2, pp125-133.

Kim, S., Lim, D.H., Lee, J., Kang, W.K., MacDonald, J.S., Park, C.H., Park, S.H., Lee, S.H., Kim, K., Park, J.O., Kim, W.S., Jung, C.W., Park, Y.S., Im, Y.H., Sohn, T.S., Noh, J.H., Heo, J.S., Kim, Y.I., Park, C.K., & Park, K. (2005). An observational study suggesting clinical benefit for adjuvant postoperative chemoradiation in a population of over 500 cases after gastric resection with D2 nodal dissection for adenocarcinoma of the stomach. *Int J Radiat Oncol Biol Phys*. Vol.63, No.5, pp1279-1285.

Kim, Y.H., Koizumi, W., Lee, K.H., Kishimoto, T., Chung, H.C., Hara, T., Cho, J.Y., Nakajima, T., Kim, H., & Fujii, M., Japan Clinical Cnacer Research Organizatoin (JACCRO) and Kkorean Cancer Study Group (KCSG) Intergroup Study. (2011). Randomized phase III study of S-1 alone versus S-1 plus docetaxel (DOC) in the treatment for advanced gastric cancer (AGC): The START trial. ASCO Gastrointestinal Cancer Symposium Abs 7.

Klaeser, B., Nitzsche, E., Schuller, J.C., Köberle, D., Widmer, L., Balmer-Majno, S., Hany, T., Cescato-Wenger, C., Brauchli, P., Zünd, M., Pestalozzi, B.C., Caspar ,C., Albrecht, S., von Moos, R., & Ruhstaller, T. (2009). Limited predictive value of FDG-PET for response assessment in the preoperative treatment of esophageal cancer: results of a prospective multi-center trial (SAKK 75/02). *Onkologie*. Vol.32, No.12, pp724-730.

Kleinberg, L., Gibson, M.K., & Forastiere, A.A. (2007). Chemoradiotherapy for localized esophageal cancer: regimen selection and molecular mechanisms of radiosensitization. *Nat Clin Pract Oncol*. Vol.4, No.5, pp282-294.

Knox, J.J., Wong, R., Visbal, A.L., Horgan, A.M., Guindi, M., Hornby, J., Xu, W., Ringash, J., Keshavjee, S., Chen, E., Haider, M., & Darling, G. (2010). Phase 2 trial of preoperative irinotecan plus cisplatin and conformal radiotherapy, followed by surgery for esophageal cancer. *Cancer*. Vol.116, No.17, pp4023-4032.

Kodera, Y., Fujiwara, M., Yokoyama, H., Ohashi, N., Miura, S., Ito, Y., Koike, M., Ito, K., & Nakao, A. (2005). Combination of oral fluoropyrimidine and docetaxel: reappraisal of synergistic effect against gastric carcinoma xenografts. *In Vivo*. Vol. 19, No.5, pp861-866.

Koizumi, W., Tanabe, S., Saigenji, K., Ohtsu, A., Boku, N., Nagashima, F., Shirao, K., Matsumura, Y., & Gotoh, M. (2003). Phase I/II study of S-1 combined with cisplatin in patients with advanced gastric cancer. *Br J Cancer*. Vol.89, No.12, pp2207-2212.

Koizumi, W., Narahara, H., Hara, T., Takagane, A., Akiya, T., Takagi, M., Miyashita, K., Nishizaki, T., Kobayashi, O., Takiyama, W., Toh, Y., Nagaie, T., Takagi, S., Yamamura, Y., Yanaoka, K., Orita, H., & Takeuchi, M. (2008). S-1 plus cisplatin versus S-1 alone for first-line treatment of advanced gastric cancer (SPIRITS trial): a phase III trial. *Lancet Oncol*. Vol.9, No.3, pp215-221.

Kulig, J., Popiela, T., Kolodziejczyk, P., Sierzega, M., & Szczepanik, A.; Polish Gastric Cancer Study Group. (2007). Standard D2 versus extended D2 (D2+) lymphadenectomy for gastric cancer: an interim safety analysis of a multicenter, randomized, clinical trial. *Am J Surg*. Vol.193, No.1, pp10-15.

Kumekawa, Y., Kaneko, K., Ito, H., Kurahashi, T., Konishi, K., Katagiri, A., Yamamoto, T., Kuwahara, M., Kubota, Y., Muramoto, T., Mizutani, Y., & Imawari, M. (2006). Late toxicity in complete response cases after definitive chemoradiotherapy for esophageal squamous cell carcinoma. *J Gastroenterol*. Vol.41, No.5, pp425-432.

Kurihara, M., Izumi, T., Yoshida, S., Ohkubo, T., Suga, S., Kiyohashi, A., Yaosaka, T., Takahashi, H., Ito, T., Sasai, T., Akiya, T., Akazawa, S., Betsuyaku, T., & Taguchi, S. (1991). A cooperative randomized study on tegafur plus mitomycin C versus combined tegafur and uracil plus mitomycin C in the treatment of advanced gastric cancer. *Jpn J Cancer Res*. Vol.82, No.5, pp613-620.

Lee, S.H., Lee, J.W., Soung, Y.H., Kim, H.S., Park, W.S., Kim, S.Y., Lee, J.H., Park, J.Y., Cho, Y.G., Kim, C.J., Nam, S.W., Kim, S.H., Lee, J.Y., & Yoo, N.J. (2003). BRAF and KRAS mutations in stomach cancer. *Oncogene*. Vol.22, No.44, pp6942-6945.

Lepage, C., Sant, M., Verdecchia, A., Forman, D., Esteve, J., & Faivre, J.; and the EUROCARE working group. (2010). Operative mortality after gastric cancer resection and long-term survival differences across Europe. *Br J Surg*. Vol.97, No.2, pp235-239.

Li, C.P., Chen, J.S., Chen, L.T., Yen, C.J., Lee, K.D., Su, W.P., Lin, P.C., Lu, C.H., Tsai, H.J., & Chao, Y. (2010). A phase II study of weekly docetaxel and cisplatin plus oral tegafur/uracil and leucovorin as first-line chemotherapy in patients with locally advanced or metastatic gastric cancer. *Br J Cancer*. Vol.103, No.9, pp1343-1348.

Li, H., Zhu, F., Cao, Y., Zhai, L., & Lin, T. (2010). Meta-analyses of randomized trials assessing the effect of neoadjuvant chemotherapy in locally advanced gastric cancer. *Proc ASCO*. Abs 4042.

Li, W., Qin, J., Sun, Y.H., & Liu, T.S. (2010). Neoadjuvant chemotherapy for advanced gastric cancer: a meta-analysis. *World J Gastroenterol*. Vol.16, No.44, pp5621-5628.

Lièvre, A., Bachet, J.B., Boige, V., Cayre, A., Le Corre, D., Buc, E., Ychou, M., Bouché, O., Landi, B., Louvet, C., André, T., Bibeau, F., Diebold, M.D., Rougier, P., Ducreux, M., Tomasic, G., Emile, J.F., Penault-Llorca, F., & Laurent-Puig, P. (2008). KRAS mutations as an independent prognostic factor in patients with advanced colorectal cancer treated with cetuximab. *J Clin Oncol*. Vol.26, No.3, pp374-379.

Liu, T.S., Wang, Y., Chen, S.Y., & Sun, Y.H. (2008). An updated meta-analysis of adjuvant chemotherapy after curative resection for gastric cancer. *Eur J Surg Oncol*. Vol.34, No.11, pp1208-1216.

Lorenzen, S., Hentrich, M., Haberl, C., Heinemann, V., Schuster, T., Seroneit, T., Roethling, N., Peschel, C., & Lordick, F. (2007). Split-dose docetaxel, cisplatin and leucovorin/ fluorouracil as first-line therapy in advanced gastric cancer and adenocarcinoma of the gastroesophageal junction: results of a phase II trial. *Ann Oncol*. Vol.18, No.10, pp1673-1679.

Lorenzen, S., Schuster, T., Porschen, R., Al-Batran, S.E., Hofheinz, R., Thuss-Patience, P., Moehler, M., Grabowski, P., Arnold, D., Greten, T., Müller, L., Röthling, N., Peschel, C., Langer, R., & Lordick, F. (2009). Cetuximab plus cisplatin-5-fluorouracil versus cisplatin-5-fluorouracil alone in first-line metastatic squamous cell carcinoma of the esophagus: a randomized phase II study of the Arbeitsgemeinschaft Internistische Onkologie. *Ann Oncol*. Vol.20, No.10, pp1667-1673.

Luu, T.D., Gaur, P., Force, S.D., Staley, C.A., Mansour, K.A., Miller, J.I. Jr, & Miller, D.L. (2008). Neoadjuvant chemoradiation versus chemotherapy for patients undergoing esophagectomy for esophageal cancer. *Ann Thorac Surg*. Vol.85, No.4, pp1217-1223.

Macdonald, J.S., Smalley, S.R., Benedetti, J., Hundahl, S.A., Estes, N.C., Stemmermann, G.N., Haller, D.G., Ajani, J.A., Gunderson, L.L., Jessup, J.M., & Martenson, J.A. (2001). Chemoradiotherapy after surgery compared with surgery alone for adenocarcinoma of the stomach or gastroesophageal junction. *N Engl J Med*. Vol.345, No.10, pp725-730.

Macdonald, J.S., Smalley, S., Benedetti, J., Estes, N., Haller, D.G., Ajani, J.A., Gunderson, L.L., Jessup, M., & Martenson, J.A. (2004). Postoperative combined radiation and chemotherapy improves disease-free survival (DFS) and overall survival (OS) in resected adenocarcinoma of the stomach and gastroesophageal junction: Update of the results of Intergroup Study INT-0116 (SWOG9008). *Proc ASCO*. Abs 6.

Maehara, Y., Hasuda, S., Koga, T., Tokunaga, E., Kakeji, Y., & Sugimachi, K. (2000). Postoperative outcome and sites of recurrence in patients following curative resection of gastric cancer. *Br J Surg*. Vol.87, No.3, pp353-357.

Mari, E., Floriani, I., Tinazzi, A., Buda, A., Belfiglio, M., Valentini, M., Cascinu, S., Barni, S., Labianca, R., & Torri, V. (2000). Efficacy of adjuvant chemotherapy after curative resection for gastric cancer: a meta-analysis of published randomised trials. A study of the GISCAD (Gruppo Italiano per lo Studio dei Carcinomi dell'Apparato Digerente). *Ann Oncol*. Vol.11, No.7, pp837-843.

Maeda, S., Sugiura, T., Saikawa, Y., Kubota, T., Otani ,Y., Kumai, K., & Kitajima, M. (2004). Docetaxel enhances the cytotoxicity of cisplatin to gastric cancer cells by modification of intracellular platinum metabolism. *Cancer Sci.* Vol.95, No.8, pp679-684.

Maher, S.G., Gillham, C.M., Duggan, S.P., Smyth, P.C., Miller, N., Muldoon, C., O'Byrne, K.J., Sheils, O.M., Hollywood, D., & Reynolds, J.V. (2009). Gene expression analysis of diagnostic biopsies predicts pathological response to neoadjuvant chemoradiotherapy of esophageal cancer. *Ann Surg.* Vol.250, No.5, pp729-737.

Malthaner, R.A., Wong, R.K., Rumble, R.B., & Zuraw, L.; Members of the Gastrointestinal Cancer Disease Site Group of Cancer Care Ontario's Program in Evidence-based Care. (2004). Neoadjuvant or adjuvant therapy for resectable esophageal cancer: a systematic review and meta-analysis. *BMC Med.* Vol.2, p35.

Malthaner, R.A., Collin, S., & Fenlon, D. (2006). Preoperative chemotherapy for resectable thoracic esophageal cancer. *Cochrane Database Syst Rev.* Vol.3, CD001556.

Maruyama, K., Okabayashi, K., & Kinoshita, T. (1987). Progress in gastric cancer surgery in Japan and its limits of radicality. *World J Surg.* Vol.11, No.4, pp418-425.

Maruyama, K., Kaminishi, M., Hayashi, K., Isobe, Y., Honda, I., Katai, H., Arai, K., Kodera, Y., & Nashimoto, A. (2006). Gastric cancer treated in 1991 in Japan: data analysis of nationwide registry. Japanese Gastric Cancer Association Registration Committee, *Gastric Cancer.* Vol.9, No.2, pp51-66.

Medical Research Council Oesophageal Cancer Working Group. (2002). Surgical resection with or without preoperative chemotherapy in oesophageal cancer: a randomised controlled trial. *Lancet.* Vol. 359, No.9319, pp1727-1733.

Minashi, K., Doi, T., Muto, M., Mera, K., Yano, T., & Ohtsu, A. (2006). chemoradiotherapy for superficial esophageal squamous cell carcinoma. *Stomach and Intestine.* Vol.41, pp1467-1474.

Minsky, B.D., Pajak, T.F., Ginsberg, R.J., Pisansky, T.M., Martenson, J., Komaki, R., Okawara, G., Rosenthal, S.A., & Kelsen, D.P. (2002). INT 0123 (Radiation Therapy Oncology Group 94-05) phase III trial of combined-modality therapy for esophageal cancer: high-dose versus standard-dose radiation therapy. *J Clin Oncol.* Vol.20, No.5, pp1167-1174.

Murad, A.M., Santiago, F.F., Petroianu, A., Rocha, P.R., Rodrigues, M.A., & Rausch, M. (1993). Modified therapy with 5-fluorouracil, doxorubicin, and methotrexate in advanced gastric cancer. *Cancer.* Vol.72, No.1, pp37-41.

Murakami, M., Kuroda, Y., Okamoto, Y., Kono, K., Yoden, E., Kusumi, F., Hajiro, K., Matsusue, S., & Takeda, H. (1998). Neoadjuvant concurrent chemoradiotherapy followed by definitive high-dose radiotherapy or surgery for operable thoracic esophageal carcinoma. *Int J Radiat Oncol Biol Phys.* Vol.40, No.5, pp1049-1059.

Nakajima, M., Fukami, T., Yamanaka, H., Higashi, E., Sakai, H., Yoshida, R., Kwon, J.T., McLeod, H.L., & Yokoi, T. (2006). Comprehensive evaluation of variability in nicotine metabolism and CYP2A6 polymorphic alleles in four ethnic populations. *Clin Pharmacol Ther.* Vol.80, No.3, pp282-297.

Nakajima, T.E., Ura, T., Ito, Y., Kato, K., Minashi, K., Nihei, K., Hironaka, S., Boku, N., Kagami, Y., & Muro, K. (2009). A phase I trial of 5-fluorouracil with cisplatin and concurrent standard-dose radiotherapy in Japanese patients with stage II/III esophageal cancer. *Jpn J Clin Oncol.* Vol.39, No.1, pp37-42.

Nakamura, T., Hayashi, K., Ota, M., Eguchi, R., Ide, H., Takasaki, K., & Mitsuhashi, N. (2004). Salvage esophagectomy after definitive chemotherapy and radiotherapy for advanced esophageal cancer. *Am J Surg.* Vol.188, No.3, pp261-266.

Nakayama, N., Koizumi, W., Sasaki, T., Higuchi, K., Tanabe, S., Nishimura, K., Katada, C., Nakatani, K., Takagi, S., & Saigenji, K. (2008). A multicenter, phase I dose-escalating study of docetaxel, cisplatin and S-1 for advanced gastric cancer (KDOG0601). *Oncology.* Vol.75, No.1-2, pp1-7.

Narahara, H., Iishi, H., Imamura, H., Tsuburaya, A., Chin, K., Imamoto, H., Esaki, T., Furukawa, H., Hamada ,C., & Sakata, Y. (2011). Randomized phase III study comparing the efficacy and safety of irinotecan plus S-1 with S-1 alone as first-line treatment for advanced gastric cancer (study GC0301/TOP-002). *Gastric Cancer.* vol.14, No.1, pp72-80.

Nashimoto, A., Nakajima, T., Furukawa, H., Kitamura, M., Kinoshita, T., Yamamura, Y., Sasako, M., Kunii, Y., Motohashi, H., & Yamamoto, S.; Gastric Cancer Surgical Study Group, Japan Clinical Oncology Group. (2003). Randomized trial of adjuvant chemotherapy with mitomycin, Fluorouracil, and Cytosine arabinoside followed by oral Fluorouracil in serosa-negative gastric cancer: Japan Clinical Oncology Group 9206-1. *J Clin Oncol.* Vol.21, No.12, pp2282-2287.

Nio, Y., Koike, M., Omori, H., Hashimoto, K., Itakura, M., Yano, S., Higami, T., & Maruyama, R. (2004). A randomized consent design trial of neoadjuvant chemotherapy with tegafur plus uracil (UFT) for gastric cancer--a single institute study. *Anticancer Res.* Vol.24, No.3b, pp1879-1887.

Nishimura, M., Daiko, H., Yoshida, J., & Nagai, K. (2007). Salvage esophagectomy following definitive chemoradiotherapy. *Gen Thorac Cardiovasc Surg.* Vol.55, No.11, pp461-464.

Nishimura, Y., Suzuki, M., Nakamatsu, K., Kanamori, S., Yagyu, Y., & Shigeoka, H. (2002). Prospective trial of concurrent chemoradiotherapy with protracted infusion of 5-fluorouracil and cisplatin for T4 esophageal cancer with or without fistula. *Int J Radiat Oncol Biol Phys.* Vol.53, No.1, pp134-139.

Oba, K., Morita, S., Tsuburaya, A., Kodera, Y., Kobayashi, M., & Sakamoto, J. (2006). Efficacy of adjuvant chemotherapy using oral fluorinated pyrimidines for curatively resected gastric cancer: a meta-analysis of centrally randomized controlled clinical trials in Japan. *J Chemother.* Vol.18, No.3, pp311-317.

Ohtsu, A., Boku, N., Muro, K., Chin, K., Muto, M., Yoshida, S., Satake, M., Ishikura, S., Ogino, T., Miyata, Y., Seki, S., Kaneko, K., & Nakamura, A. (1999). Definitive chemoradiotherapy for T4 and/or M1 lymph node squamous cell carcinoma of the esophagus. *J Clin Oncol.* Vol.17, No.9, pp2915-2921.

Ohtsu, A., Shimada, Y., Shirao, K., Boku, N., Hyodo, I., Saito, H., Yamamichi, N., Miyata, Y., Ikeda, N., Yamamoto, S., Fukuda, H., & Yoshida, S.; Japan Clinical Oncology Group Study (JCOG9205). (2003). Randomized phase III trial of fluorouracil alone versus fluorouracil plus cisplatin versus uracil and tegafur plus mitomycin in patients with unresectable, advanced gastric cancer: The Japan Clinical Oncology Group Study (JCOG9205). *J Clin Oncol.* Vol.21, No.1, pp54-59.

Oki, E., Morita, M., Kakeji, Y., Ikebe, M., Sadanaga, N., Egasira, A., Nishida, K., Koga, T., Ohata, M., Honboh, T., Yamamoto, M., Baba, H., & Maehara, Y. (2007). Salvage esophagectomy after definitive chemoradiotherapy for esophageal cancer. *Dis Esophagus*. Vol.20, No.4, pp301-304.

Okines, A.F., Norman, A.R., McCloud, P., Kang, Y.K., & Cunningham, D. (2009). Meta-analysis of the REAL-2 and ML17032 trials: evaluating capecitabine-based combination chemotherapy and infused 5-fluorouracil-based combination chemotherapy for the treatment of advanced oesophago-gastric cancer. *Ann Oncol*. Vol.20, No.9, pp1529-1534.

Overman, M.J., Kazmi, S.M., Jhamb, J., Lin, E., Yao, J.C., Abbruzzese, J.L., Ho, L., Ajani, J., & Phan, A. (2010). Weekly docetaxel, cisplatin, and 5-fluorouracil as initial therapy for patients with advanced gastric and esophageal cancer. *Cancer*. Vol.116, No.6, pp1446-1453.

Panzini, I., Gianni, L., Fattori, P.P., Tassinari, D., Imola, M., Fabbri, P., Arcangeli, V., Drudi, G., Canuti, D., Fochessati, F., & Ravaioli, A. (2002). Adjuvant chemotherapy in gastric cancer: a meta-analysis of randomized trials and a comparison with previous meta-analyses. *Tumori*. Vol.88, No.1, pp21-27.

Park, S.R., Chun, J.H., Kim, Y.W., Lee, J.H., Choi, I.J., Kim, C.G., Lee, J.S., Bae, J.M., & Kim, H.K. (2005). Phase II study of low-dose docetaxel/fluorouracil/cisplatin in metastatic gastric carcinoma. *Am J Clin Oncol*. Vol.28, No.5, pp433-438.

Park, S.R., Kook, M.C., Choi, I.J., Kim, C.G., Lee, J.Y., Cho, S.J., Kim, Y.W., Ryu, K.W., Lee, J.H., Lee, J.S., Park, Y.I., & Kim, N.K. (2010). Predictive factors for the efficacy of cetuximab plus chemotherapy as salvage therapy in metastatic gastric cancer patients. *Cancer Chemother Pharmacol*. Vol.65, No.3, pp579-587.

Pinto, C., Di Fabio, F., Siena, S., Cascinu, S., Rojas Llimpe, F.L., Ceccarelli, C., Mutri, V., Giannetta, L., Giaquinta, S., Funaioli, C., Berardi, R., Longobardi, C., Piana, E., Martoni, A.A. (2007). Phase II study of cetuximab in combination with FOLFIRI in patients with untreated advanced gastric or gastroesophageal junction adenocarcinoma (FOLCETUX study). *Ann Oncol*. Vol.18, No.3, pp510-517.

Pyrhönen, S., Kuitunen, T., Nyandoto, P., & Kouri, M. (1995). Randomised comparison of fluorouracil, epidoxorubicin and methotrexate (FEMTX) plus supportive care with supportive care alone in patients with non-resectable gastric cancer. *Br J Cancer*. Vol.71, No.3, pp587-591.

Rice, T.W., Adelstein, D.J., Chidel, M.A., Rybicki, L.A., DeCamp, M.M., Murthy, S.C., & Blackstone, E.H. (2003). Benefit of postoperative adjuvant chemoradiotherapy in locoregionally advanced esophageal carcinoma. *J Thorac Cardiovasc Surg*. Vol.126, No.5, pp1590-1596.

Rice, T.W., Rusch, V.W., Apperson-Hansen, C., Allen, M.S., Chen, L.Q., Hunter, J.G., Kesler, K.A., Law, S., Lerut, T.E., Reed, C.E., Salo, J.A., Scott, W.J., Swisher, S.G., Watson, T.J., & Blackstone, E.H. (2009). Worldwide esophageal cancer collaboration. *Dis Esophagus*. Vol.22, No.1, pp1-8.

Ries, L.A.G., Young, J.L. Jr., Keel, G.E., Eisner, M.P., Linn, Y.D., & Horner, M.D. (2007). Cancer survival among adults: U.S. SEER program, 1988-2001. Patient and tumor characteristics. National Cancer Institute, SEER Program, NIH Pub.No. 07-6215, Bethesda, MD

Roth, A.D., Fazio, N., Stupp, R., Falk, S., Bernhard, J., Saletti, P., Köberle, D., Borner, M.M., Rufibach, K., Maibach, R., Wernli, M., Leslie, M., Glynne-Jones, R., Widmer, L.,

Seymour, M., & de Braud ,F.; Swiss Group for Clinical Cancer Research. (2007). Docetaxel, cisplatin, and fluorouracil; docetaxel and cisplatin; and epirubicin, cisplatin, and fluorouracil as systemic treatment for advanced gastric carcinoma: a randomized phase II trial of the Swiss Group for Clinical Cancer Research. *J Clin Oncol.* Vol.25, No.22, pp3217-3223.

Roukos, D.H., Lorenz, M., Karakostas, K., Paraschou, P., Batsis, C., & Kappas, A.M. (2001). Pathological serosa and node-based classification accurately predicts gastric cancer recurrence risk and outcome, and determines potential and limitation of a Japanese-style extensive surgery for Western patients: a prospective with quality control 10-year follow-up study. *Br J Cancer.* Vol.84, No.12, pp1602-1609.

Roukos, D.H. (2004). Early-stage gastric cancer: a highly treatable disease. *Ann Surg Oncol.* Vol.11, No.2, pp127-129.

Roviello, F., Marrelli, D., de Manzoni, G., Morgagni, P., Di Leo, A., Saragoni, L., & De Stefano, A.; Italian Research Group for Gastric Cancer. (2003). Prospective study of peritoneal recurrence after curative surgery for gastric cancer. *Br J Surg.* Vol.90, No.9, pp1113-1119.

Ruol, A., Castoro, C., Portale, G., Cavallin, F., Sileni,V.C., Cagol, M., Alfieri, R., Corti, L., Boso, C., Zaninotto, G., Peracchia, A., & Ancona, E. (2009). Trends in management and prognosis for esophageal cancer surgery: twenty-five years of experience at a single institution. *Arch Surg.* Vol.144, No.3, pp247-254.

Safran, H., Suntharalingam, M., Dipetrillo, T., Ng, T., Doyle, L.A., Krasna, M., Plette, A., Evans, D., Wanebo, H., Akerman, P., Spector, J., Kennedy, N., & Kennedy, T. (2008). Cetuximab with concurrent chemoradiation for esophagogastric cancer: assessment of toxicity. *Int J Radiat Oncol Biol Phys.* Vol.70, No.2, pp391-395.

Sakuramoto, S., Sasako, M., Yamaguchi, T., Kinoshita, T., Fujii, M., Nashimoto, A., Furukawa, H., Nakajima, T., Ohashi, Y., Imamura, H., Higashino, M., Yamamura, Y., Kurita, A., & Arai, K.; ACTS-GC Group. (2007). Adjuvant chemotherapy for gastric cancer with S-1, an oral fluoropyrimidine. *N Engl J Med.* Vol.357, No.18, pp1810-1820.

Sano, T., Katai, H., Sasako, M., & Maruyama, K. (2002). One thousand consecutive gastrectomies without operative mortality. *Br J Surg.* Vol.89, No.1, 122-123.

Sano, T., Sasako, M., Yamamoto, S., Nashimoto, A., Kurita, A., Hiratsuka, M., Tsujinaka, T., Kinoshita, T., Arai, K., Yamamura, Y., & Okajima, K. (2004). Gastric cancer surgery: morbidity and mortality results from a prospective randomized controlled trial comparing D2 and extended para-aortic lymphadenectomy--Japan Clinical Oncology Group study 9501. *J Clin Oncol.* Vol.22, No.14, pp2767-2773.

Sasako, M., Sano, T., Yamamoto, S., Kurokawa, Y., Nashimoto, A., Kurita, A., Hiratsuka, M., Tsujinaka, T., Kinoshita, T., Arai, K., Yamamura, Y., & Okajima, K.; Japan Clinical Oncology Group. (2008). D2 lymphadenectomy alone or with para-aortic nodal dissection for gastric cancer. *N Engl J Med.* Vol.359, No.5, pp453-462.

Sasako, M. (2010). Five-year results of the randomized phase III trial comparing S-1 monotherapy versus surgery alone for stage II/III gastric cancer patients after curative D2 gastrectomy (ACTS-GC study). *Ann Oncol.* Vol.21, Suppl.8, 709PD

Sato, Y., Takayama, T., Sagawa, T., Takahashi, Y., Ohnuma, H., Okubo, S., Shintani, N., Tanaka, S., Kida, M., Sato, Y., Ohta, H., Miyanishi, K., Sato, T., Takimoto, R.,

Kobune, M., Yamaguchi, K., Hirata, K., Niitsu, Y., & Kato, J. (2010). Phase II study of S-1, docetaxel and cisplatin combination chemotherapy in patients with unresectable metastatic gastric cancer. *Cancer Chemother Pharmacol.* Vol.66, No.4, pp721-728.

Schuhmacher, C., Gretschel, S., Lordick, F., Reichardt, P., Hohenberger, W., Eisenberger, C.F., Haag, C., Mauer, M.E., Hasan, B., Welch, J., Ott, K., Hoelscher, A., Schneider, P.M., Bechstein, W., Wilke, H., Lutz, M.P., Nordlinger, B., Cutsem, E.V., Siewert, J.R., & Schlag, P.M. (2010). Neoadjuvant chemotherapy compared with surgery alone for locally advanced cancer of the stomach and cardia: European Organisation for Research and Treatment of Cancer randomized trial 40954. *J Clin Oncol.* Vol.28, No.35, pp5210-5218.

Shimada, K., & Ajani. J.A. (1999). Adjuvant therapy for gastric carcinoma patients in the past 15 years: a review of western and oriental trials. *Cancer,* Vol.86, No.9, pp.1657-1668.

Shimoyama, S. (2009). Pharmacogenetics of fluoropyrimidine and cisplatin. A future application to gastric cancer treatment. *J Gastroenterol Hepatol.* Vol.24, No.6, pp970-981.

Shimoyama, S. (2010). Pharmacogenetics of irinotecan: An ethnicity-based prediction of irinotecan adverse events. *World J Gastrointest Surg.* Vol.2, No.1, 14-21.

Shimoyama, S. (2011). Statins are logical candidates for overcoming limitations of targeting therapies on malignancy: their potential application to gastrointestinal cancers. *Cancer Chemother Pharmacol.* Vol.67, No.4, pp729-739.

Siewert, J.R., Böttcher, K., Stein, H.J., & Roder, J.D. (1998). Relevant prognostic factors in gastric cancer: ten-year results of the German Gastric Cancer Study. *Ann Surg.* Vol.228, No.4, pp449-461.

Smithers, B.M., Cullinan, M., Thomas, J.M., Martin, I., Barbour, A.P., Burmeister, B.H., Harvey, J.A., Thomson, D.B., Walpole, E.T., & Gotley, D.C. (2007). Outcomes from salvage esophagectomy post definitive chemoradiotherapy compared with resection following preoperative neoadjuvant chemoradiotherapy. *Dis Esophagus.* Vol.20, No.6, pp471-477.

Songun, I., Putter, H., Kranenbarg, E.M., Sasako, M., & van de Velde, C.J. (2010). Surgical treatment of gastric cancer: 15-year follow-up results of the randomised nationwide Dutch D1D2 trial. *Lancet Oncol.* Vol.11, No.5, pp439-449.

Sparano, J.A., Wang, M., Martino, S., Jones, V., Perez, E.A., Saphner, T., Wolff, A.C., Sledge, G.W. Jr, Wood, W.C., & Davidson, N.E. (2008). Weekly paclitaxel in the adjuvant treatment of breast cancer. *N Engl J Med.* Vol.358, No.16, pp1663-1671.

Spigel, D.R., Greco, F.A., Meluch, A.A., Lane, C.M., Farley, C., Gray, J.R., Clark, B.L., Burris, H.A. 3rd, & Hainsworth, J.D. (2010). Phase I/II trial of preoperative oxaliplatin, docetaxel, and capecitabine with concurrent radiation therapy in localized carcinoma of the esophagus or gastroesophageal junction. *J Clin Oncol.* Vol.28, No.13, pp2213-2219.

Stahl, M., Stuschke, M., Lehmann, N., Meyer, H.J., Walz, M.K., Seeber, S., Klump, B., Budach, W., Teichmann, R., Schmitt, M., Schmitt, G., Franke, C., & Wilke, H. (2005). Chemoradiation with and without surgery in patients with locally advanced squamous cell carcinoma of the esophagus. *J Clin Oncol.* Vol.23, No.10, pp2310-2317.

Stahl, M., Walz, M.K., Stuschke, M., Lehmann, N., Meyer, H.J., Riera-Knorrenschild, J., Langer, P., Engenhart-Cabillic, R., Bitzer, M., Königsrainer, A., Budach, W., & Wilke, H. (2009). Phase III comparison of preoperative chemotherapy compared with chemoradiotherapy in patients with locally advanced adenocarcinoma of the esophagogastric junction. *J Clin Oncol.* Vol.27, No.6, pp851-856.

Swisher, S.G., Wynn, P., Putnam, J.B., Mosheim, M.B., Correa, A.M., Komaki, R.R., Ajani, J.A., Smythe, W.R., Vaporciyan, A.A., Roth, J.A., & Walsh, G.L. (2002). Salvage esophagectomy for recurrent tumors after definitive chemotherapy and radiotherapy. *J Thorac Cardiovasc Surg.* Vol.123, No.1, pp175-183.

Swisher, S.G., Maish, M., Erasmus, J.J., Correa, A.M., Ajani, J.A., Bresalier, R., Komaki, R., Macapinlac, H., Munden, R.F., Putnam, J.B., Rice, D., Smythe, W.R., Vaporciyan, A.A., Walsh, G.L., Wu, T.T., & Roth, J.A. (2004). Utility of PET, CT, and EUS to identify pathologic responders in esophageal cancer. *Ann Thorac Surg.* Vol.78, No.4, pp1152-1160.

Syrigos, K.N., Zalonis, A., Kotteas, E., & Saif, M.W. (2008). Targeted therapy for oesophageal cancer: an overview. *Cancer Metastasis Rev.* Vol.27, No.2, pp273-288.

Takashima, A., Boku, N., Kato, K., Mizusawa, J., Nakamura, K., Fukuda, H., Shirao, K., Shimada, Y., & Ohtsu, A. (2010). Survival prolongation after treatment failure in patients with advanced gastric cancer (AGC): Results from combined analysis of JCOG9205 and JCOG9912. *Proc ASCO.* Abs 4061.

Tebbutt, N.C., Cummins, M.M., Sourjina, T., Strickland, A., Van Hazel, G., Ganju, V., Gibbs, D., Stockler, M., Gebski, V., & Zalcberg, J.; Australasian Gastro-Intestinal Trials Group. (2010). Randomised, non-comparative phase II study of weekly docetaxel with cisplatin and 5-fluorouracil or with capecitabine in oesophagogastric cancer: the AGITG ATTAX trial. *Br J Cancer.* Vol.102, No.3, pp475-481.

The Japan Esophageal Society. http://www.esophagus.jp/index_e.html. Accessed April, 2011.

Tachimori, Y., Kanamori, N., Uemura, N., Hokamura, N., Igaki, H., & Kato, H. (2009). Salvage esophagectomy after high-dose chemoradiotherapy for esophageal squamous cell carcinoma. *J Thorac Cardiovasc Surg.* Vol.137, No.1, pp49-54.

Tol, J., Nagtegaal, I.D., & Punt, C.J. (2009). BRAF mutation in metastatic colorectal cancer. *N Engl J Med.* Vol.361, No.1, pp98-99.

Tomimaru, Y., Yano, M., Takachi, K., Miyashiro, I., Ishihara, R., Nishiyama, K., Sasaki, Y., Ishikawa, O., Doki, Y., & Imaoka, S. (2006). Factors affecting the prognosis of patients with esophageal cancer undergoing salvage surgery after definitive chemoradiotherapy. *J Surg Oncol.* Vol.93, No.5, pp422-428.

Trivers, K.F., Sabatino, S.A., & Stewart, S.L. (2008). Trends in esophageal cancer incidence by histology, United States, 1998-2003. *Int J Cancer.* Vol.123, No.6, pp1422-1428.

Trotti, A., Pajak, T.F., Gwede, C.K., Paulus, R., Cooper, J., Forastiere, A., Ridge, J.A., Watkins-Bruner, D., Garden, A.S., Ang, K.K., & Curran, W. (2007). TAME: development of a new method for summarising adverse events of cancer treatment by the Radiation Therapy Oncology Group. *Lancet Oncol.* Vol.8, No.7, pp613-624.

Urschel, J.D., Vasan, H., & Blewett, C.J. (2002). A meta-analysis of randomized controlled trials that compared neoadjuvant chemotherapy and surgery to surgery alone for resectable esophageal cancer. *Am J Surg.* Vol.183, No.3, pp274-279.

Urschel, JD. & Vasan, H. (2003). A meta-analysis of randomized controlled trials that compared neoadjuvant chemoradiation and surgery to surgery alone for resectable esophageal cancer. *Am J Surg*. Vol.185, No.6, pp538-543.

van Cutsem, E., Moiseyenko, V.M., Tjulandin, S., Majlis, A., Constenla, M., Boni, C., Rodrigues, A., Fodor, M., Chao, Y., Voznyi, E., Risse, M.L., & Ajani, J.A.; V325 Study Group. (2006). Phase III study of docetaxel and cisplatin plus fluorouracil compared with cisplatin and fluorouracil as first-line therapy for advanced gastric cancer: a report of the V325 Study Group. *J Clin Oncol*. Vol.24, No.31, pp4991-4997.

van Cutsem, E., Shah, M., Kang, Y., Yamada, Y., Yamaguchi, K., Nishina, T., Doi, T., Wu, J., Langer, B., & Ohtsu, A. (2010). Randomized, double-blind, placebo-controlled, multicenter phase III study of capecitabine/cisplatin + bevacizumab (bev) or placebo (pl) as 1st-line therapy in patients with advanced gastric cancer (AVAGAST Update). *Ann Oncol*, Vol.21, Suppl 8, 713p.

Wagner, A.D., Grothe, W., Haerting, J., Kleber, G., Grothey, A., & Fleig, W. E. (2006). Chemotherapy in advanced gastric cancer: a systematic review and meta-analysis based on aggregate data. *J Clin Oncol*. Vol.24, No.18, pp2903-2909.

Wang, S.L., Liao, Z., Vaporciyan, A.A., Tucker, S.L., Liu, H., Wei, X., Swisher, S., Ajani, J.A., Cox, J.D., & Komaki, R. (2006). Investigation of clinical and dosimetric factors associated with postoperative pulmonary complications in esophageal cancer patients treated with concurrent chemoradiotherapy followed by surgery. *Int J Radiat Oncol Biol Phys*. Vol.64, No.3, pp692-699.

Waters, J.S., Norman, A., Cunningham, D., Scarffe, J.H., Webb, A., Harper, P., Joffe, J.K., Mackean, M., Mansi, J., Leahy, M., Hill, A., Oates, J., Rao, S., Nicolson, M., & Hickish, T. (1999). Long-term survival after epirubicin, cisplatin and fluorouracil for gastric cancer: results of a randomized trial. *Br J Cancer*. Vol.80, No.1-2, pp269-272.

Webb, A., Cunningham, D., Scarffe, J.H., Harper, P., Norman, A., Joffe, J.K., Hughes, M., Mansi, J., Findlay, M., Hill, A., Oates, J., Nicolson, M., Hickish, T., O'Brien, M., Iveson, T., Watson, M., Underhill, C., Wardley, A., & Meehan, M. (1997). Randomized trial comparing epirubicin, cisplatin, and fluorouracil versus fluorouracil, doxorubicin, and methotrexate in advanced esophagogastric cancer. *J Clin Oncol*. Vol.15, No.1, pp261-267.

Wils, J.A., Klein, H.O., Wagener, D.J., Bleiberg, H., Reis, H., Korsten, F., Conroy, T., Fickers, M., Leyvraz, S., & Buyse, M. (1991). Sequential high-dose methotrexate and fluorouracil combined with doxorubicin--a step ahead in the treatment of advanced gastric cancer: a trial of the European Organization for Research and Treatment of Cancer Gastrointestinal Tract Cooperative Group. *J Clin Oncol*. Vol.9, No.5, pp827-831.

Wilson, K.S. & Lim, J.T. (2000). Primary chemo-radiotherapy and selective oesophagectomy for oesophageal cancer: goal of cure with organ preservation. *Radiother Oncol*. Vol.54, No.2, pp129-134.

Wong, R. & Malthaner, R. (2006). Combined chemotherapy and radiotherapy (without surgery) compared with radiotherapy alone in localized carcinoma of the esophagus. *Cochrane Database Syst Rev*. Vol.25, No.1, CD002092.

Wu, A.W., Xu, G.W., Wang, H.Y., Ji, J.F., & Tang, J.L. (2007). Neoadjuvant chemotherapy versus none for resectable gastric cancer. *Cochrane Database Syst Rev*. Vol.18, No.2, CD005047.

Wu, C.W., Hsiung, C.A., Lo, S.S., Hsieh, M.C., Shia, L.T., & Whang-Peng, J. (2004). Randomized clinical trial of morbidity after D1 and D3 surgery for gastric cancer. *Br J Surg*. Vol.91, No.3, pp283-287.

Wu, C.W., Hsiung, C.A., Lo, S.S., Hsieh, M.C., Chen, J.H., Li, A.F., Lui, W.Y., & Whang-Peng, J. (2006). Nodal dissection for patients with gastric cancer: a randomised controlled trial. *Lancet Oncol*. Vol.7, No.4, pp309-315.

Yamada, Y., Koizumi, W., Takiuchi, H., Boku, N., Muro, K., Fuse, N., Komatsu, Y., & Tsuburaya, A., (2010). S-1 combined with oxaliplatin (SOX) as first-line chemotherapy against advanced gastric cancer: Updates on a multicenter phase II trial. *ASCO Gastrointestinal Cancer Symposium*, Abs 62.

Ychou, M., Pignon, J.P., Lasser, P., Conroy, T., Bouche, O., Boige, V., Segol, P., Bedenne, L., Saint-Aubert, B., & Rougier, P. (2006). Phase III preliminary results of preoperative fluorouracil)F) and cisplatin (P) versus surgery alone in adenocarcinoma of stomach and lower esophagus (ASLE): FNLCC 94012-FFCD 9703 trial. *Proc ASCO*. Abs 4026.

Yonemura, Y., Sawa, T., Kinoshita, K., Matsuki, N., Fushida, S., Tanaka, S., Ohoyama, S., Takashima, T., Kimura, H., Kamata, T., Fujimura, T., Sugiyama, K., Shima, K., & Miyazaki, I. (1993). Neoadjuvant chemotherapy for high-grade advanced gastric cancer. *World J Surg*. Vol.17, No.2, pp256-261

Yoo, J., Park, S.Y., Robinson, R.A., Kang, S.J., Ahn, W. S., & Kang, C.S. (2002). ras Gene mutations and expression of Ras signal transduction mediators in gastric adenocarcinomas. *Arch Pathol Lab Med*. Vol.126, No.9, pp1096-1100.

Yoshida, R., Nakajima, M., Nishimura, K., Tokudome, S., Kwon, J.T., & Yokoi, T. (2003). Effects of polymorphism in promoter region of human CYP2A6 gene (CYP2A6*9) on expression level of messenger ribonucleic acid and enzymatic activity in vivo and in vitro. *Clin Pharmacol Ther*. Vol.74, No.1, pp69-76.

Zang, D.Y., Kang, Y., Ryoo, B., Ryu, M., Lee, S.S., Song, H.H., Jung, J.Y., Kwon, J.H., Kim, H.S., & Choi, D.R. (2010). Phase II study with docetaxel, oxaliplatin, and S-1 combination chemotherapy for patients with metastatic gastric cancer. *Ann Oncol*, Vol.21, Abs 836.

Zhang, C.W., Zou, S.C., Shi, D., & Zhao, D.J. (2004). Clinical significance of preoperative regional intra-arterial infusion chemotherapy for advanced gastric cancer. *World J Gastroenterol*. Vol.10, No.20, pp3070-3072.

Zhang, X., Zhao, K.L., Guerrero, T.M., McGuire, S.E., Yaremko, B., Komaki, R., Cox, J.D., Hui, Z., Li, Y., Newhauser, W.D., Mohan, R., & Liao, Z. (2008). Four-dimensional computed tomography-based treatment planning for intensity-modulated radiation therapy and proton therapy for distal esophageal cancer. *Int J Radiat Oncol Biol Phys*. Vol.72, No.1, pp278-287.

Zhao, SL. & Fang, JY. (2008). The role of postoperative adjuvant chemotherapy following curative resection for gastric cancer: a meta-analysis. *Cancer Invest*. Vol.26, No.3, pp317-325.

Zhao, W., Chan, T.L., Chu, K.M., Chan, A.S., Stratton, M.R., Yuen, S.T., & Leung, S.Y. (2004). Mutations of BRAF and KRAS in gastric cancer and their association with microsatellite instability. *Int J Cancer*. Vol.108, No.1, pp167-169.

Zilberstein, B., da Costa Martins, B., Jacob, C.E., Bresciani, C., Lopasso, F.P., de Cleva, R., Pinto Junior, P.E., Junior, U.R., Perez, R.O., & Gama-Rodrigues, J. (2004). Complications of gastrectomy with lymphadenectomy in gastric cancer. *Gastric Cancer*. Vol.7, No.4, pp254-259.

5

Evidence-Based Usefulness of Physiotherapy Techniques in Breast Cancer Patients

Almir José Sarri[1] and Sonia Marta Moriguchi[2]
[1]Department of Physiotherapy
[2]Department of Nuclear Medicine
Barretos Cancer Hospital
Brazil

1. Introduction

Breast cancer is one of the most frequent causes of death among women, with high incidence in both developed and developing countries. When it is diagnosed at an advanced stage, including cases of metastatic lymph node invasion, the treatment becomes more aggressive and expensive (Johansson et al., 2002; Parkin & Fernandez, 2006), with the implication that the post-treatment complication rate will be greater (Kwan et al., 2002; Szuba et al., 2003; Goffman et al., 2004; King & Difalco, 2005).

The complications may be short or long-term, and the commonest of them include hemorrhage, infection, seroma, axillary web syndrome (AWS), chronic pain, paresthesia, reduction of the range of motion, muscle weakness in the shoulder homolateral to the surgery and lymphedema (Fig. 1). Of these, lymphedema is the most important morbid condition (Lee et al., 2008; Paskett, 2008; Fourie & Robb, 2009; Stanton et al., 2009).

Aggressive surgery, such as radical axillary dissection, may interrupt the main lymphatic drainage route in the arms, and this is the most important factor in edema formation (Bourgeois et al., 1998). Associated complementary radiotherapy induces fibrosis in lymphatic vessels in 20 to 30% of the cases, thus worsening the lymphatic flow (Paci et al., 1996; Bumpers et al., 2002; Carpentier, 2002; Kwan et al., 2002; Van Der Veen et al., 2004; Moseley et al., 2007).

This modification to the lymphatic flow induces alteration of the homeostatic equilibrium of absorption and transportation of interstitial fluid, which triggers lymphedema. This is a progressive condition characterized by four pathological factors: excess protein in tissues, edema, chronic inflammation and fibrosis. When the arm remains untreated, its volume progressively increases, as does the frequency of complications relating to this condition (Weissleder & Weissleder, 1988; Carpentier, 2002; Didem et al., 2005; King, 2006).

It is difficult to diagnose lymphedema, especially in its initial stages. Without a proper diagnosis, it always takes time to institute therapy. When the treatment is immediate, the improvement occurs quickly and progression of the condition is prevented (Szuba et al., 2003; Linnitt, 2007).

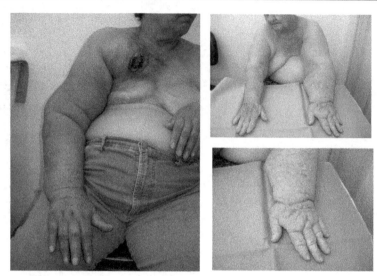

Fig. 1. Lymphedema following axillary dissection.

The pathogenesis of post-mastectomy lymphedema associated with axillary dissection is mainly attributed to greater numbers of dissected lymph nodes (Filippetti et al., 1994; Glass et al., 1999). The more extensive the axillary dissection is, the greater the risk of complications will be (Glass et al., 1999).

The desire to prevent lymphedema has led to intraoperative techniques that take a more conservative approach to the axillary chain, such as investigating the sentinel lymph node. Through this, selective, safe and less mutilating resection has become possible, with satisfactory results. Nevertheless, this is limited to patients without evidence of lymph node macrometastases (Clodius et al., 1981; Bourgeois et al., 1998; Bumpers et al., 2002; Goffman et al., 2004; Rietman et al., 2004; Ronka et al., 2004; Sakorafas et al., 2006).

When lymphedema becomes established, it is incurable. However, it can be avoided, treated and controlled with daily preventive measures (Linnitt, 2007). Studies have demonstrated that surgical and drug treatments are unsuccessful (Roucout & Oliveira, 1999; Didem et al., 2005). The aim of physical rehabilitation is to prevent and minimize the sequelae caused by oncological treatment or by the disease itself, and to improve patients' quality of life, in both its physical and its psychological aspects.

2. Physiotherapeutic approaches

Physiotherapeutic approaches for lymphedema can be divided into two parts: prophylactic and therapeutic approaches, with the aim of preventing sequelae and improving the patient's physical condition to face up to the treatment (Bergmann et al., 2006).

2.1 Prophylactic physiotherapeutic approaches

It should be started preoperatively or in the immediate postoperative period, with the aim of preventing sequelae and improving the patient's physical condition to face up to the treatment (Bergmann et al., 2006).

The focus of this evaluation aimed to identify risk factors for developing complications and morbid conditions relating to the axillary approach and to implementation of strategies for minimizing preexisting symptoms, with the aim of achieving better postoperative functional recovery (Paskett, 2008; Springer et al., 2010).

2.1.1 Preoperative physiotherapy

Limitations on shoulder range of motion, pain and diminished muscle strength are the main focuses of the assessment, since these may lead to morbid conditions that relate directly to axillary manipulation.

In the presence of limitations on shoulder range of motion and/or loss of muscle strength, passive exercises, assisted active exercises, active exercises of the scapular belt and neck relaxation exercises are indicated (Lauridsen et al., 2005; Rezende et al., 2006; Springer et al., 2010). For patients with locoregional pain, transcutaneous electrical nerve stimulation (TENS) can be applied.

Improvement of respiratory capacity through the use of apparatus to incentivize the respiratory flow or volume (incentive spirometry) is also indicated for diminishing general morbid conditions, when present (Bergmann et al., 2006).

Although preventive interventions have shown good results, the numbers of patients referred for preoperative assessments and preventive care are still very small.

2.1.2 Immediate postoperative intervention

The second step of preventive intervention starts immediately after the surgical procedure, on the first day after the operation, with guidance about positioning in bed (with the operated arm above the head), functional exercises on the limb homolateral to the surgery as shown in Fig. 2, and respiratory physiotherapy if necessary.

Guidance regarding care for the limb that underwent manipulation, with prevention of trauma and lesions that might trigger inflammation and infection in the arm homolateral to the axillary dissection, avoidance of using clothes that restrict the superficial lymphatic circulation, skin hydration and provision of kinesiotherapy limited to 90° of range of shoulder movement are administered to patients who undergo radial axillary dissection and sentinel lymph node biopsy, before hospital discharge (Roucout & Oliveira, 1999; Andersen et al., 2000; Camargo & Marx, 2000; Huit, 2000; Bergmann et al., 2006).

Additional guidance regarding early lymphatic self-massage should also be provided for patients after axillary dissection (Sarri et al., 2010).

2.2 Postoperative follow-up

A new physiotherapeutic reassessment is undertaken immediately after removal of the patient's surgical stitches and suction drain, focusing on reorientation regarding preventive measures against lymphedema and assessment of the need for early physiotherapeutic intervention, before the start of radiotherapy.

Physiotherapeutic treatment concomitant to radiotherapy is very important, because it minimizes the side effects, such as subcutaneous fibrosis, limitations on shoulder range of motion, muscle weakness and pains (Lee et al., 2008).

In outpatient rehabilitation, in addition to individualized attendance, it is also undertaken in collective groups. This has the benefit of promoting interaction among the patients, with exchanges of experiences, thus making the session more agreeable and providing encouragement towards doing the exercises (Fig. 3). Patients should be advised to continue with the treatment at home.

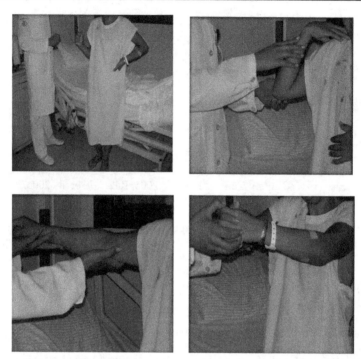

Fig. 2. Postoperative functional exercises.

In the following, we will describe the main physiotherapeutic interventions relating to specific symptoms of complications following surgical manipulation of the axillae.

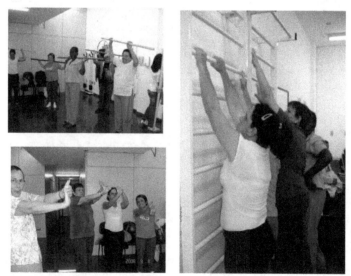

Fig. 3. Group of mastectomized patients.

3. Lymphedema

Early diagnosis and intervention, such as skincare (Kwan et al., 2002; Williams et al., 2002), kinesiotherapy and self-massage (Glass et al., 1999; Williams et al., 2002; Rietman et al., 2004), may significantly reduce the incidence of complications (Williams et al., 2002). The search for better quality of life has indicated that prevention of lymphedema is the best strategy among this group of patients. Prior knowledge of the normal lymphatic circulation and the changes that it undergoes in the presence of obstruction directs the techniques for physiotherapeutic stimulation. Several lymphatic drainage techniques are used to stimulate the lymphatic flow and treat lymphedema, such as the techniques proposed by Vodder, Leduc and Földi. Recently, we studied 22 women with breast carcinoma who underwent surgical treatment and axillary lymph node dissection. We performed early homolateral inguinal and contralateral axillary lymph node stimulation for up to 60 days after the operation, thereby simulating self-massage according to the Földi technique, and used lymphoscintigraphy to identify the immediate improvement in lymphatic flow following the stimulation (Sarri et al., 2010).

The main objective of manual lymphatic drainage is to increase lymphokinetic activity in healthy areas, before stimulating the edematous areas. There are several physiological effects, which include increased contraction of the lymphatic vessels and increased protein reabsorption, thereby reducing the microlymphatic hypertension, increasing the collateral lymphatic drainage among the lymphatic areas of the skin and improving the drainage capacity in order to direct the lymph away from the edematous area and towards lymph nodes in areas that are unaffected by lymphedema (Fritsch & Tomson, 1991; Araujo et al., 1997; Andersen et al., 2000; Huit, 2000; Williams et al., 2002; Moseley et al., 2007). As a strategy for stimulating the lymphatic circulation in cases of obstruction of the normal lymphatic flow, the collateral routes and anastomoses of the lymphatic capillaries should be taken to be the peripheral circulation. These routes deviate the lymph flow in a direction contrary to the usual flow, through the lateral cephalic lymphatic bundle and continuing over the deltoid muscle, thereby bypassing the axillary lymph node chain and draining the lymph directly to the supra and infraclavicular lymph nodes (Stanton et al., 2009; Sarri et al., 2010). Within this context, physiotherapy to treat lymphedema that has already become established and to prevent this and other comorbidities is of paramount importance for diminishing the surgical sequelae from breast cancer treatment.

3.1 Manual lymphatic drainage

The treatment for lymphedema that has already become established is based on techniques that are well accepted and described in the worldwide literature. In Brazil, treatment also known as lymph therapy or complex physical treatment is the type most used. Complete decongestive physiotherapy (CDP) is composed of four approaches: manual lymphatic drainage (MLD), compressive bandaging, skincare and lymph myokinetic exercises (Bergmann et al., 2006; Leal et al., 2009).

Lymph therapy is carried out in two phases. The first has therapeutic aims and the second consists of maintenance. The therapeutic phase aims to mobilize the accumulated protein-rich fluid and reduce the fibrosclerotic tissue, using MLD and compressive bandaging (Foldi, 1998; Camargo & Marx, 2000; Leal et al., 2009). MLD can be carried out in regions with or without edema, depending on the aim at the time of treatment. It is done in two stages: evacuation and uptake.

The evacuation maneuvers begin with a series of gentle circular movements with the therapist's palms in contact with the patient's skin. Firstly, the contralateral axillary lymph node chain is stimulated and then the inguinal region homolateral to the surgical manipulation. After these areas have been stimulated, wavelike movements are made across the anterior region of the chest, towards areas adjacent to the axilla that underwent the operation, thus stimulating first the contralateral quadrant until reaching the ipsilateral quadrant, and then making the same movement going from the ipsilateral inguinal region to the axilla, as shown in Fig. 4. These movements can be carried out both in the anterior and in the posterior region of the trunk.

After finishing the evacuation phase, the uptake process is started. This is always performed from proximal to distal regions, with wavelike maneuvers in the upper arm region and then the forearm and hand, until reaching the fingers (Fig. 5) (Foldi et al., 1985; Camargo & Marx, 2000; Williams et al., 2002; Linnitt, 2005).

The direction of lymphatic drainage should respect the anatomy of the lymphatic system, and it is very important to take into consideration the deviation in the region of the deltoid muscle (Stanton et al., 2009; Sarri et al., 2010).

After completing the manual lymphatic drainage, the arms should be hydrated using neutral cream so that compressive bandaging can be started.

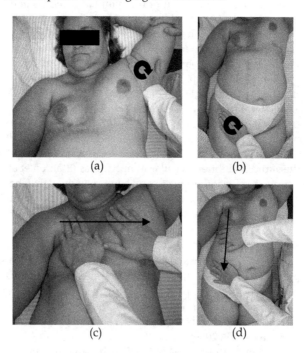

(a)   (b)

(c)   (d)

Fig. 4. Evacuation maneuvers on a patient who underwent radical right-side lymphadenectomy: a) axillary limph node chain stimulation; b) inguinal lymph node chain stimulation; c) wavelike maneuver directing the lymphatic flow towards the contralateral axillary region; d) wavelike maneuver directing the lymphatic flow towards the ipsilateral inguinal region.

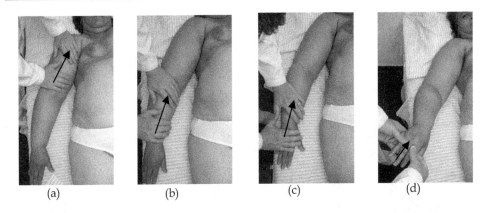

(a) (b) (c) (d)

Fig. 5. Uptake maneuver on a patient who underwent radical right-side lymphadenectomy: wavelike maneuvers directing the lymphatic flow from the proximal to the distal region: a) upper-arm region; b) forearm region; c) hand region; d) finger region.

3.2 Compressive bandaging

One of the consequences of lymphedema is that the elastic fibers are destroyed. Evacuation of the lymphatic fluid by means of manual lymphatic drainage diminishes the pressure on the tissue and increases the effective ultrafiltration pressure. Elastic bandages increase the tissue pressure and counterbalance the elastic insufficiency, thereby avoiding recurrence of lymphatic fluid accumulation in the interstices (Foldi et al., 1985).

Compressive bandaging is an important technique, because it boosts the effects achieved through the preceding lymph drainage. It should always be functional, thereby enabling all day-to-day movements and guided kinesiotherapy (Fig. 6).

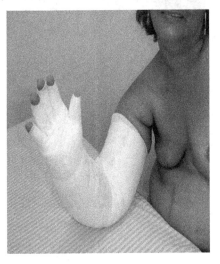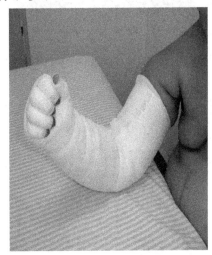

Fig. 6. Functional compressive bandaging, such that the patient was able to make movements.

After hydration, the skin and bone prominences should be protected using cotton gauze and foam, with the aim of filling in any anatomical spaces. The compressive bandaging is done using low-elasticity bandage rolls. It is started on the fingers and then the forearm and the upper arm. The pressure exerted by the bandaging is greater in the distal region and diminishes towards the root of the limb (Fig. 7). It is also important to respect the trophic conditions of the skin. The compressive bandaging is kept in place until the next physiotherapy session, i.e. for two days.

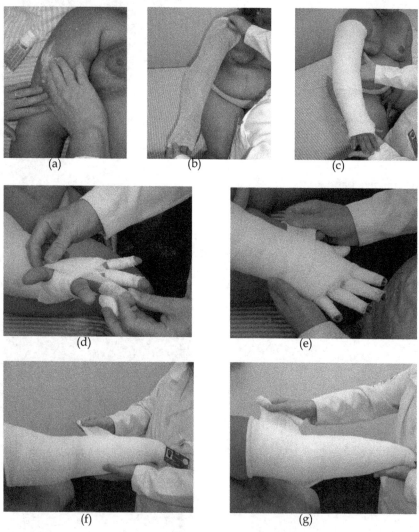

Fig. 7. Functional compressive bandaging: a) hydration; b) placement of cotton gauze; c) protection with cotton gauze; e) bandaging, starting with the fingers; f) bandaging on forearm; g) bandaging on upper arm.

The second phase, called the maintenance phase, has the aims of keeping the interstitial pressures in balance and optimizing the results obtained from the first phase of the treatment. It consists of using compression garments, skincare, hydration, kinesiotherapy and manual self-massage (Foldi et al., 1985; Camargo & Marx, 2000; Bergmann et al.; Leal et al., 2009; Sarri et al., 2010).

3.3 Compression garments
The aim of using compression garments is to maintain and optimize the results obtained from the first phase of lymphedema treatment and avoid recurrences, through keeping the interstitial pressures in balance. They should be used continuously and only be removed for personal hygiene. The model of garment and the compression used depend on the patient's needs (Fig. 8). Concomitantly with using the compression garments, the patient should also comply with the guidance previously given regarding limb care, hydration and kinesiotherapy. (Foldi et al., 1985; Roucout & Oliveira, 1999; Andersen et al., 2000; Camargo & Marx, 2000; Huit, 2000; Hampton, 2003). In our institution, we use compression garments in conjunction with self-massage and kinesiotherapy in cases of initial lymphedema, with significant improvements achieved.

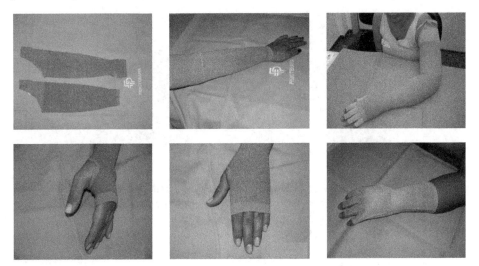

Fig. 8. Garments and gloves for elastic containment.

3.4 Lymphatic self-massage
Lymphatic self-massage, also known as simple manual lymphatic drainage, is a version of manual lymphatic drainage. The technique for this procedure is taught to the patient, who can then perform this alone, at home every day. It involves a series of gentle circular movements that begin with stimulation of the contralateral axillary lymph node chains and the inguinal chains homolateral to the surgical manipulation, followed by gentle movements starting at a place distant from the congested area and moving towards the edematous limb (Foldi et al., 1985; Camargo & Marx, 2000; Williams et al., 2002; Linnitt, 2005).

The patient should begin the self-massage with circular movements in the contralateral axillary region, with the palms in the axilla, lightly and gently moving the skin 30 times, and then repeating this in the inguinal region homolateral to the axillary dissection. After the axillary and inguinal lymph node chains have been stimulated, hand movements are made with the aim of shifting the lymph from the operated axilla to the contralateral axilla, in the region above the surgery. The same movement is then made to shift the lymph from the manipulated axilla to the homolateral inguinal region. The movement in each region is repeated 30 times (Fig. 9).

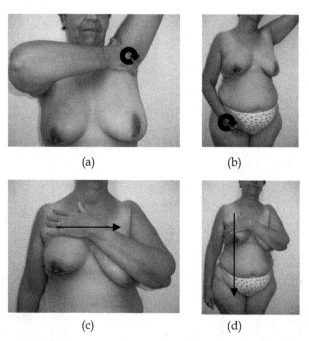

(a)   (b)

(c)   (d)

Fig. 9. Lymphatic self-massage on patient who underwent right axillary dissection:
a) axillary lymph node chain stimulation; b) inguinal lymph node chain stimulation;
c) wavelike maneuver directing the lymphatic flow towards the contralateral axillary region;
d) wavelike maneuver directing the lymphatic flow towards the ipsilateral inguinal region.

3.5 Pneumatic compression

This consists of mechanical compression with air pumps, on the edematous limb. There are basically two types of compression pumps: the segmental or sequential type and the dynamic type. Individual use of pneumatic compression has not shown satisfactory results, and high incidence of complications has been found. Several studies have combined its use with other types of treatment for lymphedema, such as the use of lymph therapy (Dini et al., 1998; Leduc et al., 1998; Camargo & Marx, 2000; Szuba et al., 2002; Leal et al., 2009).

4. Axillary web syndrome

Axillary web syndrome, also known as cording (Box et al., 2002), axillary strings (Lauridsen et al., 2005), or vascular strings (Johansson et al., 2001), is a sequela of breast cancer treatment (Fourie & Robb, 2009). It is developed between the first and fifth week after axillary dissection, as tense and painful strings under the skin of the axilla. It may extend as far as the cubital fossa or the medial face of the upper arm (Tilley et al., 2009). It is always associated with pain and limitation of shoulder and elbow movement (Lauridsen et al., 2005). Its incidence and predisposing factors are not well defined in the worldwide literature (Moskovitz et al., 2001). It is believed that interruption of the axillar lymphatic vessels has an important role in the development of this syndrome. Lymphovenous lesions with stasis, thrombophlebitis, aseptic lymphangitis and lesions in the lymphatic ducts also seem to be involved (Johansson et al., 2001; Moskovitz et al., 2001; Lauridsen et al., 2005). The literature is deficient with regard to the approach to be taken in cases of AWS. Some papers have shown that this syndrome resolves within three months, without specific treatment (Moskovitz et al., 2001; Leidenius et al., 2003). Other studies have shown benefits from implementing active range-of-motion exercises, stretching exercises and manual manipulation techniques (Moskovitz et al., 2001; Leidenius et al., 2003; Fourie & Robb, 2009; Tilley et al., 2009).

In our service, we have used string stretching with very favorable results. The maneuver consists of stretching the string with the thumbs, while applying pressure from central to distal regions, as shown in Fig. 10. This maneuver triggers tolerable local pain that is relieved as soon as the maneuver ends, thereby enabling movements that had previously been limited (Fig. 11). We have also used active and passive kinesiotherapy on the limb and light stretching.

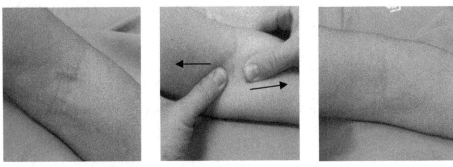

Fig. 10. Axillary Web Syndrome maneuver: a) string in anterior region of elbow; b) axillary web syndrome maneuver; c) anterior region of forearm after maneuver, without string.

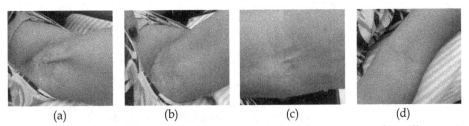

(a)   (b)   (c)   (d)

Fig. 11. Axillary Web Syndrome: a) axillary region before the maneuver; b) axillary region after the maneuver; c) anterior region of the elbow before the maneuver; d) anterior region of the elbow after the maneuver.

5. Limitation of shoulder movement

Restriction of shoulder movement, which is one of the complications following axillary lymph node dissection, may occur because of tissue and nerve lesions, with prevalence of 7-36%. This musculoskeletal disorder of the shoulder results in considerable joint debility and pain. The symptoms generally diminish within three months, but they may become chronic, thus interfering with these patients' quality of life (Kärki et al., 2001; Beurskens et al., 2007). Early physiotherapeutic treatment is effective for this disorder and promotes faster functional recovery (Kärki et al., 2001; Lauridsen et al., 2005; Beurskens et al., 2007). The treatment should be progressive, taking care in manipulating the limb so as to avoid tissue or muscle injuries. Passive exercises, assisted active exercises, active exercises of the scapular belt, neck relaxation and postural guidance should be undertaken.

6. Painful post-mastectomy syndrome

Chronic pain secondary to surgical treatment for breast cancer is of neuropathic origin or results from muscle and ligament injuries. Intercostal brachial neuralgia has been correlated most frequently in axillary treatments, in which the nerve may become injured because of its proximity (Poleshuck et al., 2006; Labreze et al., 2007; Couceiro et al., 2009). Such pain may be continuous or intermittent, with varying intensity, and it can be located in the anterior wall of the chest, the axilla or the medial face of the upper arm (Vecht et al., 1989; Caffo et al., 2003; Burckhardt & Jones, 2005). The physiotherapeutic treatment consists of specific analgesia techniques, such as transcutaneous electrical nerve stimulation (TENS), cryotherapy and kinesiotherapy. It can also be implemented in association with the use of analgesic medications.

7. Conclusion

In conclusion, physiotherapeutic interventions on patients who have undergone axillary lymph node manipulation can be implemented at any postoperative stage. However, it is increasingly certain that early intervention significantly minimizes the emergence of lymphedema.

8. Acknowledgements

The authors thank Barretos Cancer Hospital, and their coworkers Thiago Buosi and Carla Laurienzo da Cunha Andrade.

9. References

Andersen, L., Hojris, I., Erlandsen, M. & Andersen, J. (2000). Treatment of breast-cancer-related lymphedema with or without manual lymphatic drainage. A randomized study. *Acta Oncol*, Vol. 39, No. 3, pp. 399-405, ISSN 0284-186X.

Araujo, J. A., Curbelo, J. G., Mayol, A. L., Pascal, G. G., Vignale, R. A. & Fleurquin, F. (1997). Effective management of marked lymphedema of the leg. *Int J Dermatol*, Vol. 36, No. 5, May, pp. 389-92, ISSN 0011-9059 (Print), ISSN 0011-9059 (Linking)

Bergmann, A., Ribeiro, M. J. P., Pedrosa, E., Nogueira, E. A. & Oliveira, A. C. G. (2006). Physical Therapy in Breast Cancer: clinical protocol at the Cancer Hospital III/INCA. *Rev Bras Cancerol*, Vol. 52, No. 1, pp. 97-109, ISSN 0100-7203 (Print)

Beurskens, C. H., Van Uden, C. J., Strobbe, L. J., Oostendorp, R. A. & Wobbes, T. (2007). The efficacy of physiotherapy upon shoulder function following axillary dissection in breast cancer, a randomized controlled study. *BMC Cancer*, Vol. 7, pp. 166, ISSN 1471-2407 (Electronic), ISSN 1471-2407 (Linking)

Bourgeois, P., Leduc, O. & Leduc, A. (1998). Imaging techniques in the management and prevention of posttherapeutic upper limb edemas. *Cancer*, Vol. 83, No. 12 Suppl American, Dec 15, pp. 2805-13, ISSN 0008-543X (Print)

Box, R. C., Reul-Hirche, H. M., Bullock-Saxton, J. E. & Furnival, C. M. (2002). Shoulder movement after breast cancer surgery: results of a randomised controlled study of postoperative physiotherapy. *Breast Cancer Res Treat*, Vol. 75, No. 1, Sep, pp. 35-50, ISSN 0167-6806 (Print), ISSN 0167-6806 (Linking)

Bumpers, H. L., Best, I. M., Norman, D. & Weaver, W. L. (2002). Debilitating lymphedema of the upper extremity after treatment of breast cancer. *Am J Clin Oncol*, Vol. 25, No. 4, Aug, pp. 365-7, ISSN 0277-3732 (Print), ISSN 0277-3732 (Linking)

Burckhardt, C. S. & Jones, K. D. (2005). Effects of chronic widespread pain on the health status and quality of life of women after breast cancer surgery. *Health Qual Life Outcomes*, Vol. 3, pp. 30, ISSN 1477-7525 (Electronic), ISSN 1477-7525 (Linking)

Caffo, O., Amichetti, M., Ferro, A., Lucenti, A., Valduga, F. & Galligioni, E. (2003). Pain and quality of life after surgery for breast cancer. *Breast Cancer Res Treat*, Vol. 80, No. 1, Jul, pp. 39-48, ISSN 0167-6806 (Print), ISSN 0167-6806 (Linking)

Camargo, M. C. & Marx, A. G. (2000) *Reabilitação Física no Câncer de Mama*. (1ª. ed), Editora Roca, São Paulo

Carpentier, P. H. (2002). Physiopathology of lymphedema. *Rev Med Interne*, Vol. 23 Suppl 3, Jun, pp. 371s-374s, ISSN 0248-8663 (Print)

Clodius, L., Piller, N. B. & Casley-Smith, J. R. (1981). The problems of lymphatic microsurgery for lymphedema. *Lymphology*, Vol. 14, No. 2, Jun, pp. 69-76, ISSN 0024-7766 (Print)

Couceiro, T. C., Menezes, T. C. & Valenca, M. M. (2009). Post-mastectomy pain syndrome: the magnitude of the problem. *Rev Bras Anestesiol*, Vol. 59, No. 3, May-Jun, pp. 358-65, ISSN 1806-907X (Electronic), ISSN 0034-7094 (Linking)

Didem, K., Ufuk, Y. S., Serdar, S. & Zumre, A. (2005). The comparison of two different physiotherapy methods in treatment of lymphedema after breast surgery. *Breast Cancer Res Treat*, Vol. 93, No. 1, Sep, pp. 49-54, ISSN 0167-6806 (Print)

Dini, D., Del Mastro, L., Gozza, A., Lionetto, R., Garrone, O., Forno, G., Vidili, G., Bertelli, G. & Venturini, M. (1998). The role of pneumatic compression in the treatment of postmastectomy lymphedema. A randomized phase III study. *Ann Oncol*, Vol. 9, No. 2, Feb, pp. 187-90, ISSN 0923-7534 (Print), ISSN 0923-7534 (Linking)

Filippetti, M., Santoro, E., Graziano, F., Petric, M. & Rinaldi, G. (1994). Modern therapeutic approaches to postmastectomy brachial lymphedema. *Microsurgery*, Vol. 15, No. 8, pp. 604-10, ISSN 0738-1085 (Print)

Foldi, E. (1998). The treatment of lymphedema. *Cancer*, Vol. 83, No. 12 Suppl American, Dec 15, pp. 2833-4, ISSN 0008-543X (Print), ISSN 0008-543X (Linking)

Foldi, E., Foldi, M. & Weissleder, H. (1985). Conservative treatment of lymphoedema of the limbs. *Angiology*, Vol. 36, No. 3, Mar, pp. 171-80, ISSN 0003-3197 (Print)

Fourie, W. J. & Robb, K. A. (2009). Physiotherapy management of axillary web syndrome following breast cancer treatment: discussing the use of soft tissue techniques. *Physiotherapy*, Vol. 95, No. 4, Dec, pp. 314-20, ISSN 1873-1465 (Electronic), ISSN 0031-9406 (Linking)

Fritsch, C. & Tomson, D. (1991). The usefulness of lymphatic drainage. *Schweiz Rundsch Med Prax*, Vol. 80, No. 15, Apr 9, pp. 383-6, ISSN 1013-2058 (Print), ISSN 1013-2058 (Linking)

Glass, E. C., Essner, R. & Giuliano, A. E. (1999). Sentinel node localization in breast cancer. *Semin Nucl Med*, Vol. 29, No. 1, Jan, pp. 57-68, ISSN 0001-2998 (Print)

Goffman, T. E., Laronga, C., Wilson, L. & Elkins, D. (2004). Lymphedema of the arm and breast in irradiated breast cancer patients: risks in an era of dramatically changing axillary surgery. *Breast J*, Vol. 10, No. 5, Sep-Oct, pp. 405-11, ISSN 1075-122X (Print)

Hampton, S. (2003). Elvarex compression garments in the management of lymphoedema. *Br J Nurs*, Vol. 12, No. 15, Aug 14-Sep 10, pp. 925-6, 928-9, ISSN 0966-0461 (Print)

Huit, M. (2000). A guide to treating lymphoedema. *Nurs Times*, Vol. 96, No. 38, Sep 21-27, pp. 42-3, ISSN 0954-7762 (Print), ISSN 0954-7762 (Linking)

Johansson, K., Ingvar, C., Albertsson, M. & Ekdahl, C. (2001). Arm lymphoedema, shoulder mobility and muscle strenght after breast cancer treatment - a prospective 2-year study. *Adv Phys Ther*, No. 3, pp. 55-66, ISSN 2159-2896 (Electronic)

Johansson, S., Svensson, H. & Denekamp, J. (2002). Dose response and latency for radiation-induced fibrosis, edema, and neuropathy in breast cancer patients. *Int J Radiat Oncol Biol Phys*, Vol. 52, No. 5, Apr 1, pp. 1207-19, ISSN 0360-3016 (Print)

Kärki, A., Simonen, R., Mälkiä, E. & Self, J. (2001). Efficacy of physical therapy methods and exercise after a breast cancer operation: a systematic review. *Crit Rev Phys Rehab Med*, Vol. 13, pp. 159-190, ISSN 0896-2960 (Print)

King, B. (2006). Diagnosis and management of lymphoedema. *Nurs Times*, Vol. 102, No. 13, Mar 28-Apr 3, pp. 47, 49, 51, ISSN 0954-7762 (Print)

King, M. J. & Difalco, E. G. (2005). Lymphedema: skin and wound care in an aging population. *Ostomy Wound Manage*, Vol. 51, No. 11A Suppl, Nov, pp. 14-6, ISSN 0889-5899 (Print)

Kwan, W., Jackson, J., Weir, L. M., Dingee, C., Mcgregor, G. & Olivotto, I. A. (2002). Chronic arm morbidity after curative breast cancer treatment: prevalence and impact on quality of life. *J Clin Oncol*, Vol. 20, No. 20, Oct 15, pp. 4242-8, ISSN 0732-183X (Print)

Labreze, L., Dixmerias-Iskandar, F., Monnin, D., Bussieres, E., Delahaye, E., Bernard, D. & Lakdja, F. (2007). [Postmastectomy pain syndrome evidence based guidelines and decision trees]. *Bull Cancer*, Vol. 94, No. 3, Mar 1, pp. 275-85, ISSN 1769-6917 (Electronic), ISSN 0007-4551 (Linking)

Lauridsen, M. C., Christiansen, P. & Hessov, I. (2005). The effect of physiotherapy on shoulder function in patients surgically treated for breast cancer: a randomized study. *Acta Oncol*, Vol. 44, No. 5, pp. 449-57, ISSN 0284-186X (Print), ISSN 0284-186X (Linking)

Leal, N. F., Carrara, H. H., Vieira, K. F. & Ferreira, C. H. (2009). Physiotherapy treatments for breast cancer-related lymphedema: a literature review. *Rev Lat Am Enfermagem*, Vol. 17, No. 5, Sep-Oct, pp. 730-6, ISSN 0104-1169 (Print), ISSN 0104-1169 (Linking)

Leduc, O., Leduc, A., Bourgeois, P. & Belgrado, J. P. (1998). The physical treatment of upper limb edema. *Cancer*, Vol. 83, No. 12 Suppl American, Dec 15, pp. 2835-9, ISSN 0008-543X (Print), ISSN 0008-543X (Linking)

Lee, T. S., Kilbreath, S. L., Refshauge, K. M., Herbert, R. D. & Beith, J. M. (2008). Prognosis of the upper limb following surgery and radiation for breast cancer. *Breast Cancer Res Treat*, Vol. 110, No. 1, Jul, pp. 19-37, ISSN 0167-6806 (Print), ISSN 0167-6806 (Linking)

Leidenius, M., Leppanen, E., Krogerus, L. & Von Smitten, K. (2003). Motion restriction and axillary web syndrome after sentinel node biopsy and axillary clearance in breast cancer. *Am J Surg*, Vol. 185, No. 2, Feb, pp. 127-30, ISSN 0002-9610 (Print), ISSN 0002-9610 (Linking)

Linnitt, N. (2005). Lymphoedema: recognition, assessment and management. *Br J Community Nurs*, Vol. 10, No. 3, Mar, pp. S20-6, ISSN 1462-4753 (Print)

Linnitt, N. (2007). Complex skin changes in chronic oedemas. *Br J Community Nurs*, Vol. 12, No. 4, Apr, pp. S10-5, ISSN 1462-4753 (Print)

Moseley, A. L., Carati, C. J. & Piller, N. B. (2007). A systematic review of common conservative therapies for arm lymphoedema secondary to breast cancer treatment. *Ann Oncol*, Vol. 18, No. 4, Apr, pp. 639-46, ISSN 0923-7534 (Print), ISSN 0923-7534 (Linking)

Moskovitz, A. H., Anderson, B. O., Yeung, R. S., Byrd, D. R., Lawton, T. J. & Moe, R. E. (2001). Axillary web syndrome after axillary dissection. *Am J Surg*, Vol. 181, No. 5, May, pp. 434-9, ISSN 0002-9610 (Print), ISSN 0002-9610 (Linking)

Paci, E., Cariddi, A., Barchielli, A., Bianchi, S., Cardona, G., Distante, V., Giorgi, D., Pacini, P., Zappa, M. & Del Turco, M. R. (1996). Long-term sequelae of breast cancer surgery. *Tumori*, Vol. 82, No. 4, Jul-Aug, pp. 321-4, ISSN 0300-8916 (Print)

Parkin, D. M. & Fernandez, L. M. (2006). Use of statistics to assess the global burden of breast cancer. *Breast J*, Vol. 12 Suppl 1, Jan-Feb, pp. S70-80, ISSN 1075-122X (Print), ISSN 1075-122X (Linking)

Paskett, E. D. (2008). Breast cancer-related lymphedema: attention to a significant problem resulting from cancer diagnosis. *J Clin Oncol*, Vol. 26, No. 35, Dec 10, pp. 5666-7, ISSN 1527-7755 (Electronic), ISSN 0732-183X (Linking)

Poleshuck, E. L., Katz, J., Andrus, C. H., Hogan, L. A., Jung, B. F., Kulick, D. I. & Dworkin, R. H. (2006). Risk factors for chronic pain following breast cancer surgery: a prospective study. *J Pain*, Vol. 7, No. 9, Sep, pp. 626-34, ISSN 1526-5900 (Print), ISSN 1526-5900 (Linking)

Rezende, L. F., Beletti, P. O., Franco, R. L., Moraes, S. S. & Gurgel, M. S. (2006). [Random clinical comparative trial between free and directed exercise in post-operative complications of breast cancer]. *Rev Assoc Med Bras*, Vol. 52, No. 1, Jan-Feb, pp. 37-42, ISSN 0104-4230 (Print) ISSN 0104-4230 (Linking)

Rietman, J. S., Dijkstra, P. U., Geertzen, J. H., Baas, P., De Vries, J., Dolsma, W. V., Groothoff, J. W., Eisma, W. H. & Hoekstra, H. J. (2004). Treatment-related upper limb morbidity 1 year after sentinel lymph node biopsy or axillary lymph node dissection for stage I or II breast cancer. *Ann Surg Oncol*, Vol. 11, No. 11, Nov, pp. 1018-24, ISSN 1068-9265 (Print)

Ronka, R. H., Pamilo, M. S., Von Smitten, K. A. & Leidenius, M. H. (2004). Breast lymphedema after breast conserving treatment. *Acta Oncol*, Vol. 43, No. 6, pp. 551-7, ISSN 0284-186X (Print) ISSN 0284-186X (Linking)

Roucout, S. & Oliveira, V. (1999). Etiologia, prevenção e tratamento do linfedema. *Med Reab*, Vol. 49, pp. 11-15, ISSN 0103-5894

Sakorafas, G. H., Peros, G., Cataliotti, L. & Vlastos, G. (2006). Lymphedema following axillary lymph node dissection for breast cancer. *Surg Oncol*, Vol. 15, No. 3, Nov, pp. 153-65, ISSN 0960-7404 (Print) ISSN 0960-7404 (Linking)

Sarri, A. J., Moriguchi, S. M., Dias, R., Perez, S. V., Silva, E. T., Koga, K. H., Mathes, A. G. Z., Santos, M. J., Rocha, E. T. & Haikel, R. L. (2010). Physiotherapeutic stimulation: Early prevention of lymphedema following axillary lymph node dissection for breast cancer treatment. *Experimental and Therapeutic Medicine*, Vol. 1, pp. 147-152, ISSN 1792-0981 (Print). ISSN 1792-1015 (Eletronic)

Springer, B. A., Levy, E., Mcgarvey, C., Pfalzer, L. A., Stout, N. L., Gerber, L. H., Soballe, P. W. & Danoff, J. (2010). Pre-operative assessment enables early diagnosis and recovery of shoulder function in patients with breast cancer. *Breast Cancer Res Treat*, Vol. 120, No. 1, Feb, pp. 135-47, ISSN 1573-7217 (Electronic) ISSN 0167-6806 (Linking)

Stanton, A. W., Modi, S., Mellor, R. H., Levick, J. R. & Mortimer, P. S. (2009). Recent advances in breast cancer-related lymphedema of the arm: lymphatic pump failure and predisposing factors. *Lymphat Res Biol*, Vol. 7, No. 1, pp. 29-45, ISSN 1539-6851 (Print)

Szuba, A., Achalu, R. & Rockson, S. G. (2002). Decongestive lymphatic therapy for patients with breast carcinoma-associated lymphedema. A randomized, prospective study of a role for adjunctive intermittent pneumatic compression. *Cancer*, Vol. 95, No. 11, Dec 1, pp. 2260-7, ISSN 0008-543X (Print), ISSN 0008-543X (Linking)

Szuba, A., Shin, W. S., Strauss, H. W. & Rockson, S. (2003). The third circulation: radionuclide lymphoscintigraphy in the evaluation of lymphedema. *J Nucl Med*, Vol. 44, No. 1, Jan, pp. 43-57, ISSN 0161-5505 (Print)

Tilley, A., Thomas-Maclean, R. & Kwan, W. (2009). Lymphatic cording or axillary web syndrome after breast cancer surgery. *Can J Surg*, Vol. 52, No. 4, Aug, pp. E105-E106, ISSN 1488-2310 (Electronic), ISSN 0008-428X (Linking)

Van Der Veen, P., De Voogdt, N., Lievens, P., Duquet, W., Lamote, J. & Sacre, R. (2004). Lymphedema development following breast cancer surgery with full axillary resection. *Lymphology*, Vol. 37, No. 4, Dec, pp. 206-8, ISSN 0024-7766 (Print)

Vecht, C. J., Van De Brand, H. J. & Wajer, O. J. (1989). Post-axillary dissection pain in breast cancer due to a lesion of the intercostobrachial nerve. *Pain*, Vol. 38, No. 2, Aug, pp. 171-6, ISSN 0304-3959 (Print), ISSN 0304-3959 (Linking)

Weissleder, H. & Weissleder, R. (1988). Lymphedema: evaluation of qualitative and quantitative lymphoscintigraphy in 238 patients. *Radiology*, Vol. 167, No. 3, Jun, pp. 729-35, ISSN 0033-8419 (Print), ISSN 0033-8419 (Linking)

Williams, A. F., Vadgama, A., Franks, P. J. & Mortimer, P. S. (2002). A randomized controlled crossover study of manual lymphatic drainage therapy in women with breast cancer-related lymphoedema. *Eur J Cancer Care (Engl)*, Vol. 11, No. 4, Dec, pp. 254-61, ISSN 0961-5423 (Print)

6

The Evolving Role of Tissue Biospecimens in the Treatment of Cancer

Wilfrido D. Mojica
University at Buffalo, State University of New York
United States of America

1. Introduction

The field of surgical pathology is diagnostic in nature and since its inception, has always supported the treatment of cancer. The manner by which tissues are processed may vary between institutions, but the vast majority utilize formaldehyde as the fixative of choice. This fixative allows for excellent architectural tissue preservation thereby enabling optimal microscopic examination, the foundation from which surgical pathology is based upon. From fixed tissue, cancers have been categorized, sub-typed and features enumerated to help elucidate the differences that exist between them. Classification schemes that include grading and staging systems have been incorporated in their examination and, when coupled with the patient's clinical data, have been useful in prognostication and guidance of follow-up treatment. The development of immunohistochemistry has only served to further ingrain the importance of proper tissue fixation with cancer sample preparation. Yet, despite providing the basis for these invaluable contributions, the approach of fixing tissue biospecimens with formaldehyde has, in recent years, undergone criticism as being a suboptimal means of preservation when molecular analysis is desired from these specimens. Added to this are other pressures to develop novel approaches by which tissue biospecimens can be interrogated. Within the field of surgical pathology, it is becoming recognized that various pre and post fixation factors may contribute to negatively impact the overall integrity of the tissue biospecimen. Outside surgical pathology, the continually decreasing size of core biopsy specimens are minimizing the amount of tissue present for architectural evaluation. In addition, newer treatments are continually being sought in order to further personalize cancer treatment based on the type of tumor present in the tissue specimen. These forces are necessitating a re-evaluation of the entire established process of fixation, and whether alternative methods may exist or be developed that may be more amenable for both diagnosis and biospecimen integrity. In this chapter, the central role of tissue biospecimens for the support and guidance of cancer care are discussed, with an examination on how newer technologies and minimally invasive approaches will change the landscape by which these specimens will be processed.

2. The history of tissue biospecimens in cancer treatment

The examination of tissue through the microscope falls within the modern day purview of surgical pathology. Although this examination is now performed by pathologists, the emerging field of surgical pathology in the 19th century began with surgeons. Before the widespread acknowledgement that microscopic examination of tissue was compulsory for an adequate diagnosis, surgeons were limited to the gross examination of specimens and their personal assessment and experience as to whether the extirpated specimen was benign or malignant (Gal, 2001). At that time, malignant tumors often ran their course, and their examination in the living patient limited to only observation at the gross, not microscopic level. In 1856 Rudolf Virchow published the first book on histopathology, introducing the world of microanatomy to the medical community. Observations from this book and those that followed slowly led to a newfound understanding that diseases of the human body could be correlated to findings at the cellular level. A number of discoveries and inventions in the 19th century also proved instrumental in providing the basis from which tissue could be reliably and widely examined by others under the microscope. These advances, like the invention of the microtome for cutting thin tissue sections and the discovery of natural and synthetic dyes like hematoxylin for the staining of nuclei and eosin for the cytoplasm of cells, allowed for the reproducible examination of tissue and the subsequent classification of organ structure. With these advancements, excised tissue was no longer discarded, but examined and documented. The first observations between malignant and benign tissues were recorded, with malignant cells described as being different in size and shape, not connected at their margins, possessing nuclei that varied in size and number and forming irregular edges at their juxtaposition with the adjacent normal tissue. In contrast, the cells of benign epithelial growths resembled each other in size and shape, had fairly homogenous appearing nuclei, were more cohesive along the edges of their cell borders and formed straighter lines (Rosai, 1997). With time, specimen processing and evaluation of the specimen became more standardized. Through correlation over time with the clinical outcome of the patient and with observations of similar tumors from other patients, these tissue biospecimens became the first to influence the treatment of cancer in patients. With improvements in surgical techniques, anesthesia and the application of antiseptic precautions, surgeons began to broaden the degree of surgical intervention they performed on patients. The development of the frozen section, wherein a portion of the specimen was excised and sent to the pathologist for evaluation intra-operatively, burgeoned and soon became integral to the cancer patient's care. The rapid freezing and hardening of the tissue specimen enabled the cutting of thin sections that could subsequently be stained and evaluated under the microscope. The surgeon now could know if the excised margins of a tumor specimen still had tumor cells in them, allowing for an intra-operative decision as to whether additional sections were needed or not. For certain other tumors, determining the depth of invasion through the frozen section became integral in planning out the remainder of the surgical plan for the cancer patient. The processing of the biospecimen would evolve to include frozen section evaluation on some, and fixation with paraffin embedding on the majority of excised tissue specimens sent to the pathology laboratory. Through the microscopic examination of all the subsequent slides, the diagnosis that is formulated by a pathologist is based on the resemblance and similarities to an archival history of previously diagnosed specimens that have been correlated with clinical outcome. This largely empiric system has served the medical community well, with the diagnostic information rendered by the pathologist enough to guide the cancer patient's care and estimate their prognosis (Kufe, 2003).

2.1 Early tools in the assessment of tissue and tumor biospecimens

Along with hematoxylin and eosin, a number of other stains were specifically developed to help identify cell structure and determine cellular function, but in the process aided to further classify tissues and categorize tumors. Their development was spurred by the fact that, despite the enumeration of histologic criteria published and disseminated about specific diseases and tumors, reproducibility among the growing numbers of physicians that practiced pathology remained a problem. In order to engender consensus, a number of special stains were created through experimentation that would eventually serve to better delineate cellular structure, content and properties. One of these stains, the Periodic Acid Schiff stain, allowed for the detection of the presence of carbohydrate macromolecules, a feature that would prove to be a useful ancillary aid to morphology in the differentiation between different types of tumors. For example, the identification of the Periodic Acid Schiff reaction in tumors known as small round blue cells can be helpful in leading to the correct diagnosis. Positive staining material in rhabdomyosarcomas, Ewing's sarcomas, malignant peripheral neuroectodermal tumors and germinomas can help distinguish them from other tumors with similar histologic features such as desmoplastic small round cell tumors, small cell mesothelioma, and a number of other tumors with small round blue cell morphology (Leuschner, 1996). This stain is particularly helpful in identifying Ewing's sarcoma, due to the fact that over 80% of these tumors have been reported to contain glycogen within their cytoplasm. Other special stains, like the Mucicarmine and Alcian blue stains, were originally used to help characterize cells that secreted mucin, aid in the early differential diagnosis of tumors and determine if they were useful in identification of tumor origin for metastatic tumors (Johnson, 1963). These stains have persevered and have modern day utility in defining poorly differentiated tumors as being or not being adenocarcinoma and in distinguishing adenocarcinomas from poorly differentiated squamous cell carcinomas in the evaluation of lung cancers for the former stain, and as an aid in the detection of intestinal metaplasia in the medical condition known as Barrett's esophagus for the latter stain (Wallace, 2009). Yet another special stain, the reticulin stain, showed initial promise for staining specific extracellular matrix constituents, namely the collagen type III fibers that comprise the stromal network in many different organs. It can be particularly prominent in the liver, as these fibers invest the hepatocytes that make up the hepatic plates, with normal hepatic plates being two cell layers thick or less. Reticulin stains help to define hepatic adenomas and hepatocellular carcinomas from normal liver, subtle changes not so obvious when examined by hematoxylin and eosin stains alone. In hepatic adenomas, they show an expansile growth pattern whereas in hepatocellular carcinoma they demonstrate an increase in trabecular thickness. To this day, the reticulin stain continues to be recommended as part of the evaluation of nodules within the liver (Lennerz et, 2009).

Later, the development of the electron microscope, with its ability to probe sub-cellular structure, proved a boon to tissue diagnostics as it related to cancer treatment. Delivery of the correct diagnosis enabled a treating physician the opportunity to give the most clinically relevant care. Electron microscopy allowed for the visualization of subcellular organelles that could otherwise not be discerned using traditional light microscopy. When tumor tissue was examined at the electron microscopy level, the presence or absence of organelles known to be specific to certain cell types enabled the identification of poorly differentiated tumors whose cell of origin could not, at the time, be properly classified at the morphologic level. The electron microscope provided more definitive characterization of tumor subtypes than histology and special stains. In the case of Ewing's sarcoma, although it was known to be one of the tumors that possesses cytoplasmic glycogen, variability in the degree of differentiation could mean that their abundance may also be variable, and hence it was advised that the diagnosis of Ewing's sarcoma should not be based solely on the presence of glycogen detected by the Periodic Acid Schiff stain in tissue sections with the appropriate morphology. One factor may have played a role in this ambiguity, was the type of fixative being used. Eventually it was determined that the best fixative for detecting glycogen in tissue sections was alcohol, and that fixation in formaldehyde resulted in variable preservation of this macromolecule (Llombaart-Bosch, 1996). Additionally, it was also learned that specimens that were poorly fixed could lead to a complete absence of detectable glycogen. In these cases, ultrastructural evaluation would prove to be helpful in establishing the correct diagnosis. In the case of Ewing's sarcoma, examination at the ultrastructural level revealed the presence of two cell types, the primary cell referred to as the light or principal cell, and a secondary cell referred to as the dark cell. The principal cell was characterized as having homogeneously sized nuclei and ample cytoplasms, sparse numbers of organelles and abundant glycogen. The dark cells possessed elongated to ovoid nuclei with condensed chromatin, and likened to involuting principal cells. The identification of these cells have helped to characterize Ewing's sarcoma as different from other tumors possessing a similar histologic appearance, particularly olfactory neuroblastomas (Trump, 1983). Another instance where electron microscopy has impacted cancer care and proven integral to the proper identification of a tumor is in the case of poorly differentiated tumors of the pleural cavities. In these situations the differential diagnosis revolves between poorly differentiated adenocarcinoma versus mesothelioma. An incorrect diagnosis of adenocarcinoma, when in reality a tumor is a mesothelioma, can result in an expensive and time consuming work-up and legal issues. For quite a while, electron microscopy was considered the gold standard in the diagnosis of mesothelioma. The presence of long, slender, sinuous, branching and bushy microvilli found on the cell surface at the ultrastructural level were reported as being pathognomonic features for diagnosing mesothelioma (Velez, 2002). Taken altogether, the development of special stains and electron microscopy aided in leading to the further sub-classification of tumor tissue biospecimens. These tools were readily incorporated into the surgical pathology community and contributed to the early attempts to tailor patient cancer care. Despite the advances these tools brought to patient cancer care, their limitations would eventually become apparent with the development of a newer tool that would be introduced to the armamentarium of surgical pathology, immunohistochemistry.

2.2 Immunohistochemistry and the beginning of the end for empiric medicine
In the latter half of the 20th century the ability to exploit the specificity of the antibody-antigen reaction was successfully transferred from the experimental laboratory to clinical specimens. This application began with the immunofluoresence technique. However, the major liability with this approach was three-fold: the need for a specialized microscope with fluorescence capabilities; the pre-requisite for fresh frozen tissue samples; and poor morphologic resolution (Taylor, 1994). Over the period from the mid 1970's to the early 1990's these obstacles were eventually addressed with the development of alternative, non-fluoresence labels and the discovery of antigen retrieval. In the latter, the abolishment of the interfering formalin induced cross-links in fixed tissue specimens led to the widespread application of this technique, now called immunohistochemistry, to the vast archive of fixed tissue specimens banked in pathology departments. A period in the surgical pathology

community began anew, similar to the advent of special stains and electron microscopy eras, wherein panels of recently developed antibodies were tested against series of tissue and tumor specimens with the intent to identify and again better characterize human disease. This period, as with the introduction of all new tools in the fields of diagnostic pathology, was met with initial skepticism. However, one key difference that this new tool brought would emerge that would distinguish it from that of its' predecessors in the care of cancer patients. The previous tools only enabled the observation of cellular organelles and cytoplasmic or nuclear constituents. The technique of immunohistochemistry, with the specificity of the antibody-antigen relationship, allowed unprecedented access to the macromolecules integral to the functions of the cell, proteins. Through subsequent investigations of an assortment of proteins by a myriad of different investigators, the era of Personalized Medicine, in terms of its current day namesake, was unceremoniously ushered in. It now became possible to identify the presence or absence of proteins in specific cell types and tumors. In contrast to traditional empiric medicine, immunohistochemistry allowed for the identification of a specific target molecule in specific cell types. In empiric medicine, not all patients will respond to a specific drug based on the absence of the knowledge if the cancer cells in a patient contained those proteins acted upon by the drug, or had only low levels of those targeted proteins. With the advent of immunohistochemistry, proteins that were involved in or acted to drive the process of oncogenesis could now be identified. This identification allowed for rational drug treatment, with therapy based on the presence of a target protein or molecule in a cancer patient identified by immunohistochemistry on the tissue specimens. This approach represents the potential to significantly improve cancer care, taking into account the fact that the efficacy of pharmacotherapy in oncology is less than 50% (Jorgensen, 2009). In the very least, this approach will help eliminate the administration of certain therapeutic agents to those cancer patients who would not benefit from a drug, based again on the absence of the targeted molecule or protein in the patient's tissue specimen.

Possibly the first successful implementation of Personalized Medicine can be attributed to the steroid receptor estrogen in human breast cancers. The observations in preceding decades by physicians and scientists that the growth of certain reproductive organ related tumors appeared dependent on sex steroids led to further direct investigations. Eventually it was borne out that certain tumors, like those of the breast, possessed large numbers of the estrogen receptor and thus could be targeted for endocrine therapy. Later it became apparent that the amount of estrogen receptors in these tumors could be variable, and that patients with estrogen receptor positive tumors tended to have a better clinical course than those patients with estrogen receptor negative tumors. It thus became imperative to be able to determine the estrogen receptor status in these patient's tumors. The method that became the initial mainstay to assess estrogen receptor status was the steroid ligand binding assay and involved the homogenization of tumor tissue into a lysate that was then exposed to labeled estradiol. This assay however, lacked adequate specificity and sensitivity for the clinical setting. The major drawback of this assay was the fact that it was based on a tissue homogenate and was therefore without any correlative histologic picture. Thus the proportion of tumor cells to stromal cells, or the amount of necrosis present in the sample submitted could not be accounted for in the sample. Additionally, improper collection of the sample, that is, prolonged procurement time leading to artificial loss of this labile receptor, could bias the final results. With the concurrent progress in immunohistochemistry, the development of an antibody suitable to test on frozen, and then ultimately formalin fixed and paraffin embedded tissue became available that ultimately showed suitable concordance with the steroid based assay (Ottestad, 1988). Immunohistochemistry, because it enabled visualization of the receptor status on glass slides, was relatively inexpensive compared to the ligand binding assay and could evaluate small tumors, gradually gained acceptance as a means to evaluate steroid receptor status in breast cancer patients. Currently, immunohistochemistry is the standard by which estrogen and progesterone receptor status are assessed. Their assessment in the breast cancer patient is integral in guiding that patient's direction of clinical care, as endocrine therapy has proven to be of benefit only to those that have tumors that are estrogen receptor positive. However, recent emphasis on the importance of proper tissue handling has been raised again bringing back into focus the importance of the tissue biospecimen's role in cancer care. A recent collaborative effort by the American Society of Clinical Oncology and College of American Pathologists has brought to light the startling finding that up to 20% of estrogen or progesterone receptor findings by immunohistochemistry may be inaccurate, either being falsely negative or falsely positive (Hammond, 2010). These findings were determined by taking the original results and testing the same tissue blocks at an experienced immunohistochemistry central laboratory for comparison. In order to rectify this problem, this collaborative group published recommendations for the optimal handling of extirpated breast cancer specimens that under present day methods of tissue processing, would result in reproducible inter-laboratory steroid receptor studies. In this instance, breast cancer tissue biospecimens play a continuing role in the guidance of clinical care and the quality assessment of diagnosis.

The story of the Her-2 gene and the development of the humanized monoclonal antibody trastuzumab represents a case wherein tissue biospecimens aided in the rapid identification and confirmation of a targeted cancer therapy. Through the use of tissue biospecimens, researchers were able to identify a subset of patients that overexpressed the gene product of the Her-2 gene. With clinical correlation, this subset was determined to be associated with a worse overall prognosis and a relative resistance to endocrine therapy (Press, 1993). But more importantly, the presence of this overexpressed protein meant that it defined a particular group of breast cancer patients who might benefit the greatest by the creation of an anticancer agent directed specifically at that amplified gene product. The biotechnology company Genetech eventually developed a recombinant monoclonal antibody that fit within a specific extracellular cleft and effectively abrogated any further tyrosine kinase activity. An antibody was also subsequently developed that could be used on tissue biospecimens to detect this proteins presence in breast cancer cells. Through the use of banked tissue, this antibody was tested on breast cancer tissue biospecimens, the results from which produced an FDA approved assay. The publication of these results led to the ability for pathology laboratories, community in addition to academic, to incorporate this immunostain into their diagnostic regimen. The broad use of this immunostain led to the findings that the prevalence of the HER2 gene amplification in the breast cancer population was consistently between 20 to 30 percent. Similar to estrogen and progesterone receptors, continued research in the field of biospecimen science led to the conclusion that approximately one fifth of all breast cancer tissue specimens immunostained for the Her-2 protein could be inaccurate (Wolff, 2007). A number of sources for variation were identified, ranging from preanalytic (time to fixation, method of tissue processing, time of fixation, type of fixation), analytic (assay validation, equipment calibration, use of standardized laboratory procedures, training and competency assessment of staff, type of antigen retrieval, test reagents, use of standardized control material, use of automated laboratory methods) and postanalytic (interpretation criteria, use of image analysis, reporting elements, quality assurance procedures). Due to the number of sources of variation and the influence they could have on the tissue biospecimen, a number of situations were enumerated that were grounds to not use immunohistochemistry to assess Her-2 protein levels. These exclusionary criteria included the use of any fixatives other than formalin, needle biopsies fixed for less than 1 hour, excisional biopsies fixed for less than 6 hours and longer than 48 hours, core needle biopsies with edge or retraction artifact affecting the entire core or with crush artifact, tissues with strong membrane staining on internal normal ducts or lobules and tissues with controls that showed unexpected results. The initial and continued use of tissue biospecimens to assess Her-2 overexpression have been integral in creating appropriate standards aimed at establishing a uniform, reproducible result. In turn, these results continue to help further refine the clinical decision process in the care of breast cancer patients.

The use of tissue biospecimens also played a significant role in expanding the utility of certain drugs in the treatment of cancer. Imatinib mesylate (Gleevec), originally designed to target the chronic myeloid specific protein BCR-ABL, was later found to show some activity with another tyrosine kinase, notably the gene product KIT. Using tissue biospecimens, investigators were able to document that a relatively rare gastrointestinal tumor, called a Gastrointestinal Stromal and Tumor, expressed the KIT gene (Hirota, 1998). Treatment of Gastrointestinal Stromal patients with this therapeutic agent produced remarkable results. These previous examples illustrate how tissue biospecimens have helped shape the development of therapeutic agents for the treatment of cancer. A known protein that can be targeted is identified, a potentially therapeutic agent created or already is in existence, and assays developed that can identify those protein(s) on tissues. The changing paradigm is to treat a patient's tumor with an agent that is antagonistic to a protein or molecule that can be documented to be present in the tumor tissue. This is in contrast to treating the tumor based on a histologic classification and previous experience of response in a certain percentage of patient's with that tumor type. In this new era of Personalized Medicine, therapies will be given specifically to those individuals most apt to respond to them. Therefore, those who will benefit from a targeted therapy will be appropriately selected for treatment, and those who will not benefit will be treated by another regimen. Tissue biospecimens will continue to play a significant role in the new medical paradigm, however their traditional role may evolve. Whereas the current means of evaluating tissue biospecimens is after fixation and processing, with the end result a paraffin embedded specimen that is stained for visual examination either through traditional hematoxylin and eosin stains complimented by immunohistochemistry, tomorrow's biospecimen may be subjected to molecular assays. A representative scenario is the case of CD-117 positive tumors. Initially, Gastrointestinal Stromal Tumors were found to express this protein in abundance. By similar reasoning, it was assumed that other CD-117 positive tumors could also be treated by this tyrosine kinase inhibitor. A number of CD-117 positive tumors were rapidly identified that included colorectal cancers, renal cell carcinomas, thymic epithelial tumors, seminomas, Merkel cell cancers, endometrial stromal sarcoma and aggressive fibromatosis (Quek, 2009). However, the clinical community soon came to the realization after much scientific investigation that the underlying molecular alterations in Gastrointestinal Stromal Tumors, namely the gain of function mutations in the C-Kit gene in specific exons, were the underlying reason for their therapeutic responsiveness. Although other tumors may express the C-Kit gene product and can be readily identified as being CD-117 positive, without the specific mutations seen in GIST tumors, these other tumors turned out to be non-responsive to Gleevec administered therapy. This example highlights how the oncoming molecular age in medicine will play a role in the analysis of biospecimens for the rational delivery of targeted therapy.

3. Achieving personalized medicine through improved diagnostics

Although conventional light microscopy has been the stalwart of diagnostic pathology for decades, it continues to have problems with reproducibility among members of its collegium. As a continually evolving field, newly described entities go through the academic rigors of debate before consensus is reached. This can take some time, with consensus established after many years. Several examples showcase the limitations of diagnosis based solely on morphology. In the colon, preneoplastic polyps have traditionally been classified as either hyperplastic or adenomatous. In the late 1990's, two new entities were described called the serrated adenoma and the admixed polyp. Despite a decade where these entities were studied and further described, some confusion still remains regarding their correct diagnosis. When specialist gastrointestinal pathologists were shown a number of cases of these two entities, only a moderate degree of concordance was noted, and only fair inter-observer agreement evident (Wong, 2009). When cells alone are examined, that is, in the form of a cytology specimen, molecular diagnosis can be an improvement. The detection of atypical cells in sputum cells prepared for cytologic examination for the screening of lung cancer is a proven method, but suffers from low sensitivity. The addition of genomic markers can raise the sensitivity of cancer detection to 86% and specificity to 93% (Jiang, 2010). When it comes to actual tumors, interobserver agreement has had a history of similar problems with at best, modest reproducibility. One of the more difficult tumors to classify are those epithelial tumors originating from the ovary. Through decades of examination, diagnostic reproducibility based on morphology has steadily increased (Kobel, 2010). Aiding this improvement has been immunohistochemistry and molecular analysis. There are now considered to be five major subtypes of ovarian carcinoma: high grade serous, clear cell, endometrioid, mucinous and low grade serous carcinoma. The importance of this new paradigm based classification again is treatment based, with high grade serous being responsive to neoadjuvant chemotherapy whereas the others are not. From continued research utilizing all available data from the patient, the clinical outcome and most importantly the tissue, consensus in diagnosis is being achieved with diagnostic algorithms to achieving reproducible results being reported (Kalloger, 2011).

These examples demonstrate the limitation of histologic diagnosis and the increasing role molecular analysis will play in identifying, classifying and prognosticating tumors. Assays that will be developed to achieve this will most likely be used to interrogate nucleic acids, whether DNA or RNA, but may also analyze proteins. The arrival of these assays may be tied directly to therapy and hence have been given the designation companion diagnostics (Papadopoulos, 2006). The implications of using these molecular approaches are that they may eventually yield more informative data than conventional hematoxylin and eosin stained microscopic slides, even when the tissue is further worked up with immunohistochemistry. The goal is to be able to identify subgroups within a given patient population whose histology may appear similar, but end up having a different clinical course or outcome. It is hoped that through the molecular evaluation of tissue specimens, molecular signatures can be identified and assays developed that can recognize and separate these subsets of patients from the general cancer population. A realistic future scenario where molecular studies may eventually take precedence over histology is with

Stage II and III adenocarcinoma of the colon. Although histologically these tumors may appear morphologically similar and stage similarly, it is known that a certain proportion of these patients do benefit from adjuvant chemotherapy whereas for the other proportion of this group it is unnecessary. The identification of a biomarker or biomarkers capable of clearly delineating these two subpopulations would save time, effort and benefit the patients having to be and those not having to be treated. Another reason molecular analysis may be more informative than traditional hematoxylin and eosin stained sections is its objective nature. There are a number of tissue types from which human bias has been known to exist. The classification of dysplasia in the oral-pharyngeal space has for years been known to suffer from inter- and even intraobserver variability (Karabulut, 1995 and Abbey, 1995). For gliomas of the brain, histologic classification, which guides subsequent therapy, suffers from interobserver variability (Kros, 2007). Even with an updated classification scheme, diagnostic variability persists now due to the addition of newly added entities and variants (Tremblath, 2008). It would appear logical then, that another mechanism of diagnosing these types of tumors would be attempted. In fact, a recent study did find that molecular analysis did perform better than traditional histology, albeit in the realm of survival prognostication (Gravendeel, 2009). Thus it appears that with the molecular era steadily encroaching the clinical realm, the dedication of a proportion of tissue from excised tumor biospecimens may be needed as part of the standard of care for the cancer patient. The tissue biospecimen will still be integral in patient care, but the manner by which it is examined will evolve.

4. Barriers to the molecular profiling of clinical specimens - formalin fixation

Several barriers exist that limit the application of molecular techniques to tissue biospecimens. Since the main goal of extirpated tissue is the establishment of a diagnosis, the priority for such specimens is the optimal preparation of a tissue section for morphologic evaluation. In order to do this, tissue preparation involves fixation and processing, followed by sectioning and staining for microscopic examination. In the vast majority of community and academic pathology departments, the fixation used is 10% neutral buffered formaldehyde. Whereas this fixative results in a reliable and reproducible end product for histologic examination, it has been shown to be detrimental to the recovery and examination of cellular molecules. Formaldehyde interacts with DNA to create hydroxymethyl groups, forms methylene bridges between amino acids, generates apurinic and apyrimidic sites that lead to highly unstable cyclic carboxonium ions that hydrolyze into 2-deoxy-D-ribose, and cause the slow hydrolysis of phosphodiester bonds that result in short chains of polydeoxyribose with intact pyrimidines. In short, the chemical reaction between formaldehyde and deoxyribose nucleic acids leads to the denaturation of these molecules as well as the formation of cross links with proteins. The result is the recovery of shortened segments or fragmented DNA and decreased recovery. For certain high throughput downstream molecular based assays, like array comparative genomic hybridization that are designed to evaluate the copy numbers of genes from the entire genome, the absence of gene segments may lead to erroneously biased conclusions relating to genetic deletions. Several reports have noted that DNA extracted from formalin fixed, paraffin embedded tissue blocks and run on an array comparative genomic hybridization platform, tended to yield data prone to spurious changes in genetic copy number in addition to copy number loss when compared to matched fresh frozen tissue (McSherry,

2007). To complicate matters worse, the presence of formaldehyde results in the presence of high background 'noise' on array comparative genomic hybridization data, making the determination of legitimate significant molecular alterations problematic (Johnson, 2006 and Mojica, 2008). At the nucleotide level, formaldehyde has been documented to result in random changes in amplified sequences relative to the original DNA sequence. Formalin fixation is thought to cause base damage, but the overall template can still be read by polymerases. When PCR is performed using *Taq* polymerase, errors in translesional synthesis can occur (Quach, 2004). Although this error rate is low, it can be a factor when small amounts of originating material are used. This has grave implications at the clinical level, as the reporting of non-existent mutations may severely impact a patient's care altering the treatment regimen from which the fixed tissue originated from.

RNA is another potential biomarker that can be assayed from tissue biospecimens, and in the past decade has already influenced the realm of pathologic diagnostics in the field of breast cancer. Through expression array analysis, breast cancers now are considered to comprise a number of subgroups (normal-like, luminal, basal-like, HER-2(+)) within the broad spectrum of what was originally only considered part of one entity, ductal adenocarcinoma. Work is currently progressing on finding the most appropriate therapeutic regimen for each subtype. Based on the clinical success of this molecular based classification, other tumors are being probed for their molecular signature. However, it must be noted that the original work that defined these breast cancer subtypes was based on fresh frozen material. Any subsequent discoveries on such tissue must be able to be translated to clinical material, which again routinely undergoes formalin fixation and processing. Similar to DNA, mRNA recovery from FFPE tissue is encumbered by the crosslinking of molecules and poor recovery (Cox, 2006). But since mRNA is a more labile molecule than DNA, degradation of the RNA molecule impacts the overall recovery more with significantly reduced quantities and poor quality obtained from fixed tissue specimens when compared to matched frozen material (Specht, 2001). This negatively impacts the consideration of using FFPE tissue biospecimens for gene expression on cancer samples. RNA extracted from FFPE tissue is partially degraded resulting in gene expression data with low signal intensity data. In one study, only a quarter of unselected samples that were FFPE provided enough starting material for subsequent gene expression assays (Penland, 2007). In another study, gene expression values differed by a value greater than two fold in almost 20% of the genes studied between matched FFPE and frozen tissue samples (Mojica, 2007). This rather significant discrepancy can be accounted for by either a decrease in gene expression due to degradation or an increase in gene expression due to changes in the tissue microenvironment and the cells subsequent reaction prior to fixation. The major implication however, in regards to human tissue that could be potentially assayed for mRNA expression levels that may influence clinical care, is to determine beforehand which mRNA transcripts are stable, and remain stable. It is these transcripts that would be of clinical value, as opposed to those more labile ones prone to either degradation or biased due to *ex vivo* conditions (Lee, 2005). This obviously would require an in depth investigation into which transcripts are most stable and least resistant to the external pressures associated with the tissue fixation process, so that those that are susceptible to degradation during the process of fixation are excluded from further consideration and studies (Opitz, 2010).

Proteins are the last major molecule to be mentioned here that are routinely assayed from clinical tissue biospecimens. The formalin-fixed, paraffin-embedded tissue specimens routinely examined in surgical pathology departments currently undergo proteomic evaluation in the form of immunohistochemistry. However, this analysis is often limited to evaluating only one, or at most two proteins in the tissue section. When tissue biospecimens are exceedingly small, the tissue may get exhausted, limiting the number of proteins that can be examined through immunohistochemistry. An approach that may see increased use, especially when a number of proteins will need to be evaluated in a tissue biospecimen, is mass spectrometry. Currently, mass spectrometry is finding initial success as a diagnostic modality for amyloidosis, and its integration into other pathologic conditions most likely will soon follow suit. However, as with DNA and RNA, the analysis of the traditionally formalin-fixed, paraffin-embedded tissue biospecimen by mass spectrometry will present with problems once again associated with formaldehyde. The cross links formed in proteins increase the complexity of data analysis and peptide identification through the addition of 12 and 30 Dalton changes in the peptide mass (Metz, 2006). Adding to the complexity of this reaction is the finding that with time, more methylene bridges (cross-links) are formed creating increases in the molecular weight of a peptide by multiples of 12 Daltons (Toews, 2008). Chemical reactions that occur with cross-linked peptides can result in incomplete fragments upon collision-induced dissociation, requiring additional targeted experiments to correctly identify those peptide fragments (Sutherland, 2008). This necessitates the creation of specialized software that takes into consideration these mass effect changes before correct peptide identification can be made, a daunting task considering the multitude of combinations possible due to fixation (Leitner, 2010). The presence of cross links may also result in intra-protein peptide combinations as well as portions of peptides between different proteins, making an already difficult task even more complicated. Research into the mass spectrometry analysis of formalin-fixed, paraffin-embedded tissue has shown that comparable data with matched fresh frozen material can be done using principles learned from antigen retrieval and immunohistochemistry. The original findings that compared the numbers of proteins identified by mass spectrometry analysis between matched formalin fixed, paraffin embedded and frozen tissue sections showed the former to consistently be quantitatively less than the latter (Crockett, 2005, Bagnato, 2007 and Guo, 2007). Despite claims touting the feasibility of mass spectrometric analysis on formalin-fixed paraffin-embedded tissue, complete concordance of protein inventories with matched frozen tissue has yet to be achieved, leading to speculation that material not detected from formalin-fixed, paraffin-embedded tissue may be due to incomplete lysis of cross links and either incomplete or biased protein extraction (Nirmalan, 2008). Research on fixed biospecimen material continues with the goal that either a mechanism of improved recovery will be found, a more molecular friendly method of fixation developed, or an alternative means of diagnostics created that is compatible with both surgical pathology and molecular assays.

4.1 Barriers to the molecular profiling of clinical specimens - preanalytical variables
Complicating the implementation of molecular analysis on fixed tissue biospecimens is the growing awareness that a number of preanalytical factors may unduly influence the characteristics of certain molecules prior to fixation. Since the intent of assaying a tissue biospecimen is the characterization of molecules reflective of a cancer cells' *in vivo* state, it stands that any factor that alters that state is undesirable. Unfortunately, a number of factors have now been recognized that may introduce unintended molecular variation to the biospecimen and include the type of surgical procedure, warm and cold ischemia, time to fixation, tissue thickness and rate of fixative penetration. These variables predominantly

affect the most labile molecules, namely mRNA and protein phosphorylation status (Sprussel, 2004 and Espina, 2008) and occur early in the procedure (Miyatake, 2004 and Schlomm, 2008). The first of these variables, the type of surgical procedure, can influence a cell's molecular signature due to the initiation of hypoxia. As the specimen is being excised, vessels are sequentially ligated before the entire specimen is ready to be extirpated. The type of procedure can influence the molecular signature, as the shorter, quicker procedure will have less of an influence than procedures that take longer, time wise. An approach that is becoming more popular because it is less invasive and therefore results in a shorter hospital stay, is laparoscopic surgery. For resections of colon cancer specimens, the durations of surgery increases 55 minutes from that of an open surgical resection (COSTG, 2004). With the introduction of robotic assisted surgery, a procedure rising in popularity because of benefits like less blood loss for the patient, the duration of ischemia can increase between 30 minutes to 1.5 hours in prostatectomy specimens. These short changes in time may not be significant enough to change the levels of proteins, but can unduly influence the expression profile signatures of the more labile mRNA transcripts (Ricciardelli, 2010). This increase is attributable to a reversal in the sequence of vessel ligation, where in robotic assisted prostatectomy procedures they are done earlier as opposed to later, as in open prostatectomies. Whereas these changes occur prior to the acquisition of the tissue by the department of pathology, other variables influence the molecular signature of cells within tissue post-acquisition. Cold ischemia, or the time the tissue is outside of the body and either frozen or fixed, is the major factor in determining the adequacy of the tissue for further analysis. Although not incorporated into many protocols, the time from receipt to freezing has a strong negative impact on the molecular profile of the tissue specimen (De Cecco, 2009). For tissue that undergoes fixation, the cold ischemia time is longer. For these specimens, once they are received within the department of pathology, they are immersed in 10% neutral buffered formalin. The cells within the tissue however, will remain viable for a limited time, most likely until they become fixed. The cells are now enduring a loss of their blood supply, accumulation of lactic acid with the subsequent decrease in their cellular pH, and changes in temperature (room temperature vs. *in vivo* body temperature), all resulting in biologic stress. In response to this biologic stress, they will react, and in the process their molecular signature will be altered to some degree to this stress. The obvious conundrum is to determine what of the molecular signature can be considered artifactual, i.e., as a complication of this artificially induced stress, and what can be characteristic of the neoplastic state. An added layer complicating these changes is the fact that tissue thickness can lead to regional differences in the specimen's molecular profile. Formalin infuses into tissue at 1 mm an hour. If specimens are not sectioned before they are placed in a container of formalin, the tissue at the center of the specimen will be fixed last relative to the exterior of the specimen. Since the cells in the tissue are still viable until fixation, the cells within the center of the specimen will be responding to their new environment (Stan, 2006). Depending on their distance from the fixative, these cells will experience progressively hypoxic, acidic and nutrient depleted conditions over time (Espina, 2008 and van Maldegem, 2008). As viable cells now under biologic stress, their molecular profile may alter leading to falsely elevated or decreased levels of a putative biomarker relative to those cells in direct initial contact with formaldehyde. The basic tenet when working with clinical specimens is to realize that excised tissue is viable and not only vulnerable but reactive to *ex vivo* stressors, and that an understanding as to their location within the specimen with respect to exposure to fixative should be considered in the data analysis (Espina, 2008).

These preanalytical factors have the potential to lead to significant variability in the molecular signature of cells within a tissue specimen. Although there exists numerous tissue biorepositories within the United States, a major problem with each is the wide variation in tissue collection, processing and storage of these samples and an absence of standardized procedures for each step (National Biospecimen Network Blueprint, 2003). The development of a sample preanalytical code proposed by the International Society of Biospecimen and Environmental Repositories represents a good start towards standardization (Betsou, 2010). Through the compilation of data from tissue biospecimens, and correlation with this proposed grading system of specimen integrity, the factors that play into macromolecule integrity can be identified. Each organ may exhibit differences in the stability of the molecules within their cells, with those possessing digestive type enzymes (e.g., the pancreas) more labile than those without (e.g. skeletal muscle). A previous study indicated that the biopsy, based on the smaller tissue size and exposure to the shorter periods of warm or cold ischemia, to be the optimal tissue biospecimen for molecular analysis. The small size of the biopsy allows for even exposure to fixative, while the actual procedure of acquiring small pieces of tissue are not encumbered by extensive periods of surgically induced ischemia required to excise a diseased organ nor intraoperative procedures that are deemed clinically imperative to the needs of biospecimen collection (Schlomm, 2008 and Espina, 2008).

4.2 Barriers to the clinical profiling of clinical specimens - tissue heterogeneity

Another barrier to molecular profiling of clinical tissue biospecimens is tissue heterogeneity. Human tissue specimens are increasingly being used as the primary source of investigational material for cancer related studies. They offer advantages over cells lines because they are more representative of the diagnosed condition and reflective of the *in vivo* condition, not having undergone numerous passages and the resultant phenotypic and genetic drift. Properly collected and annotated, they can avert the problems of misidentification, a relatively widespread situation wherein certain cell lines actually correspond to other cell types than what they are designated to be (Buehring, 2004)). Despite extensive work on cell lines, the realization that the cell of origin may actually be a contaminant would be disastrous for any investigator. However, using tissue itself is fraught with problems. The integrated architecture of tissue means that the targeted cell of interest will vary with respect to the overall cell volume, even in normal tissue (Figure 1). In tumor samples, the same problem exists (Enkemann, 2010). Depending on the type of tumor, the percentage of non-tumor cells can also be less than 50%. Although in grossly solid areas of tumor tissue colon cancer, lung cancer and breast cancer can compromise over 80% of the tumor, prostate cancer is notable for interdigitating between normal glands, possibly biasing any subsequent findings based on such a tissue biospecimen (Figure 2). The presence of contaminating normal cells in a tumor sample can have the affect of dampening a signal or mask the detection of a potential biomarker molecule. The presence of segments of nucleic acids originating from contaminating normal cells can have the untoward affect of decreasing the amplitude of a deleted gene in a tumor sample (Mojica, 2007). Ideally, any work done on a sample should ensure that it is a pure, or close to pure cell population of the desired cell type, so that retrospective analysis trying to deconvolute the data does not have to be performed (Tureci, 2003 and Shen-Orr, 2010). The development of the laser capture micro-dissection tool has provided an answer to tissue heterogeneity. With this machine or one of its congeners, specific cell types can be visualized, identified and then procured,

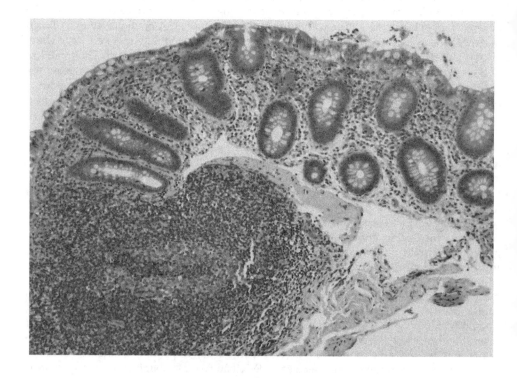

Fig. 1. Histology of normal colonic mucosa. The glands and surface consist of epithelial cells, while the lamina propria contains chronic inflammatory cells. Interspersed in the mucosa are lymphoid aggregates (left side of figure), which cannot be readily discerned at the gross examination level. Without microscopic examination, the proportion of targeted cells, in this case colonic epithelial cells, could account for less than 50% of the cells in sample. Hematoxylin and Eosin stain, 10X

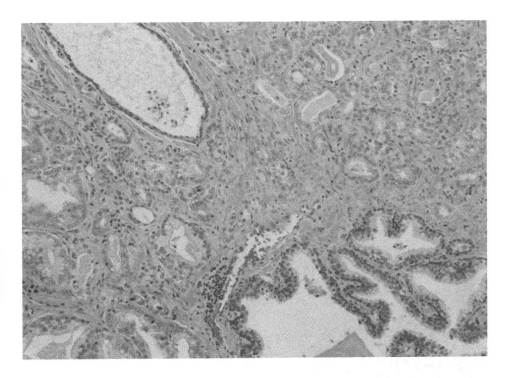

Fig. 2. Histology of prostate cancer. Tumor is in the upper right hand corner, while normal glandular prostatic cells and stroma make up the remainder of the specimen. Hematoxylin and Eosin stain, 10X.

leaving the unwanted contaminating cells with the tissue. It works for both frozen tissue specimens and formalin fixed paraffin embedded tissue. A major drawback with its use however, is the time consuming nature of manually procuring the wanted cells. This issue has been addressed with the development of automated programs, that coupled with cell recognition software, have alleviated the overall time needed to select cells from tissue specimens. The other major drawback with this instrument has been its high start-up cost. Most machines have a six figure price tag, but newer, cheaper versions have been developed. An alternative method has been the use of immunomagnetic beads for the recovery of targeted cells (Mojica, 2006).This approach starts with fresh tissue specimens, that is, before they are fixed, and after a series of manipulations, recovers a highly enriched collection of cells. This method is cost effective, and does not involve any significant expenditure. It has advantages over using straight (un-enriched) biopsy samples in that it can enrich for a targeted cell population. Simple adjustments to the procedure can

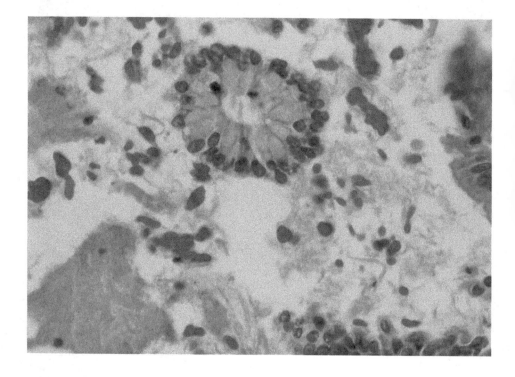

Fig. 3. Cells exfoliated from colonic tissue with no enrichment. Note presence of red blood cells and mucus. Hematoxylin and Eosin stain , 40X.

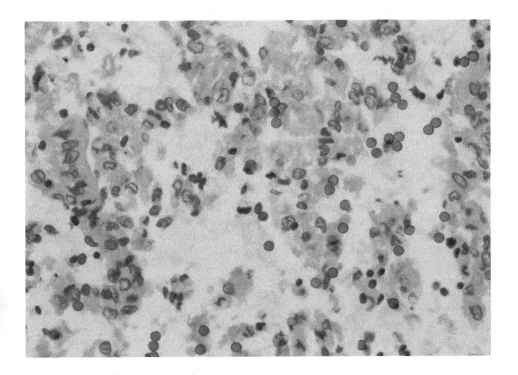

Fig. 4. Recovered cells from enrichment described in text. Yellow dots are immunomagnetic beads. Hematoxylin and Eosin stain 40X

targeted cell population. Simple adjustments to the procedure can be made to eliminate the presence of red blood cells, whose presence is significant in tissue biospecimens (Figure 3). This is particularly important for proteomic, and not so much for nucleic acid studies, as red blood cells have a number of proteins within their cytosol that may contribute to complicate any subsequent un-enriched lysate (Pasini, 2006, and D'Alessandro, 2010). The result of such enrichment is an expansion in the detection of the proteins from the targeted cell (dePetris, 2010). The use of several washes helps eliminate the presence of other contaminating substances, using as an example, excess mucus from colon specimens. Mucus itself is not detrimental to downstream analysis, since it is the secreted product of certain types of colonic epithelial cells. It is however, the location whereby commensal organisms like bacteria habitate, and their inclusion in any sample for downstream analysis could lead to confounding genetic or proteomic results (Qin, 2010). Since the technique can be done on fresh tissue specimens, the problems associated with formalin enumerated earlier are not encountered. Finally, the use of the ber-Ep4 immunomagentic beads are commercially available and have been for several years. As ber-Ep4 recognizes an epitope in epithelial cells, this method works nicely as a means for their procurement from specimens with the intent to isolate epithelial cells from the underlying tissue (Figure 4). The overall technique however, is not restricted to ber-EP4, as other antibodies with specificities to other cell surface membrane proteins can be conjugated to the magnetic beads. One of the limiting factors however, is the relative paucity of antibodies available to select from that may be used to positively enrich for a specific cell type from a heterogeneous population. This dearth is attributable to the limited knowledge of the proteome of the plasma membrane, which in turn is due to the difficulties associated with examining molecules with hydrophilic and hydrophobic properties. When the plasma membrane proteome is not known for a specific cell type, an alternative but reportedly equally effective approach would be through negative enrichment, where contaminating cells are targeted and removed from the sample population. This has been used for the examination of sputum with respect for lung cancer diagnosis (Qui, 2008). In cytology, the presence of pulmonary macrophages is essential to document that the material has cells from the lung, and not just the oral cavity. These same cells however, would contribute to the heterogeneity of the sample for any subsequent molecular analysis. Their selection, and that of neutrophils using anti-CD-14 and anti-CD-16 immunomagnetic beads can lead to a significant improvement in the numbers of bronchial epithelial cells recovered. An alternative to using antibodies are aptamers. Aptamers are short single stranded nucleic acid oligomers that can take on a variety of three dimensional shapes, thus allowing them to bind to a wide variety of molecules, with binding affinities similar to monoclonal antibodies (Kim, 2009). One advantage of using aptamers over antibodies is their relative stability. Another is the ability to work with cells without knowing specific proteins. This approach would thus be an alternative to the extensive plasma membrane profiling that would be required in order to identify differentially expressed proteins between normal and tumor cell populations.

5. The advent of molecular analysis in cancer tissue specimens

Despite all these roadblocks to using clinically derived tissue specimens for molecular analysis, their use in clinical cancer care already exists. A perfect example is the use of monoclonal antibodies created to antagonistically bind and inhibit the plasma membrane protein Epidermal Growth Factor Receptor (EGFR) in colorectal cancer and non-small cell lung cancer (Plesec, 2009 and Wang, 2010). Although the EGFR receptor can be recognized by immunohistochemistry in tissue specimens, this assay has been found to not be a reliable means of determining those likely to respond to this type of therapy. However, the identification of those patients most likely to respond is imperative in order to avoid any unnecessary side effects, treatment related costs and delays in the administration of a more effective therapy. Since immunohistochemistry was deemed unreliable as a mechanism that could select patients for EGFR therapy, downstream components of the EGFR signaling cascade were examined. The result of these investigations was the finding that mutations in the KRAS gene could identify those patients who would not be responsive to monoclonal antibody therapy directed at the EGFR receptor. In unselected patients, the number of patients that responded to cetuximab, the antibody directed against EGFR, was between 10-20%, but when patients were selected for treatment based on the criteria of no KRAS mutations, this percentage rose to 60%. The detection of these mutations can be accomplished by a number of different methods, the common denominator being that they evaluated the DNA sequence of the KRAS gene within tumor cells. The issues previously described associated with DNA and formalin fixation now have practical clinical relevance. Again, these issues relate mostly to template degradation and tissue purity. For the former, the amplified product must be designed to be small enough to account for degradation yet long enough to enable specificity. For tissue purity, most laboratories require the tumor component in the tissue to be equal to or greater than 75%. The presence of contaminating normal cells raises the possibility that the DNA from these cells may be assayed instead of the tumor cell's DNA, resulting in a normal sequencing electropherogram or false negative finding for the relevant mutations. In some specimens the amount of contaminating normal cells is significant, and although laser capture microdissection can be used, the transference of this predominantly research tool to the clinical setting is prohibitive due to its labor intensive nature. A promising approach is the technique of "cold-PCR", wherein mutant alleles in tumor cell can be amplified and subsequently sequenced when specific alleles from these tumor cells comprise only a minority population in a tissue sample (Li, 2008). A recent report documented the ability to detect mutations in tumor cells when they constitute only 20% of the tissue sample using the technique of Cold-PCR (Yu, 2011). If no other developments in tissue preparation are introduced, this method may represent an approach that may become a standard assay for tissue biospecimens.

6. Changes in the clinical arena warranting changes in biospecimen preparation

Although the technique of cold-PCR will prove very useful in the evaluation of tumor specimens for specific mutations, its application or modification to whole genome profiling is unknown. Despite an ever expanding database of information that is characterizing oncogenesis, there still remains a significant amount of knowledge to be gained. A recent initiative to correlate the molecular signatures of tumor tissue specimens with the corresponding cancer patient's clinical parameters underscores the need to identify biomarkers that will aid in cancer care. As such, the tissue biospecimen will continue to play a significant role in cancer diagnosis and treatment. One lesson that is becoming increasingly more apparent is that material that is not fixed serves as the best medium from which to start (De Rienzo, 2010 and Jimeno, 2010). This is a reiteration of what has previously been documented, but applied to actual biospecimens. The nature of the unfixed specimen in the form of fine-needle aspirates however, has one major drawback. The technique of fine needle aspiration involves inserting a needle into a mass, and pulling the needle in and out of the mass so that tissue fragments are obtained. Since the tool is a needle, the tissue fragments are minute. Obtaining a diagnosis based on cytology requires extensive training in pathology and its subspecialty, cytopathology. Without the architecture, the presence of malignant cells can be diagnosed, but the diminutive nature of the specimen sometimes precludes assigning what type of tumor it is. This is particularly true for tumors of the lung, where a process similar to fine needle aspiration, in terms of quantities of cells recovered, is performed. Whether the procedure is a bronchoscopy with material obtained as washings or brushings, or a trans-thoracic needle biopsy, the material recovered will be diminutive. Again, the diagnosis of malignancy can be made, but for poorly differentiated tumors, the classification into adenocarcinoma, squamous cell carcinoma or large cell undifferentiated carcinoma, which is now often requested to help guide therapy, will be extremely difficult if next to impossible without a large enough piece of tissue to showcase architecture (Wallace, 2009). For adenocarcinoma, the presence of five or more vacuoles in two consecutive high power fields is required to differentiate adenocarcinoma from large cell undifferentiated carcinoma. However, the diminutive nature of these specimens may not even fulfill this size criterion. If not enough material is available to make a definitive diagnosis, the patient may require another invasive procedure that may aim to get tissue instead of cells. A similar situation is occurring with the biopsy of small kidney tumors where cryoablation instead of resection will be performed. Although attempts to obtain tissue so that a histologic diagnosis can be made, often times the specimen is too small and not recovered after tissue processing. The absence of an established diagnosis means that should another mass lesion arise in a patient treated by cryoablation, it will not be known if the mass represents a metastatic or primary tumor Although tumors of unknown origin can be worked up through conventional immunohistochemistry, the absence of a previous diagnosis incurs additional costs for this work-up. Thus, at today's medical environment, a histologic diagnosis is still imperative, and thus in order to optimally process any specimens in the near future, tools will need to be developed that are capable of allowing the evaluation of these cells at both the cytologic and molecular level.

In order to circumvent the problem of enabling a diagnosis on small biopsy specimens all the while providing some material for molecular analysis, investigators have begun designing platforms capable of recovering specific subsets of cells from clinical specimens (Weigum, 2010, Wan, 2010, and Sun, 2010). These platforms are ideal for taking on the problems of small amounts of cells or tissues. Although immunohistochemistry is an extremely useful diagnostic tool in the laboratory, the amount of tissue used per assay is significant. When a battery of stains is needed to be performed, each 4 or 5 micron thick section may end up exhausting the amount of recoverable tissue. Precious tissue can also be lost at the microtome step, where some material may be lost just due to the process of aligning the block and blade. Flow cytometry has been used extensively for years for hematologic malignancies, but its requirement for ample amounts of starting material negate its consideration as a tool for biopsy specimens. Thus, platforms based on microfluidics appear to be best suited to interrogate these small biopsy specimens. Using techniques similar to the one previously described above that help enrich for targeted cells, these enriched cell populations can then be introduced to a microfluidic platform for subsequent evaluation. One noticeable limitation of these platforms however, is the absence of the ability to visually evaluate these cells. Although the enrichment approach previously described is capable of selecting for epithelial cells from the heterogeneous cell population that comprises tissue, the epitope recognized by the ber-EP4 antibody can be present in both non-neoplastic and malignant epithelial cells. Thus, until plasma membrane proteins are identified and characterized that are specific for either normal or neoplastic epithelial cells, enrichment is limited to epithelial cells. This is not so much a limitation in certain tumors like colonic adenocarcinomas, where the tumor mass effaces the surrounding tissue so that it is composed of tumor epithelial cells and surrounding stroma, but will not be as effective in other tumors like the prostate, where the tumor cells infiltrate between normal prostatic glands and stroma. For microfluidic platforms, the need to visualize cells will allow investigators whether to attribute molecular findings appropriately to neoplastic cells or not. At the clinical level, the ability to visualize cells allows for a diagnosis, and determination whether the biopsy contains tumor cells and thus is representative of a mass versus no tumor cells and therefore not representative of a mass.

In the development of such a platform, cytologic examination plays the vital role of stratifying whether the cells are tumor or not. Identifying the type of tumor is not so vital as the cells, or specifically their contents, can be interrogated through a variety of downstream assays. The platform needs to be designed such that the cells are not permanently immobilized on the glass slide. Once visualized, they should either be able to be eluted out as intact cells, lysed so that the molecules from them can be assayed, or have a lab-on-a chip assay integrated to a portion of the slide. Thus, such a microfluidic platform should allow for conventional cytologic based examination for screening purposes, followed by molecular interrogation for tumor designation. A period of molecular annotation will take place within the next decade wherein reliable biomarkers will be discovered and validated for specific tumor types. The transition to molecular identification of tumor tissue has already begun and has shown early success in helping determine the site of origin in several instances (Ismael, 2006, Greco, 2010, and Monzon, 2010). Molecular tumor classification is not yet a reality, with histologic examination still the gold standard for diagnosis (Kotsakis, 2010). However, in the next decade, when molecular analysis of tumor specimens will occur concurrent with histologic examination, a gradual shift in emphasis may occur. With Personalized Medicine, the identification of target molecules may eventually become more important for cancer treatment than histology.

6.1 An integrated approach to optimize the biospecimen for cancer care

Taking into consideration all the factors that may bias the macromolecular profiles of a specimen, a tentative approach can be postulated that would recover cells bearing the most similar molecular disposition to their *in vivo* counterparts from clinical material. To address preanalytical bias, the specimen most suited for analysis may be the biopsy. Clinically, the patient undergoing a biopsy of a tumor would not be subjected to the depth of anesthesia that the patient undergoing a surgical resection would be for the same tumor. The degree of preparation of the patient is less, with the process most often an out-patient procedure. Therefore, confounding issues that potentially could influence, but are hard to confirm, the molecular profile of a cell, like administration of intravenous fluids, antibiotics and anxiety to name just a few, are not introduced (Compton, 2006). For issues related to warm ischemia, the short time required to obtain a biopsy is also preferred to the comparatively longer time required to excise a portion of organ with tumor (Schlomm, 2008). Once the biopsy is obtained, the next step would be sample stabilization, an attempt to immediately try to preserve the molecules within the cells. For the more labile molecules like RNA, this can be achieved by immersing the specimen in RNA Later (Mutter, 2004) or for proteins, through heat denaturation (Svensson, 2008). For the latter, the use of heat inactivation helps to preserve post-translational modifications, a form of intercellular signaling with a transient time frame within proteins that can be lost or altered during cold ischemia, or the period after extirpation (Rountree, 2010). Once stabilized, the cells should be disaggregated from the tissue and unwanted elements and contaminating normal cells eliminated through some form of enrichment. It should be noted that at no point in this proposed procedure fixation with formaldehyde is involved. The cells then should be examined cytologically, to confirm that the targeted cells are indeed present, that they are enriched and to what percentage they constitute the sample. This should be done on some fluidic based platform, so that these same cells can be further examined at the molecular level after microscopic diagnostic evaluation. The cells are then eluted and their contents extracted for downstream molecular analysis. Alternatively, other methods may develop wherein diagnostics can be performed on the immobilized cell. Through the development of the above protocol, the maximal amount of informative data can be extracted from the biospecimen, with a combination of traditional anatomic (cytologic) related diagnostics and future molecular interrogation for treatment guidance obtained from an optimally recovered specimen.

6.2 Biospecimens as the focal point of cancer care
The development of a platform capable of enriching unfixed, preserved tumor cells from tissue specimens will enhance clinical research. For some years now it has been known that one of the major obstacles to progression in the post-genomic era has been the absence of high quality biospecimens. An attempt in the previous decade to obtain 500 cases each of specific types of brain, lung and ovarian cancer for gene sequencing initially failed at the accrual stage. Although archives in pathology departments have numerous amounts of preserved tissue specimens, issues with percentage of tumor content, necrosis or even proper consent have become factors preventing their use at a national level. Differences in the procurement, handling and storage of samples may also play a role in the differences noted between similar tumors from different institutions. Nevertheless, the National Cancer Institute has embarked on an initiative to address those issues related to poor biospecimen procurement and to rectify them. The need for high quality biospecimens is reflected in their incorporation in innovative study designs for clinical trials, like the new phase 0 trial. In this new type of study, the need for patient tumor tissue is necessary in order to determine the biological effectiveness of the therapeutic agent being tested. In phase 1 trials the need for high quality biospecimens is also warranted, to match the administration of specific agents to patients possessing a specific molecular signature, deemed through previous experimentation, to be the target of those agent(s). This approach identifies useful therapeutic agents in a subset cohort from the general cancer population, where if an empiric approach had been used, the agent may not have resulted in a significant enough number of patients to warrant further testing. Molecular testing should also be able to identify patients who will be resistant to certain agents, thus guiding the clinician to alternative approaches and avoiding any unwarranted side effects and unnecessary costs. In the future, the tissue biospecimen will serve many roles, with two being the basis of future molecular, proteomic and/or metabolomic research and the other being the starting point for the treatment of the cancer patient. The development of newer biotechnological tools will certainly result in a continuing evolution of the tissue biospecimen's role in the treatment of cancer.

7. Conclusions

The role of tissue biospecimens in cancer care has evolved over time from observation and little impact, to anatomic and molecular diagnostics with high impact on guidance of clinical treatment. This evolution has come about based on the changes in the evaluation of the specimen, from humble beginnings wherein only the gross anatomic features were noted in malignant tissue and the patient's clinical course observed, to the biotechnological revolution and the high throughput capabilities created that can profile molecular alterations within cells, identify therapeutic targets and selectively lead to the administration of reagents best suited for each individual cancer patient. Advances in science continue to influence the evaluation of the biospecimen, with an urgent need to develop and adapt newer approaches capable of maximizing the amount of informative data that can be derived from these samples. The importance of the tissue biospecimen in the care of the cancer patient has grown dramatically. It is safe to assume its role in the care of the cancer patient of the near future will become even more vital than it is today.

8. References

Abbey, L.M., Kaugars, G.E., Gunsolley, J.C., et al. (1995) Intraexaminer and interexaminer reliability in the diagnosis of oral epithelial dysplasia. *Oral Surgery, Oral Medicine, Oral Pathology, Oral Radiology and Endodontology.* Vol.80, No.2, (August, 1995), pp188-191

Bagnato, C., Thumar, J., Mayya, V., et al. (2007)Proteomic analysis of human coronary atherosclerotic plaque: a feasibility study of direct tissue proteomics by liquid-chromatography and tandem mass spectrometry. *Molecular and Cellular Proteomics,* Vol.6, No.6, (June, 2007), pp.1088-1102

Betsou, F., Lehmann, S., Ashton, G., et al. (2010) Standard preanalytical coding for biospecimens: Defining the sample PREanalytical code. *Cancer Epidemiology, Biomarkers and Prevention,* Vol.19, No.4, (April 2010), pp.1004-1011

Compton, C. (2006) The Biospecimen Research Network of the National Cancer Institute. Accessioned May 2008. Available at http://biospecimens.cancer.gov/sciences/compton.pdf

COSTSG (The Clinical Outcomes of Surgical Therapy Study Group). (2004) A comparison of laparoscopically assisted and open colectomy for colon cancer. *New England Journal of Medicine,* Vol.350, No.20, (May 2004), pp.2050-2059

Cox, M.L., Schray, C.L., Luster, C.N., et al. (2006). Assessment of fixatives, fixation, and tissue processing on morphology and RNA integrity. *Experimental and Molecular Pathology,* Vol.80, No.2, (April 2006) pp.183-189

Crockett, D.K., Lin, Z., Vaughn, C.P., et al. (2005) Identification of proteins from formalin-fixed paraffin-embedded cells by LC-MS/MS. *Laboratory Investigation,* Vol.85, No.11 (November 2005) pp.1405-1415

D'Alessandro, A., Righetti, P.G. Zolla. L. (2010) The red blood cell proteome and interactome: An update. *Journal of Proteome Research* Vol.9, No.1 (January 2010), pp.144-163

De Cecco, L., Musell, V., Venoeroni, S., et al. (2009) Impact of biospecimens handling on biomarker research in breast cancer. *BMC Cancer* Vol.9:409. Accessioned January 2011. Available at http://biomedcentral.com/1471-2407/9/409

De Petris, L., Pernemalm, M., Elmberger, G., et al. (2010) A novel method for sample preparation of fresh lung cancer tissue for proteomics analysis by tumor cell enrichment and removal of blood contaminants. *Proteome Science* Vol.8 (February 2010) pp.8e. Accessioned January 2011. Available at http://www.proteomesci.com/content/8/1/9

De Rienzo, A., Dong, L., Yeap, B.Y. et al. (2011) Fine needle aspiration biopsies for gene expression ratio-based diagnostic and prognostic tests in malignant pleural mesothelioma. *Clinical Cancer Research* Vol.17, No.2, (January 2011) pp:310-316

Enkemann, S.A. (2010) Standards affecting the consistency of gene expression arrays in clinical applications. *Cancer, Epidemiology, Biomarkers and Prevention* Vol.19, No.4, (April 2010), pp.1000-1003

Espina, V., Edmiston, K.H., Heiby, M., et al. (2008) A portrait of tissue phosphoprotein stability in the clinical tissue procurement process. *Molecular and Cellular Proteomics,* Vol.7, No.10, (October 2008), pp. 1998-2018

Gal, A. (2001). In search of the origins of modern surgical pathology. *Advances in Anatomic Pathology,* Vol.8, No.1, (January 2001), pp.1-13

Gravendeel, L.A.M., Kouwenhoven M.C.M., Gevaert, O., et al. (2009) Intrinsic gene expression profiles of gliomas are a better predictor of survival than histology. *Cancer Research,* Vol.69, No.23, (December 2009) pp.9065-9072

Greco, F.A., Spigel, D.R., Yardley, D.A., et al. (2010) Molecular profiling in unknown primary cancer: accuracy of tissue of origin prediction. *Oncologist* Vol.15, No.5, (April 2010), pp.500-506

Guo, T., Wang, W., Rudnick, P.A. et al. (2007) Proteome analysis of microdissected formalin-fixed and paraffin-embedded tissue specimens. *Journal of Histochemisty and Cytochemistry.* Vol.55, No.7, (July 2007) pp.763-772

Hammond, M.E.H., Hayes, D.F., Dowsett, M., et al. (2010)American Society of Clinical Oncology/ College of American Pathologists guideline recommendations for immunohistochemical testing of Estrogen and Progesterone receptors in breast cancer. *Archives of Pathology and Laboratory Medicine,* Vol.134 (July 2010), pp.48-72.

Hirota, S, Isozaki, K., Moriyama, Y., et al. (1998). Gain-of-function mutations of c-kit in human gastrointestinal stromal tumors. *Science,* Vol.279, No.5350 (January 1998), pp.577-580

Ismael, G., de Azambuja, E., Awadu, A., (2006) Molecular profiling of a tumor of unknown origin. *New England Journal of Medicine* Vol.355, No.10, (September 2006), pp.1071-1072

Jiang, F., Todd, N.W., Li, R, et al. (2010). A panel of sputum-based genomic marker for early detection of lung cancer. *Cancer Prevention Research,* Vol.3, No.12, (December, 2010), pp:1571-1578

Jimeno, A., Rubio-Viqueira, B., Rajeshkumar, N.V., et al. (2010). A fine-needle aspirate-based vulnerability assay identifies polo-like kinase 1 as a mediator of gemcitabine resistance in pancreatic cancer. *Molecular Cancer Therapeutics,* Vol.9, No.2, (February 2010), pp.311-318

Johnson, N.A., Hamoudi, R., Ichimura, K., et al. (2006). Application of array CGH on archival formalin-fixed paraffin-embedded tissues including small numbers of microdissected cells. *Laboratory Investigation,* Vol.86, No.9 (September 2006) pp.968-978

Johnson, W.C., Helwig, E.B. (1963). Histochemistry of primary and metastatic mucus-secreting tumors. *Annals of the New York Academy of Sciences,* Vol.106, (March 1963) pp.794-803, ISSN 0077-8923

Jorgensen, J.T., Winther, H. (2009) The new era of personalized medicine: 10 years later. *Personalized Medicine,* Vol.6, No.4, (July 2009), pp.423-428

Kalloger, S.E., Kobel, M., Leung, S., et al. (2011). Calculator for ovarian carcinoma subtype prediction. *Modern Pathology,* Vol.24, No.4, (April 2011), pp. 512-521

Karabulut, A., Reibel, J., Therkildsen, M.H., et al.(1995). Observer variability in the histologic assessment of oral premalignant lesions. *Journal of Oral Pathology and Medicine.* Vol.24, No.5, (May 1995), pp.198-200

Kim, Y., Liu, C., Tan, W. (2009). Aptamers generated by Cell SELEX for biomarker discovery. *Biomarkers in Medicine* Vol.3, No.2, (April 2009), pp.193-202

Kobel, M., Kalloger, S.E., Baker, P.M., et al. (2010). Diagnosis of ovarian carcinoma cell type is highly reproducible: a Transcanadian study. *American Journal of Surgical Pathology* Vol.34, No.7, (July 2010), pp.984-993

Kotsakis, A., Yousem, S. and Gadgeel, S.M. (2010) Is histologic subtype significant in the management of NSLCLC? *The Open Lung Cancer Journal* Vol. 3, pp.66-72

Kros, J.M., Gorlia, T., Kouwenhoven, M.C., et al. (2007). Panel review of anaplastic oligodendroglioma from European Organization for Research and Treatment of Cancer Trial 26951: assessment of consensus in diagnosis, influence of 1p/19q loss, and correlations with outcome. *Journal of Neuropathology and Experimental Neurology,* Vol.66, No.6, (June 2007), pp.545-551

Kufe DW, Pollock RE, Weichselbaum RR, et al (Eds.). 2003. *Role of the surgical pathologist in the diagnosis and management of the cancer patient.* Holland-Frei Cancer Medicine, Hamilton(ON).

Lee, J., Hever, A., Willhite, D., et al. (2005). Effects of RNA degradation on gene expression analysis of human postmortem tissues. *The FASEB Journal* Vol.19, No.10, (August 2005), pp.1356-1358

Leitner, A., Walzthoeni, T., Kahraman, A., et al. ((2010) Probing native protein structures by chemical cross-linking, mass spectrometry, and bioinformatics. *Molecular and Cellular Proteomics,* Vol.9, No.8, (August 2010), pp.1634-1649

Lennerz J.K.M., Crippin, J.S. & Brunt, E.M. (2009). Diagnostic considerations of nodules in the cirrhotic liver. *Pathology Case Reviews,* Vol.14, No.1, (January/February 2009), pp.3-12, ISSN 1082-9784/09/1401-0003

Li, J., Wang, L.L., Mamon, H., et al. (2008). Replacing PCR with OL-PCR enriches variant DNA sequences and redefines the sensitivity of genetic testing. *Nature Medicine* Vol.14, (April 2008), pp.579-584

Llombart-Bosch, A., Contesso, G. & Peydro-Olaya, A. (1996). Histology, immunohistochemistry, and electron microscopy of small round cell tumors of bone. *Seminars in Diagnostic Pathology,* Vol.13, No.3, (August 1996), pp.153-170

Leuschner, I., Radig, K. & Harms, D. (1996). Desmoplastic small round cell tumor. *Seminars in Diagnostic Pathology,* Vol.13,No.3, (August 1996), pp.204-212, ISSN 0740-2570/96/1303-0005

McSherry, E.A., McGoldrick, A., Kay, E.W., et al. (2007). Formalin-fixed paraffin-embedded clinical tissue show spurious copy number changes in aCGH profiles. *Clinical Gentics.*Vol.72, No.5, (November 2007), pp.441-447

Metz, B., Kersten, G.F.A., Baart, G.J.E., et al. (2006). Identification of formaldehyde-induced modifications in proteins : Reactions with insulin. *Bioconjugate Chemistry* Vol.17, No.3 (May-June 2006), pp.815-822

Miyatake, Y., Ikeda, H., Michimata, R., et al. (2004). Differential modulation of gene expression among rat tissues with warm ischemia. *Experimental and Molecular Pathology,* Vol.77, No.3, (December 2004), pp.222-230

Mojica, W.D., Stein, L., Hawthorn, L.A. (2007). An exfoliation and enrichment strategy results in improved transcriptional profiles when compared to matched formalin fixed samples. *BMC Clinical Pathology*, Vol.7. e

Mojica, W.D., Sykes, D., Conroy, J., et al. A comparative analysis of two tissue procurement approaches for the genomic profiling of clinical colorectal cancer samples. *International Journal of Colorectal Disease*, Vol.23, No.11, pp.1089-1098.

Monzon, F.A., Medeiros, F., Lyons Weiler, M., et al. (2010). Identification of tissue of origin in a carcinoma of unknown primary with a microarray-based gene expression test. *Diagnostic Pathology* Vol.5:3, Accessioned August 2010. Available at http://www.diagnosticpathology.org/content/5/1/3

Mutter, G.L., Zahrieh, D., Liu, C., et al. (2004) Comparison of frozen and RNALater solid tissue storage methods for use in RNA expression microarrays. *BMC Genomics* Vol.5:88. Accessioned December 2009. Available from http://www.biomedcentral.com/1471-2164/5/88

National Biospecimen Network Blueprint (2003). Accessioned June 2009. Available at http://biospecimens.cancer.gov/global/pdfs/FINAL_NBN_Blueprint.pdf

Nirmalan, N.J., Harnden, P., Selby, P.J. & Banks, R.E. (2008). Mining the archival formalin-fixed paraffin-embedded tissue proteome: opportunities and challenges. *Molecular BioSystems*, Vol.4,No.7, (July 2008), pp.712-720

Opitz, L., Salinas-Riester, G., Grade, M., et al.(2010) Impact of RNA degradation on gene expression profiling. *BMC Genomics* Vol.3, e36. Accessioned February 2011. Available at http://www.biomedcentral.com/1755-8794/3/36

Papadopoulos, N., Kinzler, K.W., & Vogelstein, B. (2006). The role of companion diagnostics in the development and used of mutation-targeted cancer therapies. *Nature Biotechnology* Vol.24, No.8 (August, 2006), pp.985-995

Pasini, E.M., Kirekegaard, M., Mortensen, P., et al. (2006) In depth analysis of the membrane and cytosolic proteome of red blood cells. *Blood* Vol.108, No.3 (August 2006), pp.791-801

Penland, S.K., Keku, T.O., Torrice, C., et al. (2007). RNA expression analysis of formalin-fixed, paraffin-embedded tumors. *Labortaory Investigation*, Vol.87, No.4, (April 2007), pp.383-391

Plesec, T.P. and Hunt, J.L. (2009). KRAS mutation testing in colorectal cancer. *Advances in Anatomic Pathology* Vol.16, No.4 (July 2009), pp.196-203

Press, M., Pike, M., Chazin, V., et al. (1993). Her-2/neu expression in node-negative breast cancer: Direct tissue quantitation by computerized image analysis and association of overexpression with increased risk of recurrent disease. *Cancer Research*. Vol.53, No.20, (October 1993), pp.4960-4970

Qin, J., Li, R., Raes, J., et al. (2010). A human gut microbial gene catalogue established by metagenomic sequencing. *Nature* Vol.464, No.7285 (March 2010), pp. 59-65

Quach, N., Goodman, M.F., & Shibata, D. (2004), In vitro mutation artifacts after formalin fixation and error prone translesional synthesis during PCR. *BMC Clinical Pathology* Vol4:1. Accessed August 2010. Available at http://www.biomedcentral.com/1472-6890/4/1

Quek, T.P.L., Yan, B., Yong, W.P.P., et al. (2009). Targeted therapeutic-oriented tumor classification: a paradigm shift. *Personalized Medicine*, Vol.6, No.5, pp.465-468

Qui, Q., Todd, N.W., Li, R., et al. (2008) Magnetic enrichment of bronchial epithelial cells from sputum for lung cancer diagnosis. *Cancer* Vol.114, (August, 2008), pp.275-283

Ricciardelli, C., Bianco-Miotto, T., Jindal, S., et al. (2010). Comparative biomarker expression and RNA integrity in biospecimens derived from radical retropubic and robot-assisted laparoscopic prostatectomies. *Cancer Epidemiology, Biomarkers and Prevention* Vol.19, No.7 (July, 2010), pp.1755-1765.

Rosai, J. (Ed.). 1997. *Guiding the surgeon's hand.* American Registry of Pathology, ISBN 1-881041-42-5, Washington, D.C.

Rountree, C.B., Van Kirk, C.A., You, H., et al. (2010) Clinical application for the preservation of phosphoproteins through in-situ tissue stabilization. *Proteome Science* Vol.8:61. Accessioned April 2011. Available at http://www.proteomescie.com/cpmtent/8/1/61

Schlomm, T., Nakel, E., Lubke, A., et al. (2008). Marked gene transcript level alterations occur early during radical prostatectomy. *European Journal of Urology.* Vol.53, No.2, (February 2008), pp.333-346

Scicchitano, M.S., Dalmas, D.A., Boyce, R.W., et al. (2009). Protein extraction of formalin-fixed, paraffin-embedded tissue enables robust proteomic profiles by mass spectrometry. *Journal of Histochemistry and Cytochemistry.* Vol.57, No.9, (September 2009), pp.849-860

Shen-Orr S.S., Tishirani, R., Khatri, P., et al. (2010) Cell type-specific gene expression differences in complex tissues. *Nature Methods* vol.7, No.4 (April 2010), pp.287-289

Specht, K., Muller, U., Walch, A., et al.(2001). Quantitative gene expression analysis in microdissected archival formalin-fixed and paraffin-embedded tumor tissue. *American Journal of Pathology*, Vol.158, No.2, (February 2001) pp.419-429

Spruessel, A., Steimann, G., Jung, M. et al. (2004). Tissue ischemia time affects gene and protein expression patterns within minutes following surgical tumor excision. *Biotechniques.* Vol.36, No.6, (June 2004), pp.1030-1037

Stan, A.D., Ghose, S., Gao, X., et al. (2006). Human postmortem tissue: What quality markers matter? *Brain Research*, Vol.1123, No.1, (December 2006), pp.1-11

Sun, J., Masterman-Smith, M.D., Graham, N.A. et al. (2010). A microfluidic platform for systems pathology: Multiparameter single cell signaling measurements of clinical brain tumor specimens. *Cancer Research*, Vol.70, No.15, (August 2010), pp.6128-6138

Svensson, M., Boren, M., Skold, K., et al.(2009). Heat stabilization of the tissue proteome: A new technology for improved proteomics. *Journal of Proteome Research* Vol.8, No.2 (February 2009), pp.974-981

Sutherland, B.W., Toews, J., Kast, J. (2008) Utility of formaldehyde cross-linking and mass spectrometry in the study of protein-protein interactions. *Journal of Mass Spectrometry* Vol.43, No.6 (June 2008), pp.699-715

Taylor, CR.. & Cote, R.J. (Eds.) 1994. *Immunomicroscopy: A diagnostic tool for the surgical pathologist.* W.B. Saunders Company, ISBN 0-7216-6462-8, Philadelphia, PA

Thomas, G.(2008). Practical applications of biospecimen science in biobanking. In: *2008 BRN Symposium.* Accessed March 2010, Available from: http://brnsymposium.com/meeting/brnsymposium/2008/

Toews, J., Rogalski, J.C., Clark, T.J. et al. Mass spectrometric identification of formaldehyde-induced peptide modifications under *in vivo* protein cross-linking conditions. *Analytica Chimica Acta* Vol.618, No.2 (June, 2008), pp.16-183.

Tremblath, D., Miller, C., Perry, A. (2008). Gray zones in brain tumor classification: Evolving concepts. *Advances in Anatomic Pathology* Vol.15, No.5 (September, 2008), pp.287-297

Trump, B.F. & Jones R.T. (Eds.) 1983. *Diagnostic electron microscopy.* John Wiley and Sons, ISBN 0-471-015149-7, New York.

Tureci, O., Ding, J., Hilton, H., et al.(2003). Computational dissection of tissue contamination for identification of colon cancer-specific expression profiles. *FASEB,* Vol.17 (March, 2003), pp.376-385

Van Maldegem, F., de Wit, M., Mosink, F., et al. (2008). Effects of processing delay, formalin fixation, and immunohistochemistry on RNA recovery from formalin-fixed paraffin-embedded tissue sections. *Diagnostic Molecular Pathology* Vol.17, No.1 (March 2008), pp.51-58

Velez, E., Turbat-Herrera, E.A. & Herrera, G.A. (2002). Malignant epithelial mesothelioma versus pulmonary adenocarcinoma – a pathologic dilemma with medicolegal implications. *Pathology Case Reviews,* Vol.7, No.5 (September/October 2002), pp.234-243

Wallace, WAH. (2009). The challenge of classifying poorly differentiate tumours in the lung. *Histopatology,* Vol.54, (January 2009), pp.28-42

Wan, Y., Kim, Y., Li, N., et al.(2010),. Surface-immobilized aptamers for cancer cell isolation and microscopic cytology. *Cancer Research,* Vol.70, No.22, (November 2010), pp.9371-9380

Wang, H.L., Lopategui, J., Amin, M.B., et al. (2010). KRAS mutation testing in human cancers: The Pathologist's role in the era of Personalized Medicine. *Advances in Anatomic Pathology* Vol.17, No.1 (January 2010), pp.23-31

Weigum, S.E., Floriano, P.N., Redding, S.W., et al. (2010). Nano-Bio-Chip sensor platform for examination of oral exfoliative cytology. *Cancer Prevention Research,* Vol.3, No.4, (April 2010), pp.518-528.

Wong, N.A.C.S., Hunt, L.P., Novelli, M.R., et al. Observer agreement in the diagnosis of serrated polyps of the large bowel. *Histopathology,* Vol.55, No.1, (July 2009), pp.63-66

Yu, S., Xie, L, Hou, Z., et al. (2011) Co-amplification at lower denaturation temperature polymerase chain reaction enables selective identification of K-*Ras* mutations in formalin-fixed, paraffin-embedded tumor tissues without tumor-cell enrichment. *Human Pathology* (in press)

7

Negative Impact of Paclitaxel Crystallization on Hydrogels and Novel Approaches for Anticancer Drug Delivery Systems

Javier S. Castro[1,2], Lillian V.Tapia[1], Rocio A. Silveyra[1],
Carlos A. Martinez[1] and Pierre A. Deymier[2]
[1]Materials Science and Engineering, Institute of Engineering and Technology,
Autonomous University of Juarez City, Juarez City, Chih.
[2]Department of Materials Science and Engineering,
University of Arizona, Tucson AZ 85721
[1]Mexico
[2]USA

1. Introduction

Paclitaxel, better known as Taxol® its original name and now trade mark, and its direct derivatives, has been one of the most effective drugs used against tumors and cancer (Rowinsky et al., 1990; Rowinsky & Donehower, 1995) due to its ability to stabilize microtubules in the mitotic spindle and thus stopping the cell cycle in eukaryotic cells (Wani et al.,1971). The stabilization of microtubules is due to the specific bond between Taxol® and beta tubulin preventing microtubule depolymerization (Schiff et al., 1979). It has also been reported that Taxol® inhibits the process of angiogenesis (Wang et al., 2003). These Taxol® qualities have been taken as an advantage for the usage of this drug in killing carcinogenic cells in tumors.

One of the main drawbacks of this molecule is its high hydrophobicity; making it practically insoluble in water which hinders their use in treatments inside the human body. In order to overcome such inconveniences, several strategies have been developed such as the use of adjuvants like Cremofor/Etanol (CrEL), solubilizant agent that facilitates the intravenously administration of the drug, process termed as chemotherapy. This technique has brought many disadvantages such as the fact of reducing considerably the drug's diffusion capacity, making that a limited quantity of the drug be reached into the target site (Marupudi et al., 2007), and therefore limiting the concentration level needed to eliminate tumors. To solve these inconveniences it has been resolved to increase the delivery cycles. The usage of Taxol® in CrEL and the high doses have produced undesired consequences with a numerous of hypersensitivity reactions and side effects including nausea, vomiting, urticaria, abdominal pain, diaphoresis, and other (Weiss et al., 1990; Wiernik et al., 1987). Looking for minimizing such secondary reactions, new options in the field of drug delivery are being explored. In the last decade a variety of drug delivery systems have been proposed as carriers of hydrophobic anticancer drugs. The list of these systems includes drug loaded hydrogels, drug loaded nanoparticles, functionalized nanoparticles and some combined systems. Through this chapter we review the current trends for the transport and delivery of the most common anticancer drugs. Based in facts we point a delicate issue, Taxol crystallization in hydrogels and its negative impact, and finally we make a discussion about novel approaches for drug delivery against cancer.

2. Hydrogels for drug delivery systems

Currently the development of smart hydrogels that can respond to external stimuli such as variations in temperature, pH, and electric fields or hydrogels with controlled biodegradability has been used in biomedical applications. As such hydrogels are used in a wide range of applications including tissue engineering and regenerative medicine (Lee & Mooney, 2001), diagnosis (Van Der Linden et al., 2003), cell immobilization (Jen et al., 1996), bimolecular and cell separation (Wang et al., 1993), barriers to regulate the biological adhesion (Bennett et al., 2003). Hydrogels can be made, in theory, from any water-soluble polymer, encompassing a wide range of chemical compositions and physical properties. The polymer forms aggregates that form a three-dimensional matrix with interconnected pores in which the solvent (usually water or aqueous solutions) and other particles can diffuse (Figure 1). Some hydrogels have a high capacity to contain compounds that can be released in a controlled manner for therapeutic purposes. Its porosity allows the loading of drugs within the polymer matrix and their subsequent release at a rate that depends on the coefficient of diffusion of drug through the gel matrix in the case of hydrophilic drugs. For hydrophobic drugs, the rate of release depends on the rate of degradation of the gel. Besides their biodegradability can be designed to be via enzymatic, hydrolytic, or environmental (pH, temperature or electric fields).

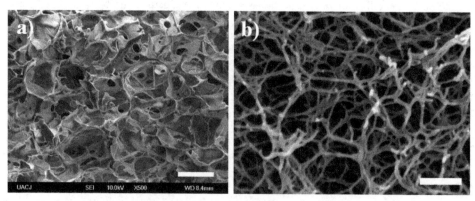

Fig. 1. Hydrogel structures observed by FESEM (Field Emission Scanning Electron Microscope). a) Chitosan-Glycerophosphate termosensitive hydrogel. Bar 40μm. b) Agarose hydrogel. Bar 250 nm.

2.1 Thermosensitive hydrogels for anticancer drug delivery

Commonly hydrogels gelatinize when their temperature drops; in other words they are present in a liquid state at higher temperatures, and they solidify when it drops. However, there are hydrogels that exhibit the phenomenon of reverse thermal gelation, also known as thermally induced hydrogels. In this case they are liquid at lower temperatures, but they solidify when their temperature rises (Klouda & Mikos, 2008). This property has been exploited to create hydrogels that remain liquid at temperatures below 30 ° C, but they solidify at temperatures close to physiological temperature (37 °C). Therefore, they are better injected subcutaneously as a liquid and solidify when they reach body temperature. Some of these hydrogels are tri-block copolymer synthesized by open-ring polymerization such as poly (ethylene glycol)-poly(epsilon-caprolactone)-poly (ethylene glycol) (PEG-PCL-PEG) (ChangYang et al., 2009; Yu, 2009), tri-block copolymer poly(ethylene oxide)-poly (oxidopropileno) -poly (ethylene oxide) (PEO-PPO-PEO) (Li & Li, 2008), and biopolymer chitosan (C) neutralized with b-glycerophosphate (GP) (Ruel-Gariépy et al., 2004). Most of these hydrogels are studied for drug delivery and some have already been used successfully for this purpose. For example, PEO-PPO-PEO-name Poloxamer 407 has been used to prolong the release of lidocaine (Chen et al., 2004). Also, some natural polymers exhibit the phenomenon of reverse thermal gelation such as those based on chitosan, which have reported positive results; for instance, a solution of chitosan with 40% weight of PEG has been tested on the release of serum bovine holding a sustained release of at least 70 hours (Bhattarai et al., 2005). Other organic hydrogels with this property are hydroxypropyl cellulose (Cai et al., 2003; Uraki et al., 2004) and methyl cellulose (Kumar et al., 1993).

Among the new methods aimed to replace intravenous chemotherapy for the treatment of tumors there are certain proposals which emphasize the use of temperature-sensitive hydrogels loaded with anticancer drugs. They suggest the injection of the thermosensitive hydrogels containing drug directly into the affected area (tumor), due to its reverse thermal behavior it solidifies inside the body and then the drug is released gradually. The most common proposed systems for Taxol® delivery have been those that offer direct incorporation of the drug into the thermosensitive hydrogel (Chun et al., 2009; Dai et al., 2006; Kasala et al., 2008; Livnat et al., 2005; Marupudi et al., 2007; Ruel-Gariépy et al., 2004; Shi & Burt, 2004; Woo Sun et al., 2007). Just to mention some examples, the alginate hydrogel with polyethylene glycol (PEG) (Livnat et al., 2005), the hydrogel Dx-g-PCL result of the synthesis of polycaprolactone (PLC) and Dextran (Dextran70 and Dextran 500) (Shi & Burt, 2004), so as the thermosensitive chitosan-based hydrogel BST-Gel liquid (Marupudi et al., 2007).

2.2 Paclitaxel crystallization in hydrogels

We have studied Taxol® crystallization in aqueous solutions and hydrogels (Castro et al., 2010). In both environments Taxol® forms needle-like crystals that grow concentrically forming complex morphologies such as spherulites, in the case of heterogeneous nucleation, or sheaves (axialites) when they are formed by homogeneous nucleation. In solution or gel these crystals can be observed by DIC (Differential Interference Contrast) microscopy or by fluorescent microscopy when they are labeled with a fluorescent dye such as rhodamine, as described in (Castro et al. 2009). Dried they can be analyzed by scanning electron microscopy (Figure 2). solution by heterogeneous nucleation with a Taxol concentration of 50 µM. Sample was prepared by drying a drop in a TEM (Transmission Electron Microscope) cooper grid and then metalized by sputter coating with a gold-palladium target. a) Bar 2.5 µm, b) bar 10 µm.

The process of crystallization in aqueous solutions and hydrogels is quite similar and we can describe it in few words, Taxol crystallization follows the classical homogeneous nucleation theory. For low supersaturation (low Taxol concentrations), only a small number of crystals nuclei may form whereas for high supersaturation (>20 µM) the number of nuclei increases drastically with increasing Taxol® concentration.

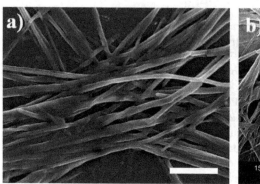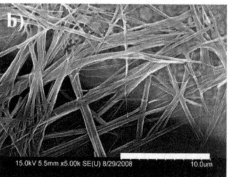

Fig. 2. Taxol crystals observed by FESEM. These crystals were obtained in aqueous solution.

As we mentioned before, the most common Hydrogel-based Taxol® delivery systems reported in literature suggest the direct incorporation of the drug into the thermosensitive hydrogel (Chun et al., 2009; Dai et al., 2006; Kasala et al., 2008; Livnat et al., 2005; Marupudi et al., 2007; Ruel-Gariépy et al., 2004; Shi & Burt, 2004; Woo Sun et al., 2007). But nobody, except Shi & Burt (2004), has reported Taxol crystallizacion in their systems. We claim that this phenomenon is present in most of these works, unfortunately this problem has been a neglected topic by many researchers and may go unnoticed because Taxol® crystals are not detectable by commonly used techniques for the characterization of the hydrogels. Perhaps, researchers have been concerned primarily in designing a good delivery system, neglecting other aspects of the drug, such as its crystallization. In studies reported in the literature that follow this line, no one takes into account, neither they mentioned nor reported studies of crystallization of Taxol® in hydrogels, despite that the use of the drug concentrations is greatly exceeded in its limit of solubility in aqueous solutions (0.77µM) (Shi & Burt 2004).

In order to provide evidence of Taxol crystallization in these hydrogels we have performed several experiments following similar conditions to that reported in the papers mentioned before. For instance we used similar hydrogels such as agarose, chitosan, poly (L-lactic acid) PLLA and thermosensitive Chitosan-Glycerophosphate and we also used Taxol concentrations similar, or even lower, to that reported in that works. As result we have found that Taxol® crystallization is always present in hydrogels and thermosensitive hydrogels (Figure 3). According to our observations Taxol® crystallization follows the behavior of the classical homogenous nucleation theory, as mentioned before. That means that at low Taxol concentrations (<30 µM) few but big (15-25 µm) axialites are present, while at higher many and smaller axialites are observed (Castro et al., 2011). Moreover paclitaxel crystals are very stable in aqueous environments. We have observed these crystals up to two months of formation without any noticeable change. Hence we can speculate that Taxol crystals inside the body probably would last for long time activating immune reactions.

Direct incorporation of paclitaxel into hydrogels can lead to crystallization of the drug which can dramatically decrease the therapeutic effects and effectiveness of paclitaxel delivery systems. Supporting our theory, we find in the work of Chun (2009) who reported that *in vivo* experiments with rats, contrary to what would be expected, the hydrogel with a lower concentration of Taxol® was more effective at tumor inhibition than hydrogel with the highest concentration. Although the authors did not provide explanations for such unexpected results, for us a good reason of this fact is the phenomenon of Taxol® crystallization, which is enhanced at higher concentrations. All this experimental evidence could be enough reason to believe that these systems do not meet the desired expectations and require major rethinking.

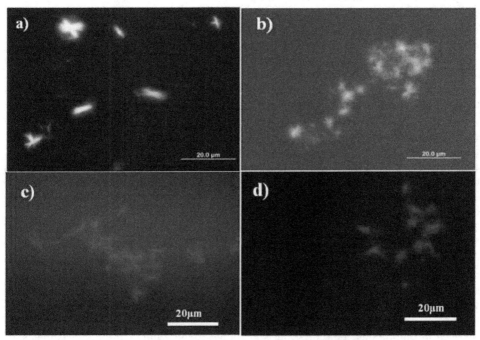

Fig. 3. Taxol crystals formed in hydrogels. a) in aqueous solution, b) in agarose hydrogel, c) in poly (L-lactic acid) hydrogel, d) Chitosan-Glycerophosphate hydrogel. All samples prepared at a paclitaxel concentration of 100 μM.

3. Nanoparticles for drug delivery

In order to minimize the inconvenient of the hydrophobicity many authors have proposed the encapsulation of hydrophobic drugs in nanoparticles, this would allow increasing the amount of drug administered without using nasty solvents such as CrEL in the case of paclitaxel. Thus it is being explored new types of delivery systems based in nanocarriers such as micelles (You et al., 2008), nanoparticles (Liang et al., 2006), thin films (Shi & Burt, 2004), and microspheres (Liu et al., 2007) among others (Ferrari & Downing, 2005), whose effectiveness is related to its size, modification of pharmacokinetics, biodistribution, delivery control and toxicity reduction (Jun et al., 2008). Each one of these particles has unique characteristics that should be carefully analyzed taking into account the type of drug and the desired interaction to obtain the adequate system delivery. The liposome usage for delivery agent of the anticancer drugs is very broad, such as Doxil®, this drug is commercially distributed and used in several ovarian cancer treatments (Gordon et al., 2001). However, the liposomes present several disadvantages due to their high permeability and stability *in vivo* (Conlin et al., 2009). Dendrimers are macromolecules characterized by their structural monodispersivity and symmetry. They consist of a central nucleus and its diverse ramifications. It contains different functional groups generally located on the exterior, which play an important role in their properties (Caminade et al., 2005). A disadvantage is its difficulty to be synthesized (Tomalia et al., 1990). The dendrimers are used in research studies for the prevention of sexually transmitted diseases (Zolnik & Sadrieh, 2009), as contrasting agents in Magnetic Resonance Imaging (Zolnik & Sadrieh, 2009), combined with anticancer drugs (Malik et al., 1999), among other usages. The nanocapsules are vesicular systems with colloidal size, in which the drug is located inside and surrounded by a polymeric membrane (Soppimath et al., 2001). In this system, the nucleus consists of oily liquid and a simple polymeric layer covers it, this system has shown to be effective in encapsulating and releasing certain types of hydrophobic drugs (Ameller et al., 2003). Nanospheres are solid colloidal particles in which the drug can be dissolved, encapsulated, conjugated or absorbed (Gref et al., 1995; Soppimath et al., 2001). They are generally larger than micelles and although its elimination is slow due to its hydrophobicity, are susceptible to renal filtration and the mono nuclear phagocyte system (MPS), It is therefore necessary to modify its surface (Letchford & Burt, 2007). Good stability has been achieved in nanospheres using amphiphilic copolymers (Gref et al., 1995), so it is possible the encapsulation of the bioactive molecule at the core of the nanosphere (Yanasarn et al., 2009), for example, it has been observed that the nanoparticles synthesized from emulsion of lecithin / water loaded with paclitaxel are more effective in attacking cancer cells than pure paclitaxel (Hu et al., 2009). In another study, gold nanoparticles encapsulated in nanospheres of chitosan and poly (acrylic acid) CS-PAA-Au have been used as delivery system drugs as well as for observation of cells (Latere et al., 2002).

Within this range of particles could not miss the micelles, which have had a great interest in the issue of drug delivery and location into tumors (Lee et al., 2003; Yokoyama et al., 1999). Micelles are amphiphilic molecules consisting of hydrophilic and hydrophobic segments. Its outer layer, which is highly hydrated, provides stability in aqueous environments, while the hydrophobic core allows the incorporation of water-insoluble drugs. Moreover, if the polymeric micelles have a diameter ranging from 10 to 100nm allows long circulation in the bloodstream avoiding defenses of the mono nuclear phagocyte system and suppressing renal clearance. They can be large enough to avoid being excreted by the kidneys but small enough to pass the interendothelial cell filtration (Yang et al., 2009).

As a result, drug activity continues after a single application over a long period of time. In addition, these micelles remain intact at levels below the critical micelle concentration (CMC), so they retain their structure and preferentially accumulate in solid tumors via the permeability and retention effect (EPR) (Nakayama et al., 2007; Saez et al., 2004). Its amphiphilic nature gives them a central place in the area of the release of hydrophobic drugs, due to its excellent drug storage capacity in its core.

The hydrophobic core also has other important features such as protecting the drug from being deactivated by enzymes or other bioactive species from the aqueous medium (blood fluid) (Wilhelm et al., 1991; (Yokoyama et al., 1990). Also, this medium affects the rate of drug release, in many cases declining it, as the release rate is controlled both by the stability of the micelles as the hydrophobicity of their core and the chemical species used to attach the drug to the polymer backbone. These factors may be independent of the properties of the drug.

While each system has its advantages and disadvantages, micelles and nanospheres formed by amphiphilic copolymers have greater flexibility in their synthesis and uses, and they have had good results with hydrophobic drugs. The difference lies in the method of preparation and length of the hydrophobic segment. Although for some authors the nanospheres are systems that perform in vivo by presenting better retention properties of the drug, they have a burst effect when the drug is readily released; in this sense, the nanospheres are overcome by the micelles who exhibit more stable behaviors (Gaucher et al., 2010; Kwon, 2003). We can mention some examples of micelles made of different polymers used to carry drugs. We cite a few micelles synthesized from copolymer PEG-PASP-DMEDA loaded with ammonium glycyrrhizate (AMG) poorly water soluble drug used against Hepatitis C (Yang et al., 2009). Copolymer polylactide / polyethylene glycol is synthesized by polymerization of ring-opened was used to encapsulate paclitaxel without the presence of an organic solvent (Kim et al., 2009). Also, some micelles are sensitive to changes in pH, this feature can be used to control drug release as self-assembled micelles of copolymer PEG-b-PMA with divalent metals loaded with doxorucibin (Li et al., 2009). Tamoxifen and paclitaxel have also been charged in micelles with a hydrophilic block of poly [2 - (ethyl methacriloyloxi) phosphorylcholine] (MPC), hydrophobic block and a pH sensitive poly [2 - (diisopropylamine)ethyl methacrylate] (DPA) (FA-MPC-DPA) (Licciardi et al., 2008). Doxorubicin was loaded using thermosensitive blocks such as poly (N-isopropylacrylamide-co-N, N-dimethyl-acrylamide) in which the hydrophobic part was synthesized from poly (D, L-lactide), poly(epsilon-caprolactone) or poly (D, L-lactide-co-ε-caprolactone) (Masamichi et al.; 2006). Another type of thermosensitive micelles have been synthesized from poly (N-isopropylacrylamide) and poly (butyl methacrylate) also loaded with doxorubicin (Chung et al., 1999). Similarly, micelles have been developed and modified in the copolymer as synthesized from poly (ethylene glycol)-poly (aspartateester groups heptyl, nonyl, phenyl propyl benzyl and for greater stabilization of the drug N-(4 - hydroxifenil) retinamide (Tomoyuki et al., 2008).

Encapsulation of paclitaxel in nanoparticles is very promising and results have been favorable, judging by the reports in the literature. However, most authors suggest the use of nanoparticles to be injected into the bloodstream, following the route of traditional chemotherapy, which somehow still has the disadvantage of low specificity in which the problem is attacked. But that's not all, perhaps the main problem is not the lack of specificity of the method, but the risk involved in the use of nanoparticles in the bloodstream. Currently, no one knows for sure the adverse effects of the use of nanoparticles in the bloodstream, since its size could pass biological membranes or barriers and it has unknown effects on areas of the body, becoming a health risk factor , as noted by experts on the subject of the risks of nanotechnology in medicine (Scott et al., 2008). To this, we must add that the nanoparticles contain a highly cytotoxic drug.

3.1 Functionalization of nanoparticles

Particle functionalization with specific ligands for cancer cells has gained considerable attention for those looking for more specificity in their systems carrying the drug. Work is being currently done to prove their effectiveness with different ligand-receptor systems in a variety of cancer cell lines to test the efficiency of the functionalization of these systems. The effectiveness of the functionalization of nanoparticles lies in the premise of the existence of certain molecules in tumors are different from those found in normal tissues and can be identified as biomarkers of tumorogenesis (Mohd & Mohammad, 2009). Depending on its test site, they may be biomarkers of tissue or circulatory. Tissue biomarkers have different categories such as membrane receptors, oncogenes, tumor suppressor genes, nucleic antigens, growth factors and components of degradation. Circulatory biomarkers include a broad category of tumor-associated antigens (TAA). Selective biomarkers can identify risks and help tumor detection, and an early diagnosis allows appropriate therapeutic interventions for an effective treatment. In addition to these biomarkers, it is also common to find an over expression of certain proteins membrane in cancer cells, which has been used for the use of specific ligands or molecules to these proteins, such as folic acid to folate receptors, to obtain greater interaction of nanoparticles to cancer cells. In this case, the effectiveness of the functionalization is more a matter of statistics than specificity by itself, since having the over expression of these receptors will increase the likelihood of attracting a greater number of drug-loaded nanoparticles to diseased cells.

Micelles have been recently reported to have been functionalized with folic acid as a specific ligand , which is strongly attracted to its receptor in the cell membrane. The folate receptor is a protein that is generated in large quantities during cell proliferation in several types of cancer cells such as ovarian, breast, brain and lung (Ross et al., 1994).

Also, peptides have been used for the functionalization of micelles as locators of cancer cells. The nature of polypeptides allows performance optimization of specific ligands by adjusting the sequence or conformation of the peptides. One example is the peptide cRGD (cyclic Arg-Gly-Asp-D-Phe-Lys) specific for $\alpha v \beta 3$ receptor produced in large amounts in tumor endothelial cells (Nasongkla et al., 2004). These receptors are a cell membrane protein that is affected with the growth of tumors, local invasiveness and potentially in metastasis, but it is not detected in quiescent vessels (Rueg et al., 2002; Teti et al., 2002; Vamer & Cheresh, 1996). This membrane receptor increases its levels in vascular angiogenesis, thus making tumor treatment specific for the generation of new blood vessels (Wermuth et al., 1997). Carbohydrate functionalized micelles, asialoglycoprotein receptor (ASGPR) is a recipient of lecithin membrane commonly found in liver cells (Ashwelland & Harford, 1982). In hepatocellular carcinoma are high levels of (ASGPR), which helps the specificity of chemotherapy for liver (Wands & Blum, 1991). Carbohydrate molecules such as galactose and mannose are specific ligands of this receptor (Goto et al., 1994; Jansen et al., 1991).

The use of antibodies as specific ligands is promising as they are able to bind to a range of specific antigens in cancer cells. The combination of a brain-specific antibody increased to 5-fold the neuroleptic action in charged micelles than in non-functionalized micelles, and it is 20 times greater than for the free drug (Kabanov et al., 1989). Micelles have been reported (PEG-PE) functionalized with 2 antibodies, a monoclonal anti-cancer antibody (mAb2C5) and anti-myosin (mAb2G4). Both antibodies have great ability to bind to the substrates after conjugation of the micelles. The antibody 2C5 in micelles loaded with paclitaxel increased 4 times the drug accumulation in the tumor after 2 hours (Torchilin et al., 2003). Furthermore, there is the functionalization of micelles with aptamers. The aptamers are DNA and RNA oligonucleotides that can identify a large number of specific molecules (Torchilin et al., 2003; Tuerkand & Gold, 1990). We have seen that PEG-PLA micelles with an RNA aptamer specifically bind to an antigen on the membrane of prostate tumor (PSMA). Nanoparticles with the induction of aptamer showed 77 times more specificity to PSMA receptor than non-functionalized particles (Ellingtonand & Szostak, 1990). The use of ligands has yielded promising results for the location of cancer cells. This will allow drug release systems based on nanoparticles using different ligands that recognize different types of cancer. There is further research to look for future and further specific treatments with low or no side effects. Instead of using a single ligand, nanoparticles' specificity can be potentiated using multiple ligands in a single particle. Sooner or later, these systems will have the ability to attack different cancers at once or they will be designed to exchange specific ligands in an easy way, having a generic nanoparticle system capable of receiving any desired ligand presenting a universal binding system.

4. Combined systems based on hydrogels and nanoparticles

There are few studies that have integrated particles or micelles loaded with Taxol® in thermosensitive hydrogels. As good examples we can mention the system proposed by Jiang Liu et al. (2007) (Liu et al., 2007). This system consists of a biodegradable gelatin sponge containing PLGA-PTX microspheres (polylactide-co-glycolic acid-paclitaxel) in order to provide continuous local release of PTX (paclitaxel). They obtained a more prolonged release rate for up to 19 days, in contrast to simple systems where the paclitaxel was released within a range less than one hour. In another study presented by Yang Yang et al. (2009) joined Docetaxol (DTX) in a pluronic gel F127(PF127) injectable thermosensitive mixed micelles prepared with the same material (PF127) and loaded with Taxol® (system GMM). During a test of 156 hours, it was found that the proposed system maintains a prolonged release of DTX compared with other control systems (Yang et al., 2009).

The development of combined drug delivery systems based on efficient and innovative drug encapsulation in functionalized nanoparticles to detect and attack cancer cells, using thermosensitive hydrogels as vehicles that can be injected locally can be an excellent option for the treatment of cancerous tumors, thereby eliminating the supply of intravenous drugs and consequently the severe side effects. Specifically for Taxol®, its encapsulation in nanoparticles would prevent crystallization when deposited in the hydrogel. In addition, the release rates could be controlled in a double form, both by the action of the degradation of gel particles released and at the same time by the degradation of the particle containing the Taxol®. Achieving prolonged drug release would increase the therapeutic effects for longer periods. An added value to these systems is the funcionalization or even multifuncionalization of nanoparticles with ligands or antibodies for high specificity to cancer cells, which should increase the efficiency and the therapeutic effectiveness of the system. Even today very few researchers have worked with Taxol® delivery systems with the characteristics listed above; making this theme of the project attractive and innovative for study.

5. Conclusions

Researchers are currently exploring new methods for transport and controlled release of drugs for cancer treatment, thereby seeking to reduce the side effects the of currently applied chemotherapy as well as looking for battling more efficiently and accurately such disease. Although there are a number of published research focused on this issue, the fact is that so far no systems have emerged to prove conclusively its efficacy, although always positive progress has been shown, each proposed system suffers from certain drawbacks that slows down the progress towards real applications. The disadvantages found in the systems of transport and release of anticancer drugs proposed in recent years can be overcome by taking advantage of each method and combining them into drug delivery systems composed with more sophistication and complexity than their predecessors. This idea has already begun to be implemented by some researchers who have integrated drug-loaded nanoparticles on thermosensitive hydrogels (Liu et al., 2007), but these authors have not exploited the alternative of functionalization or multi-functionalization of nanoparticles. So, there is still much room for much improvement in these drug delivery systems and it is where researchers could find novel ideas. For example we can think in to make functionalized or multifunctionalized nanoparticles loaded with a anticancer drug, then incorporate them into a thermosensitive hydrogel. With this proposed system, the hydrogel may be injected into the tumor area (in the case of solid tumors) and gradually functionalized nanoparticles will be released. Due to its functionalization, they will be attracted mainly to diseased cells, nanoparticles will be biodegraded and drug will be released surrounding the cell. There are several advantages of using combined systems. For example, the highly localized application by avoiding the bloodstream, in the case of solid tumors; an improved release profile with a slow and steady dose that highly favored the drug's effectiveness in eliminating cells. The effectiveness of the functionalization of nanoparticles will be favored by the close application to malignant cells; in general, we will expect to acquire treatments where the typical collateral damage observed in common chemotherapies would be considerably lower as well as the required dose.

6. Acknowledgment

We want to express our gratitude to Alejandro Martinez and Jorge A. Perez Leon for access to their laboratory and fluorescent microscope supported by CONACYT, Selene Sandoval for sample preparation, Rodolfo Avitia for language assistance and corrections, the University of Arizona and the Autonomous University of Juarez City (UACJ) for the backup and the financial support from PROMEP (Programa para el mejoramiento del profesorado) grant UACJ-EXB-131 and NSF/NIRT grant 0303863.

7. References

Ameller,T.; Marsaud, V.; Legrand, P.; Gref, R.; Barratt, G. & Renoir, J.M. (2003). Polyester-Poly(Ethylene Glycol) Nanoparticles Loades with the Pure Antiestrogen RU 58668: 0 Pysicochemical and Opsonization Properties. *Pharm. Res.*, Vol.20, pp. (1063-1070).

Ashwelland, G. & Harford, J. (1982). Carbohydrate-specific receptors of the liver. *Ann. Rev. Biochem*, Vol. 51, pp.(531-554).

Bennett, S.L.; Melanson, D.A.; Torchiana, D.F.; Wiseman, D.M. & Sawhney, A.S. (2003). Next-Generation HydroGel Films as Tissue Sealants and Adhesion Barriers. *Journal of Cardiac Surgery*, Vol.18, No. 6, pp.(494-499).

Bhattarai, N.; Ramay, H.R.; Gunn, J.; Matsen, F.A. & Zhang, M.Q. (2005). PEG-grafted chitosan as an injectable thermosensitive hydrogel for sustained protein release. *Journal of Controlled Release*, Vol.103, No.3, pp.(609-624).

Cai, T.; Hu, Z.B.; Ponder, B.; St John, J. & Moro, D. (2003). Synthesis and study of and controlled release from nanoparticles and their networks based on functionalized hydroxypropylcellulose. *Macromolecules*.Vol.36, No.17, pp. (6559-6564).

Caminade, A.M.; Laurent. R. & Majoral, J.P. (2005). Characterization of dendrimers. *Advanced Drug Delivery Reviews*, Vol.57, pp.(2130-2146).

Castro, J.S. ; Deymier, P.A. ; & Trzaskowski, B. (2011). Paclitaxel Crystals: Molecular Interactions, Nucleation and Growth, and Possible Implications on Cell Studies. *Horizons in Cancer Research*, Vol. 45, 5, Editor: Hiroto S. Watanabe, ISBN:978-1-61209-377-2, Nova Science Publishers, Inc. Hauppauge, New York.

Castro, J. S.; Deymier, P. A.; Trzaskowski, B. & Bucay, J. (2010). Heterogeneous and homogeneous nucleation of Taxol crystals in aqueous solutions and gels: effect of tubulin proteins. Submitted to Colloids and Surfaces B: Biointerfaces, Vol.76, pp. (199-206)

Castro, J. S.; Trzaskowski B.; Deymier, P. A.; Bucay j.; Adamowicz L.; and Hoying, J. B. (2009). Binding Affinity of Fluorochromes and Fluorescent Proteins to Taxol Crystals. *Materials Science and Engineering:C*, Vol. 29, pp. (1609-1615).

ChangYang, G.; Shuai, S.; PengWei, D.; Bing, K.; MaLing, G.; XianHuo, W.; XingYi, L.; Feng, L.; Xia, Z.; YuQuan, W. & ZhiYong, Q. (2009). Synthesis and characterization of PEG-PCL-PEG thermosensitive hydrogel. *International Journal of Pharmaceutics*, Vol. 365, pp. (89–99).

Chen, P.C., Kohane, D.S., Park, Y.J., Bartlett, R.H., Langer, R. & Yang, VC. (2004). *Journal of Biomedical Materials Research Part A*, Vol.70, No.3, pp. (459-466).

Chun, C.; Lee, S.M.; Sang, Y.,K.; Kim, Y.H., & Song, S.C. (2009). Thermosensitive poly(organophosphazene)-paclitaxel conjugate gels for antitumor applications. *Biomaterials*, Vol.30, pp.(2349-2360).

Chung, J.E.; Yokoyama M., Yamato M., Aoyagi T., Sakurai Y., Okano T. (1999) Thermo-responsive drug delivery from polymeric micelles constructed using block copolymers of poly(N-isopropylacrylamide) and poly(butylmethacrylate). *Journal of Controlled Release*, 62, pp.(115-127).

Conlin, P.; O'Neil, S. T.; Demurtas, D.; Finka, A. & Hubbell, J. A. (2009). A Novel Method for the Encapsulation of Biomolecules into Polymersomes via Direct Hydration. *Langmuir*, Vol.25, No.16, pp.(9025–9029).

Dai, P.H; Woo Sun, S.; Ji Heung, K. & Doo Sung, L. (2006). pH/temperature sensitive poly(ethylene glycol)-based biodegradable polyester block copolymer hydrogels. *Polymer*, Vol.47, pp. (7918-7926).

Ellingtonand A. D. & Szostak, J. W. (1990). In vitro selection of Rna molecules that bind specifc ligands. *Nature*, Vol.346, pp.(818-822).

Ferrari, M. & Downing, G. (2005). Medical nanotechnology: shortening clinical trials and regulatory pathways. *BioDrugs*, Vol.19, pp.(203–210).

for the controlled release of paclitaxel. *International Journal of Pharmaceutics*, Vol.271, pp.(167–179).

Gaucher, G.; Marchessault, R.H. & Leroux, J.C. (2010). Polyester-based micelles and nanoparticles for the parenteral delivery of taxanes. *Journal of Controlled Release,* Vol.143, pp. (2-12).

Gordon, A.N.; Fleagle, J.T.; Guthrie, D.; Parkin, D.E.; Gore, M.E. & Lacave, A.J. (2001). Recurrent epithelial ovarian carcinoma: a randomized phase III study of pegylated liposomal doxorubicin versus topotecan. *J Clin Oncol,* Vol.19, pp.(3312–3322).

Goto, M.; Yura, H.; Chang, C.W.; Kobayashi, A.; Shinoda, T.; Maeda, A.; Kojima, S.; Kobayashi, K. & Akaike, T. (1994). Lactose-carrying plystyrene as a drug delivery carrier-investigation of body distribution to parenchymal liver-cells using I-125 labeled lactose-carrying polystyrene. *J. Control. Release,* Vol. 28, pp.(223-233)

Gref, R.; Domb, A.; Quellec, P.; Bluk, T.; Mueller, R.H.; Verbavatz, J.M. & Langer, R. (1995). The controlled intravenous delivery of drugs using PEG-coated sterically stabilized nanospheres. *Adv. Drug Deliv. Rev.,* Vol.16, pp. (215-233).

Hu, Y.; Chen, Q.; Ding, Y.; Li, R.; Jiang, X. & Liu, B. (2009). Entering and Lighting Up Nuclei Using Hollow Chitosan–Gold Hybrid Nanospheres. *Advanced Materials,* Vol.21, pp. (3639–3643).

Jansen, R. W.; Molema, G.; Ching, T. L.; Oosting, R.; Harms, G.; Moolenaar, F.; Hardonk, M, J. & Meijer, D. K. (1991). Hepatic endocytosis of various types of mannose-terminated albumins. What is important, sugar recognition, net charge, or the combination of these features. *J. Biol. Chem.,* Vol.266, pp(3343-3348).

Jen, A.C.; Wake, M.C. & Mikos, A.G. (1996). Review: Hydrogels for cell immobilization. *Biotechnology and Bioengineering,* Vol.50, No.4, pp.(357-364).

Jun, Y. J.; Min, J. H.; Ji, D. E.; Yoo, J. H.; Kim, H. H.; Lee, H. J.; Byeongmoon, J. & Youn, S.S. (2008). A micellar prodrug of Paclitaxel conjugated to cyclotriphosphazene. *Biorganic & Medical Chemistry Letters,* Vol.18, pp.(6410-6414).

Kabanov, A.V.; Checkhonim, V. P.; Alakhov, V. Y.; Batrakova, E. V.; Lebedev, A. S.; Meliknubarov, N. S.; Arzhakov, S. A.; Levashov, A. V.; Morozov, G. V.; Severin E. S. & Kabanov, V. A. (1989). The neuroleptic activity of haloperidol increases after its solubilization in surfantant micelles-micelles as microcontainers for drug targeting. *FEBS Lett.,* Vol. 258, pp.(343-345).

Kasala, D.; Chaoliang, H. & Doo Sung, L. (2008). In situ gelling aqueous solutions of pH- and temperature-sensitive poly(ester amino urethane). *Polymer,* Vol.49, pp.(4620–4625).

Kim, J. O.; Kabanov, A. V. & Bronich, T. K. (2009). Polymer micelles with cross-linked polyanion core for delivery of a cationic drug doxorubicin. *Journal of Controlled Release,* Vol.138, pp. (197–204).

Klouda, L. & Mikos, A. G.. (2008) Thermoresponsive hydrogels in biomedical applications. European Journal of Pharmaceutics and Biopharmaceutics (68), pp.(34–45)

Kumar, G.N.; Walle, U.K.; Bhalla, K.N. & Walle, T. (1993). Binding of taxol to human plasma, albumin and α 1-acid glycoprotein. *Res. Commun. Chem. Pathol Pharmacol,* Vol. 80, No.3, pp. (337-334).

Kwon, G.S. (2003). Polymeric micelles for delivery of poorly watersoluble compounds. *Crit. Rev. Ther. Drug Carr. Syst.,* Vol.20, pp. (357– 403).

Latere, J.P.; Lecomte, P.; Dubois, P. & Jerome, R. (2002). 2-Oxepane-1,5-dione: A Precursor of a Novel Class of Versatile Semicrystalline Biodegradable (Co)polyesters. *Macromolecules,* Vol.35, No.21, pp. (7857–7859).

Lee, E.S.; Na, K. & Bae, Y.H. (2003). Polymeric micelles for pH and foalte-mediated targeting. *J. Controlled Release*, Vol. 91, pp. (13-103).

Lee, K.Y. & Mooney, D.J. (2001). Hydrogels for tissue enginnering. *Chemical Reviews*, Vol.101, No.7, pp.(1869-1880).

Letchford, K. & Bur,t H. (2007). A review of the formation and classification of amphiphilic block copolymer nanopaticulate structures: micelles, nanospheres, nanocapsules and polymersomes. *European Journal of Pharmaceutics and Biophamaceutics.*, Vol.65, pp. (26-259).

Li, J.; Zhan, Y.; Chen, J.; Wang, C. & Lang, M. (2005). Preparation, Characterization and Drug Release Behavior of 5-Fluorouracil Loaded Carboxylic Poly(-caprolactone) Nanoparticles. *Journal of Macromolecular Science*, Part A, Vol.104, No.3, pp. (477-488).

Li X. and Li J. (2008). Supramolecular hydrogels based on self-assembly betweenPEO-PPO-PEO triblock copolymers and a-cyclodextrin. *Journal of Biomedical Materials Research Part A*, Vol. 86A, No. 4, pp. (1055-1061).

Liang, H.F., Chen, S.C., Chen, M.C., Lee, P.W., Chen, C.T., Sung, H.W., (2006)Paclitaxel-Loaded Poly(γ-glutamic acid)-poly(lactide) Nanoparticles as a Targeted Drug Delivery System against Cultured HepG2 Cells. *Bioconjugate Chemistry*. Vol.17, No.2, pp.(291-299).

Licciardi, M.; Craparo, E. F. ; Giammona, G. ; Armes, S. P. ; Tang, Y. ; Lewis, A.L. (2008). In vitro Biological Evaluation of Folate-Functionalized Block Copolymer Micelles for Selective Anti-Cancer Drug Delivery. *Macromol. Biosci.* Vol. 8, (615-626).

Liu, J.; Meisner, D.; Kwong, E.; Xiao Y. W. & Johnston, M.R. (2007). A novel trans-lymphatic drug delivery system: Implantable gelatin sponge impregnated with PLGA–paclitaxel microspheres. *Biomaterials*, Vol.28, pp.(3236–3244).

Livnat, M.; Beyar, R. & Dror, S. (2005). Endoluminal hydrogel films made of alginate and polyethylene glycol: Physical characteristics and drug-eluting properties. *Wiley InterScience*. Vol. 75, No.3, pp. (710-722).

Malik, N.; Evagorou, E.G., Duncan, R. (1999). Dendrimer–platinate: a novel approach to cancer chemotherapy. *Anticancer Drugs*, Vol. 10, pp. (76–767).

Marupudi, N.I.; Han, J.E.; Li, K.W., Renard, V.M.; Tyler, B.M. & Brem, H. (2007. Paclitaxel: a review of adverse toxicities and novel delivery strategies. *Expert Opin. Drug Saf.* Vol.6, No.5, pp.(609-621).

Masamichi, N.; Teruo,O.; Takanari, M.; Fukashi, K.; Kiyotaka,S. & Masayuki, Y. (2006). Molecular design of biodegradable polymeric micelles for temperature-responsive drug release. *Journal of Controlled Release*, Vol. 115, pp.(46-56).

Nakayama, M.; Chung, J.E.; Miyazaki, T., Yokoyama, M.; Sakai, K. & Okano, T. (2007). Thermal modulation of intracellular drug distribution using thermoresponsive polymeric micelles. *Reactive & Functional Polymers*, Vol. 67, pp. (1398-1407).

Nasongkla, N.; Shuai, X.; Ai, H.; Weinberg, B.D.; Pink, J.; Boothman, D.A. & Gao, J. M. (2004) cRGD-functonalized polymer micelles for target doxorubicin delivery. *Angewandle chemie-international Edition*, Vol.43, pp.(6323-6327).

receptor isoforms in normal and malignant tissues *in vivo* and in establish cell-lines physiological and clinical implications. *Cancer*, Vol.73, pp.(2432-2443).

Ross, J. F.; Chaudhuri, P. K. & Ratnam, M. (1994). Differential regulation of folate receptor isoforms in normal and malignant tissues in vivo and in establish cell-lines physiological and clinical implications. *Cancer.*73, pp.(2432-2443).

Rowinsky, E.K., Donehower, R.C. (1995). Paclitaxel (Taxol). *New Engl. J. Med,* Vol.332, No.15, pp.(1004-1014).

Rowinsky, E.K.; Cazenave, L.A. & Donehower, R.C. (1990). Taxol: A Novel Investigational Antimicrotubule Agent. *J. Natl. Cancer I.* Vol.82, pp.(1247-1259).

Ruegg, C.; Dormond, O. & Foletti, A. (2002). Suppression of tumor angiogenesis through the inhibition of integrin function and signaling in endothelial cells: which side to target? Endotheliun. *Journal,* Vol.9, pp.(151-160).

Ruel-Gariépy, E.; Shive, M.; Bichara, A.; Berrada, M.; Le Garrec, D.; Chenite, A. & Leroux, J.C. (2004). A thermosensitive chitosan-based hydrogel for the local delivery of paclitaxel. *European Journal of Pharmaceutics and Biopharmaceutics,* Vol.57, pp. (53-63).

Schiff, P.B.; Fant, J.; Hortwitz S.B. (1979) Promotion of microtubule assembly in vitro by taxol. Nature, 227, 5698, (665).

Scott, W.; Balbus, J. M.; Denison, R.; & Florinim, K. (2008). Nanotechnolgoy: getting it right the first time. *Journal of cleaner production,* Vol.16, pp.(1018-1020).

Shi, R. & Burt, H. M. (2004). Amphiphilic dextran-graft-poly(epsilon-caprolactone) films *International journal of pharmaceutics.* Vol. 271, No. 1-2, pp.(167-179).

Soppimath, K.S.; Aminabhavi, T.M.; Kulkarni, A.R. & Rudzinski, W.E. (2001). Biodegradable polymeric nanoparticles as drug delivery devices. *J. Controlled Release,* Vol. 70, pp. (1-20).

Teti, A.; Migliaccio, S. & Baron. R. (2002). The role of the alphaVbeta3 integrin in the development of osteolityc bone metastases: a pharmacological target for alternative therapy? Calcif.Tissue Int.*Journal,* Vol.71, pp.(293-299).

Tomalia, D.A.; Naylor, A.M. & Goddard, W.A. (1990). Starburst dendrimers: molecular-level control of size, shape, surface chemistry, topology and flexibility in the conversion of atoms to macroscopic materials. *Angew, Chem. Int.,* Vol.102, No.2, pp.(119-157).

Tomoyuki, O.; Shigeru, K.; Masayuki, Y.; Tatsuhiro, Y.; Fumiyoshi, Y. & Mitsuru, H. (2008). Block copolymer design for stable encapsulation of N-(4-hydroxyphenyl)retinamide into polymeric micelles in mice. *International Journal of Pharmaceutics,* Vol.37, pp.(318-322).

Torchilin, V. P.; Lukyanov, A, N.; Gao, Z. & Papahadjopoulos-Sterberg, B. (2003). Immunomicelles: targeted pharmaceutical carriers for poorly soluble drugs. *Proc. Natl. Acad. Sci. USA.,* Vol. 100, pp.(6039-6044).

Tuerkand, C. & Gold, L. (1990). Systematic evolution of ligands by exponential enrichment-Rna Ligands to Bacteriophage-T4 DNA-Polymerase. *Science,* Vol. 249, pp.(505-510).

Uraki, Y.; Imura, T.; Kishimoto, T. & Ubukata, M. (2004). Body temperature-responsive gels derived from hydroxypropylcellulose bearing lignin. *Carbohydrate Polymers.* Vol.58, No.2, pp.(123-130).

Van Der Linden, H.J.; Herber, S.; Olthuis, W. & Bergveld, P. (2003). Stimulus-sensitive hydrogels and their applications in chemical (micro) analysis. *Analyist,* Vol. 128, No.4, pp. (325-331).

Varner, J. A. & Cheresh, D. A. (1996). Tumor angiogenesis and the role of vascular cell integrin alphavbeta3. *Important Adv. Oncol.,* pp.(69-87).

Wands, J. R. & Blum, H. E. (1991). Primary Hepatocelluar carcinoma. N. Engl. *J. Med.,* Vol. 325, pp(729-731).

Wang, J.; Loup, P.; Lesnieswki, R. & Henkin, J. (2003). Placlitaxel at ultra low concentrations inhibits angiogenesis without affecting cellular microtubule assembly. *Anticancer Drugs*. Vol.14, No.1, pp.(13-19).

Wang, K.; Burban, J. & Cussle, E. (1993). Hydrogels as separation agents. *Advances in polymer science*. Vol. 110, pp.(67-79).

Wani., M.C., Taylor, H.L., Wall, M.E., Coggon, P., McPhail. A.T., (1971) Plant antitumor agents. VI. Isolation and structure of taxol, a novel antileukemic and antitumor agent from Taxus brevifolia. J. Am. Chem. Soc., Vol. 93, pp.(2325).

Weiss, R.B.; Donehower, R.C. & Wiernik, P.H. (1990). Hypersensitivity reactions from taxol. *J. Clin. Oncol.* Vol.8, No.7, pp.(1263-1268).

Wermuth, J.; Goodman, S. L.; Jonczyk, A. & Kessler, H. (1997). Stereoisomerism and biological activity of the selective and superactive alpha(v)beta(3) integrin inhibitor cyclo(-RGDfV-) and its retro-inverso peptide. *J. Am. Chem. Soc.*, Vol.119, pp.(1328-1335).

Wiernik, P.H.; Schwartz, E.L. & Strauman, J.J. (1987) Phase I clinical and pharmacokinetic study of taxol. *Cancer Res*. Vol. 47, No.9, pp.(2486-2493).

Wilhelm, M.; Zhao, C.L.; Wan, Y.; Xu, R. & Winnik, M.A. (1991). Poly(styrene-ehylene oxide) Block Copolymer Micelle Formation in Water: A Fluorescence Probe Study. *Macromolecules*, Vol.24, pp. (1033-1040).

Woo Sun, S.; Jong-Ho, K.; Kwangmeyung, Kim.; Yoo-Shin, Kim.; Rang-Woon, Park.; In-San, Kim.; Ick Chan, Kwon. & Doo Sung, Lee. (2007). pH-and temperature sensitive injectable biodegradable block copolymer hydrogels as carriers for paclitaxel. *International Journal of Pharmaceutics*, Vol.331, pp. (11-18).

Yanasarn, N.; Sloat, B.R. & Cui, Z. (2009). Nanoparticles engineered from lecithin-in-water emulsions as a potential delivery system for docetaxe. *International Journal of Pharmaceutics.*, Vol. 379, pp. (174–180).

Yang, D.; Zhang, X.; Yuan, L. & Hu, J. (2009). PEG-g-poly(aspartamide-co-N,N-dimethylethylenediamino aspartamide): Synthesis, characterization and its application as a drug delivery system. *Progress in Natural Science.*, Vol.19, pp. (1305–1310).

Yang, L.; Wu, X.; Liu, F.; Duan, Y. & Li, S. (2009). Novel Biodegradable Polylactide/poly(ethylene glycol) Micelles Prepared by Direct Dissolution Method for Controlled Delivery of Anticancer Drugs. *Pharmaceutical Research*, Vol.26, No.10, pp. (2332-2342).

Yang, Y.; JianCheng, W.; Xuan, Z.; WangLiang, L. & Qiang, Z. (2009). A novel mixed micelle gel with thermo-sensitive property for the local delivery of docetaxel. *Journal of Controlled Release*, Vol.135, pp.(175–182).

Yokoyama, M.; Okano, T.; Sakuri, Y.; Fukushima, S.; Okamoto, K. & Kataoka, K. (1999). Selective delivery of adriamicin to a solid tumor using a polymeric micelle carrier system. *J. Drug Targeting,*Vol. 7, pp. (86-171).

Yokoyama, M.; Miyauchi, M.; Yamada, N.; Okano, T. & Sakuri, Y. (1990). Polymer Micelles as novel drug carrier: Adriamycin-conjugated Poly(ethylene glycol)-Poly(aspartic acid) block copolymer. *Journal of Controlled Release*, Vol.11, pp. (269-278).

You, J.; Li, X. ; Cui, F. ; Du, Y.Z. ; Yuan, H. &Hu, F.Q. (2008). Folate-conjugated polymer micelles for active targeting to cancer cells: preparation, *in vitro* evaluation of targeting ability and cytotoxicity. *Nanotechnology*. Vol.19, pp.(9), ISSN 045102.

Yu, Tang. (2009). Jagdish Singh.Biodegradable and biocompatible thermosensitive polymer based injectable implant for controlled release of protein. *International Journal of Pharmaceutics*, Vol. 365. (34–43).

Zolnik, B. S. & Sadrieh, N. (2009). Regulatory perspective on the importance of ADME assessment of nanoscale material containing drugs. *Advanced Drug Delivery Reviews*, Vol.61, pp.(422–427).

Permissions

The contributors of this book come from diverse backgrounds, making this book a truly international effort. This book will bring forth new frontiers with its revolutionizing research information and detailed analysis of the nascent developments around the world.

We would like to thank Assoc. Prof. Dr. Öner Özdemir, for lending his expertise to make the book truly unique. He has played a crucial role in the development of this book. Without his invaluable contribution this book wouldn't have been possible. He has made vital efforts to compile up to date information on the varied aspects of this subject to make this book a valuable addition to the collection of many professionals and students.

This book was conceptualized with the vision of imparting up-to-date information and advanced data in this field. To ensure the same, a matchless editorial board was set up. Every individual on the board went through rigorous rounds of assessment to prove their worth. After which they invested a large part of their time researching and compiling the most relevant data for our readers. Conferences and sessions were held from time to time between the editorial board and the contributing authors to present the data in the most comprehensible form. The editorial team has worked tirelessly to provide valuable and valid information to help people across the globe.

Every chapter published in this book has been scrutinized by our experts. Their significance has been extensively debated. The topics covered herein carry significant findings which will fuel the growth of the discipline. They may even be implemented as practical applications or may be referred to as a beginning point for another development. Chapters in this book were first published by InTech; hereby published with permission under the Creative Commons Attribution License or equivalent.

The editorial board has been involved in producing this book since its inception. They have spent rigorous hours researching and exploring the diverse topics which have resulted in the successful publishing of this book. They have passed on their knowledge of decades through this book. To expedite this challenging task, the publisher supported the team at every step. A small team of assistant editors was also appointed to further simplify the editing procedure and attain best results for the readers.

Our editorial team has been hand-picked from every corner of the world. Their multi-ethnicity adds dynamic inputs to the discussions which result in innovative outcomes. These outcomes are then further discussed with the researchers and contributors who give their valuable feedback and opinion regarding the same. The feedback is then collaborated with the researches and they are edited in a comprehensive manner to aid the understanding of the subject.

Apart from the editorial board, the designing team has also invested a significant amount of their time in understanding the subject and creating the most relevant covers. They scrutinized every image to scout for the most suitable representation of the subject and create an appropriate cover for the book.

The publishing team has been involved in this book since its early stages. They were actively engaged in every process, be it collecting the data, connecting with the contributors or procuring relevant information. The team has been an ardent support to the editorial, designing and production team. Their endless efforts to recruit the best for this project, has resulted in the accomplishment of this book. They are a veteran in the field of academics and their pool of knowledge is as vast as their experience in printing. Their expertise and guidance has proved useful at every step. Their uncompromising quality standards have made this book an exceptional effort. Their encouragement from time to time has been an inspiration for everyone.

The publisher and the editorial board hope that this book will prove to be a valuable piece of knowledge for researchers, students, practitioners and scholars across the globe.

List of Contributors

Júlio César Nepomuceno
Universidade Federal de Uberlândia/Instituto de Genética e Bioquímica, Brazil

Ana Catarina Pinto and Sérgio Simões
Bluepharma, Indústria Farmacêutica S.A., S. Martinho do Bispo, Coimbra, Portugal

João Nuno Moreira and Sérgio Simões
Laboratory of Pharmaceutical Technology, Faculty of Pharmacy, University of Coimbra, Coimbra, Portugal

João Nuno Moreira and Sérgio Simões
Center for Neurosciences and Cell Biology, University of Coimbra, Coimbra, Portugal

Zahra Tayarani-Najaran
Department of Pharmacology and Pharmacological Research Centre of Medicinal Plants, School of Medicine, Mashhad, University of Medical Sciences, Mashhad, Iran

Seyed Ahmad Emami
Department of Pharmacognosy, School of Pharmacy, Mashhad, University of Medical Sciences, Mashhad, Iran

Shouji Shimoyama
Gastrointestinal Unit, Settlement Clinic, Japan

Almir José Sarri
Department of Physiotherapy, Barretos Cancer Hospital, Brazil

Sonia Marta Moriguchi
Department of Nuclear Medicine, Barretos Cancer Hospital, Brazil

Wilfrido D. Mojica
University at Buffalo, State University of New York, United States of America

Javier S. Castro, Lillian V.Tapia, Rocio A. Silveyra and Carlos A. Martinez
Materials Science and Engineering, Institute of Engineering and Technology, Autonomous University of Juarez City, Juarez City, Chih, Mexico

Javier S. Castro and Pierre A. Deymier
Department of Materials Science and Engineering, University of Arizona, Tucson AZ 85721, USA

Printed in the USA
CPSIA information can be obtained
at www.ICGtesting.com
JSHW011358221024
72173JS00003B/328

9 781632 410092